EXTREME WEIGHT LOSS HYPNOSIS

*4 in 1. All You Need to Reclaim your Body, and Self-Esteem. Powerful Hypnosis with Daily Meditations &
Affirmations for Autopilot Fat Burn & Rapid Weight Loss*

CAROLINE LEAN

Copyright 2020 - All rights reserved.

THIS BOOK INCLUDES

BOOK 1: 8 (FIRST PAGE)
RAPID WEIGHT LOSS HYPNOSIS
Start Your Body Transformation and Lose Weight Fast with Guided Powerful Hypnosis and Daily Meditations. A Personalized Journey Towards Your New Beautiful Shape

BOOK 2: 146 (FIRST PAGE)
RAPID WEIGHT-LOSS HYPNOSIS FOR WOMEN
The Ultimate Collection of Powerful Self-Hypnosis and Meditations for Weight Loss at Any Age. Transform Your Body Naturally and Feel Amazing in Just 30 Days

BOOK 3: 304 (FIRST PAGE)
WEIGHT LOSS HYPNOSIS AND AFFIRMATIONS:
Harness the Power of Your Mind to Reshape Your Body. Burn Fat, Stop Cravings and Control Emotional Eating with Powerful Guided Meditations and Affirmations.

BOOK 4: 460 (FIRST PAGE)
GASTRIC BAND HYPNOSIS
Proven Hypnosis to Lose Weight and Transform Your Body. Control Sugar Cravings and Food Addiction with Guided Meditations for Rapid, Massive and Lasting Weight Loss

RAPID WEIGHT LOSS HYPNOSIS

Start Your Body Transformation and Lose Weight Fast with Guided Powerful Hypnosis and Daily Meditations.
A Personalized Journey Towards Your New Beautiful Shape

CAROLINE LEAN

Table of Contents

Introduction

Hypnosis plays an important role in medicinal solutions. In modern-day society, it is recommended for treating many different conditions, including obesity or weight loss in individuals who are overweight. It also serves patients who have undergone surgery extremely well, particularly if they are restricted from exercising after surgery. Given that it is the perfect option for losing weight, it is additionally helpful to anyone who is disabled or recovering from an injury. Once you understand the practice and how it is conducted, you will find that everything makes sense. Hypnosis works for weight loss because of the relationship between our minds and bodies. Without proper communication being relayed from our minds to our bodies, we would not be able to function properly. Since hypnosis allows the brain to adopt new ideas and habits, it can help push anyone in the right direction and could potentially improve our quality of living.

Adopting new habits can help to eliminate fear, improve confidence, and inspire you to maintain persistence and a sense of motivation on your weight loss journey. Since two of the biggest issues society faces today are media-based influences and a lack of motivation, you can easily solve any related issues by simply correcting your mind.

Correcting your mind is an entirely different mission on its own, or without hypnosis, that is. It is a challenge that most get frustrated with. Nobody wants to deal with themselves. Although that may be true, perhaps one of the best lessons hypnosis teaches you is the significance of spending time focusing on your intentions. Practicing hypnosis daily includes focusing on certain ideas. Once these ideas are normalized in your daily routine and life, you will find it easier to cope with struggles and ultimately break bad habits, which is the ultimate goal.

In reality, it takes 21 consecutive days to break a bad habit, but only if a person remains persistent, integrating both a conscious and consistent effort to quit or rectify a habit. It takes the same amount of time to adopt a new healthy habit. With hypnosis, it can take up to three months to either break a bad habit or form a new one. However, even though hypnosis takes longer, it tends to work far more effectively than just forcing yourself to do something you don't want to do.

Our brains are powerful operating systems that can be fooled under the right circumstances. Hypnosis has been proven to be effective for breaking habits and adopting new ones due to its powerful effect on the mind. It can be measured in the same line of consistency and power as affirmations. Now, many would argue that hypnosis is unnecessary and that completing a 90-day practice of hypnotherapy to change habits for weight loss is a complete waste of time. However, when you think about someone who needs to lose weight but can't seem to do it, then you might start reconsidering it as a helpful solution to the problem. It's no secret that the human brain requires far more than a little push or single affirmation to thrive. Looking at motivational video clips and reading quotes daily is great, but is it really helping you to move further than from A to B?

It's true that today, we are faced with a sense of rushing through life. Asking an obese or unhealthy individual why they gained weight, there's a certainty that you'll receive similar answers.

Could it be that no one has the time to, for instance, cook or prep healthy meals, visit the gym or simply move their bodies? Apart from making up excuses as to why you can't do something, there's actual evidence hidden in the reasons why we sell ourselves short and opt for the easy way out.

Could it be that the majority of individuals have just become lazy?

Regardless of your excuses, reasons or inabilities, hypnosis debunks the idea that you have to go all out to get healthier. Losing weight to improve your physical appearance has always been a challenge, and although there is no easy way out, daily persistence and 10 to 60 minutes a day of practice could help you to lose weight. Not just that, but it can also restructure your brain and help you to develop better habits, which will guide you in experiencing a much more positive and sustainable means of living.

Regardless of the practice or routine, you follow at the end of the day, the principle of losing weight always remains the same. You have to follow a balanced diet in proportion with a sustainable exercise routine.

By not doing so is where most people tend to go wrong with their weight loss journeys. It doesn't matter whether it's a dietary supplement, weight loss tea, or even hypnosis. Your diet and exercise routine still playing an increasingly important role in losing weight and will be the number one factor that will help you to obtain permanent results.

There's a lot of truth in the advice given that there aren't any quick fixes to help you losing weight faster than what's recommended.

Usually, anything that promotes standard weight loss, which is generally about two to five pounds a week, depending on your current Body Mass Index (BMI), works no matter what it is. The trick to losing weight doesn't necessarily lie in what you do, but rather in how you do it.

When people start with hypnosis, they may be very likely to quit after a few days or weeks, as it may not seem useful or it isn't leading to any noticeable results. Nevertheless, if you remain consistent with it, eat a balanced diet instead of crash dieting, and follow a simple exercise routine, then you will find that it has a lot more to offer you than just weight loss.

Even though weight loss is the goal of this book, it's important to keep in mind that lasting results don't occur overnight. There are no quick fixes, especially with hypnosis.

Adopting the practice, you will discover many benefits, yet two of the most important ones are healing and learning how to activate the fat burning process inside of your body.

Healing the Body With Hypnosis

Hypnosis is a practice used for losing weight, but since healing forms an essential part of retraining both the body and mind to perform in perfect harmony, it needs to be treated as a tool to calm the mind. Once you've mastered the art of self-control, you can move on and easily convince yourself that you are capable of losing weight, reaching your goal weight, and achieving many other fitness goals that you once thought wasn't possible.

Losing weight is a time-consuming process. The more weight you have to lose, the more patience and persistence you need to become successful. In that same breath, if you've got a lot of weight to lose, it's most likely that you will also have to address certain health issues. Integrating hypnosis into your daily routine can reduce stress and help obtain a sense of regularity and balance, which is required to lose weight. Medically speaking, since hypnosis treats stress too, it is perfect for anyone suffering from obesity, eating disorders, an overactive or underactive thyroid, or anyone who struggles to follow a healthy, balanced diet.

Fat Burning Activation With Hypnosis

Hypnosis is not a diet, nor is it a fast-track method to get you where you want to go. Instead, it is a tool used to help individuals reach their goals by implementing proper habits. These habits can help you achieve results by focusing on proper diet and exercise. Since most weight-related issues are influenced by psychological issues, hypnosis acts as the perfect tool, laying a foundation for a healthy mind.

Hypnosis is not a type of mind control, yet it is designed to alter your mind by shifting your feelings toward liking something that you might have hated before, such as exercise or eating a balanced diet. The same goes for quitting sugar or binge eating. Hypnosis identifies the root of the issues you may be dealing with and works by rectifying it accordingly. Given that it changes your thought pattern, you may also experience a much calmer and relaxed approach to everything you do.

Hypnosis works by maintaining changes made in mind because of neuroplasticity. Consistent hypnotherapy sessions create new patterns in the brain that result in the creation of new habits. Since consistency is the number one key to losing weight, it acts as a solution to overcome barriers in your mind, which is something the majority of individuals struggle with. Hypnosis can also provide you with many techniques to meet different goals, such as gastric band hypnosis, which works by limiting eating habits, causing you to refrain from overeating.

CHAPTER 1:

What is Hypnosis?

Hypnosis is the art of using imagination to lead someone into an "alternative" reality and to have experiences there that are helpful in dealing with current problems or symptoms. The more intensely this alternative reality is experienced—in a "therapy in a trance"—the higher the likelihood that these imagined experiences will also be implemented in the concrete reality of life.

Various techniques and rituals have been developed over 250 years to enable and facilitate the initiation of a trance. Not all people can get involved equally well. So we can talk of high, medium, or low hypnotic suggestibility or hypnotizability. Unfortunately, there is still no independent method for determining hypnotizability; that's why you just have to try it out.

The sole induction of a hypnotic trance is not sufficient. Building an inner "different" reality to change clinically relevant symptoms requires in-depth therapeutic knowledge.

A simple suggestion "Do this or not!"—even if the trance is so deep and the suggestion is repeated often and impressively—it is usually not enough to change the symptoms that have existed for decades.

Trances

Hypnosis is a form of communication in a verbal and non-verbal level. It aims to help the patient get into various forms of trances. Trances are changed, natural states of consciousness that differ from everyday thinking and in which, for example, attention can be concentrated, feelings can be strengthened or weakened, perceptions such as pain can be changed, and the patient's creativity can be increased and more sensory-related. An opening for new solutions is possible.

The patient is helped with selected-adapted-to-the-situation forms of communication to go into a trance state of different depths, in which he or she can experience problems and symptoms on a different level of consciousness: not rational, analytical, and dependent on the will, but sensory-related, imaginative, and intuitive. The patient's conscious will is in no way broken but rather set aside so that the patient can more easily discover and activate idle unconscious resources. Hypnosis can be combined with any conventional form of psychotherapy, whether behavioral or analytical, which increases the effectiveness of both. The special form of communication of hypnosis deepens the doctor-patient relationship in a positive sense, and it is possible to significantly promote the self-help potential and the creative abilities of the patient.

What Is Hypnosis in Weight Loss?

Losing weight with hypnosis is about changing firmly anchored behavioral habits. It's mostly like hidden snacks in between hearty meals that you use to treat yourself as a reward. In contrast to a diet, people should not be given the feeling that something is being taken away from them. Hypnosis makes it possible to prevent this negative effect. When you lose weight with hypnosis, you don't lose the pleasure of eating what you like but gain something, which is for you to lose that unwanted weight. The hypnotherapist guides the patient through his voice and with the help of visualizations through everyday life and various realistic situations. In doing so, he tracks down the very individual habits and needs and can anchor healthy eating and a lot of exercise as new behaviors, and all that is what you get in this eBook.

When you experience sessions with hypnosis, you lie or sit very relaxed. Using certain formulas or concentrating on a laydown process, you will be put in a trance. Hypnosis is often described as the state between waking and sleeping, like in a dream phase, when one is fully conscious. In the meantime, you are particularly receptive to positive messages. For example: to only eat in the future if you are really hungry. Or that it is just so much fun to be active for at least thirty minutes every day. Most people find hypnosis to be extremely pleasant and relaxing. Sessions usually last between thirty and ninety minutes. For some people, a single session can have a big impact, but most often, a series of treatments over a few weeks is advantageous.

Losing weight with hypnosis has the advantage that you can lose weight without changing your diet. At the University of Texas, it was proven that one could lose as many pounds with hypnosis as with a diet—while the side effects are much less.

Everyone can try to lose weight with hypnosis. Hypnotherapy is useful for anyone who is very overweight or is a yoga candidate. So, if you have been on a diet for over two years and then you realize that you always put on the pounds again, you could try the power of hypnosis to tackle the problem.

If you don't want to try self-hypnosis, a hypnotherapist can be a good option. A good hypnotherapist starts with a detailed discussion, explaining the process and the possibilities that arise from the treatment. All that is what we are going to deal with in this handy guide.

Hypnosis and Weight Loss - Why Do They Go Together Perfectly?

Have you tried various diets? Are you familiar with all the common nutritional concepts from calorie counting to low-carb? Perhaps you have already lost weight, but have not been able to sustain your new weight?

Then hypnosis offers you a new approach that makes lasting success possible.

But let's first look at the technique of hypnosis and why it goes hand in hand with weight loss:

Because of its two halves, our brain specializes in different functions. During the day, the area of linguistic analysis thinking is usually activated. This is usually the left brain for right-handed people.

The right brain, on the other hand, captures more complex relationships, images, sounds, and experiences already made. Holistic, intuitive processes are laid out in this half, while the left-hand side separates ideas conceptually and linearly, i.e., step by step.

Unfortunately, in our time, there is a tendency to emphasize the logical-analytical side. This can lead to imbalance and one-sidedness.

By using hypnosis, i.e., creating a trance, the two halves of the brain are harmonized, and the less-used intuitive half is activated.

A trance is characterized by the improved receptivity to ideas and meanings, as well as the increased willingness to react to them and to try new behaviors.

In this state, you are also more receptive to suggestions. These are short guidelines that lead to a kind of programming. For example, new eating behavior can be "suggested" in a trance, which can then be intuitively tried out and used later when awake.

Ultimately, the aim is to improve communication between consciousness and subconscious and to become more familiar with the visual and symbolic language of the subconscious.

Since the logic of consciousness is overridden in the trance state, not only an "either-or" but always an "and" applies.

In this way, new perspectives can be learned and old beliefs restructured.

For weight loss, this means:

Since excess weight is ultimately the result of our eating behavior, the use of hypnosis offers an excellent opportunity to look at the behavior in a trance, so to speak, "from the outside." With this, certain behavioral patterns become clear, often also in connection with certain everyday situations.

With that being said, recommendations are developed that suggest a change in eating behavior to the subconscious without excluding certain foods or limiting quantities. It is primarily about using your wisdom and creating a better body awareness (e.g., developing the feeling of satiety).

If necessary, hypnosis is used to train others to deal with stressful living conditions and stress factors, which often have a major influence on our eating behavior and, thus, on our weight.

Furthermore, depending on your wishes, you can work in a trance on the desired target to move on or on the motivation to tackle and persevere with changes.

Instead of a long, time-consuming diet, hypnosis can help you lose weight without much effort. Being overweight is mostly based on psychological problems or established behavior patterns. The subconscious mind reacts with food to frustration, constant dissatisfaction, or a lack of self-esteem. This always leads us to eat without discipline. Losing weight with hypnosis is about changing deep patterns. Hypnosis for weight loss enables you to solve your psychological problems yourself and get your life back under control. And once these problems are under control, nothing stands in the way of becoming slim. Hypnosis can have a very positive effect on losing weight, but how does it work? Stay tuned and enjoy.

During the treatment, you will be put into a hypnotic trance by your physician or your weight-loss trainer. In this relaxation, the therapist can communicate with you subconsciously, respecting your requirements, agreements, and self-determination at all times.

Deep thoughts, beliefs, and behaviors can be positively influenced and "reprogrammed."

Under hypnosis, you are in a trance-like, changed state of consciousness. Meanwhile, your subconscious mind is more responsive and more receptive to positive messages.

Hypnosis takes advantage of this condition, intending to influence the difficulty of accessing mental areas for your benefit.

A study by the Milton Erickson Society in collaboration with the University of Texas shows that hypnosis—and especially weight loss— works with hypnosis. In some weight loss training programs (ten sessions each), men and women were hypnotized.

The different causes of being overweight were considered. For comparison and also with the aim of reducing weight, a control group was utilized in which no hypnotherapeutic elements were used.

In summary, the result of the study indicates:

"Especially in the long term, hypnotherapy appears to be superior to other psychotherapies and dietary therapies and has a particularly long-term positive impact on the quality of life."

The Milton Erickson Society's academy sees the success of hypnosis as:

"In the hypnotic trance, the patient perceives his inner images and feelings more intensely; thereby, the therapist draws attention to overlooked experiences, behavioral options, and positive attitudes to biographically-related obstacles and how they can be overcoming. Through intensive re-experience of the resources or the problem solution presented and the transfer to everyday life, current difficult situations can be perceived and dealt with differently."

For example, hypnosis can be used for a deep hypnotic relaxation to reduce stress or to change your eating habits. Unhealthy foods are then of no interest to you, and your dietary levels up in a healthy way. Step by step, you approach your weight loss goal. Without having to forego eating pleasure, you develop new body awareness, zest for life, satisfaction, and joy in losing weight.

Induction Techniques to Get Self-Hypnosis

Make yourself as comfortable as possible in your bed. Please have all the light's turned off and distractions put away. You have already put in a full, hard day of work.

Think of sleeping sound and comfortable through the night as a reward for working so hard.

- How was your day today?

- Were you productive?

- How did you feel?

I want you to think about these questions as you settle further into the bed. Gently tuck yourself under the cover, and we will begin our journey. Ready?

Inhale deeply. Hold onto that breath for a moment, and then let it go. To begin, I am going to lead you through an induction script for self-hypnosis. By allowing yourself to slip into this state of mind, it will help you let go of any stress you may be holding onto, even if it is in your subconscious. I am going to help you tap into these emotions so you can let them go and sleep like you never have before.

All of us are stressed. Honestly, who can sleep when they are worried? In this state of mind, you probably feel too alert to even think about sleeping. When you are stressed, the adrenal glands in your body release adrenaline and cortisol. Both of these hormones keep you awake and stop you from falling asleep.

We will go now over letting go your worries, even if it is just for the night. You are in a safe place right now. Anything you need to get done can wait until tomorrow. It is important you take this time for yourself. We all need a break from our responsibilities at some point or another. I invite you now to take another deep breath so we can focus on what is important right now; sleep.

To start, I would like you to close your eyes gently as you do this, wiggle slightly until your body feels comfortable in your bed. When you find your most comfortable position, it is time to begin breathing.

As you focus on your breath, remind yourself to breathe slow and deep. Feel as the air fills your lungs and release it in a comfortable way. Feel as your body relaxes further under the sheets. You begin to feel a warm glow, wrapping your whole body in a comfortable blanket.

Before you let go into a deep hypnotic state, listen carefully to the words I am saying at this moment.

Everything is going to happen automatically.

At this moment, there is nothing you need to focus on. You will have no control over what happens next in our session. But you are okay with that. At this moment, you are warm and safe. You are preparing your body for a full night's rest and letting go of any thoughts you may have. There is no need to think of the future or the past. The only thing that matters right now is your comfort, your breath, and the incredible sleep you are about to experience.

Now, feel as the muscles around your eyes begin to relax. I invite you to continue breathing deeply and bring your attention to your eyes. They are beginning to feel heavy and relaxed. Your eyes worked hard for you today. They watched as you worked, they kept you safe as you walked around, and they showed other people you were paying attention to them as you spoke. Thank your eyes at this moment and allow them to rest for the night so they will be prepared for tomorrow.

Your breath is coming easy and free now. Soon, you will enter a hypnotic trance with no effort. This trance will be deep, peaceful, and safe. There is nothing for your conscious mind to do at this moment. There are no activities you need to complete. Allow for your subconscious mind to take over and do the work for you.

This trance will come automatically. Soon, you will feel like you are dreaming. Allow yourself to relax and give in to my voice. All you need to focus on is my voice.

You are doing wonderfully. Without noticing, you have already changed your rate of breath. You are breathing easy and free. There is no thought involved. Your body knows what you need to do, and you can relax further into your subconscious mind.

Now, you are beginning to show signs of drifting off into this peaceful hypnotic trance. I invite you to enjoy the sensations as your subconscious mind takes over and listens to the words I am speaking to you. It is slowly becoming less important for you to listen to me. Your subconscious listens, even as I begin to whisper.

You are drifting further and further away. You are becoming more relaxed and more comfortable. At this moment, nothing is bothering you. Your inner mind is listening to me, and you are beginning to realize that you don't care about slipping into a deep trance.

This peaceful state allows you to be comfortable and relaxed. Being hypnotized is pleasant and enjoyable. This is beginning to feel natural for you. Each time I hypnotize you, it becomes more enjoyable than the time before.

You will enjoy these sensations. You are comfortable. You are peaceful. You are completely calm.

As we progress through the relaxing exercises, you will learn something new about yourself. You are working gently to develop your own sleep techniques without even knowing you are developing them in the first place.

On the count of three, you are going to slip completely into your subconscious state. When I say number three, your brain is going to take over, and you will find yourself in the forest. This forest is peaceful, calm, and serene. It is safe and comfortable, much like your bed at this moment.

As you inhale, try to bring more oxygen into your body with nice, deep breaths. As you exhale, feel as your body relaxes more and more into the bed. Breathing comes easy and free for you. As you continue to focus on your breath, you are becoming more peaceful and calmer without even realizing it.

As we continue, you do not care how relaxed you are. You are happy in the state of mind. You do not have a care in the world. Your subconscious mind is always aware of the words I am saying to you. As we go along, it is becoming less important for you to listen to my voice.

Your inner mind is receiving everything I tell you. Your conscious mind is relaxed and peaceful. As you find your own peace of mind, we will begin to explore this forest you have found yourself in, together.

Now, I want you to imagine you are lying near a stream in this beautiful and peaceful forest. It is a sunny, warm summer day. As you lay comfortably in the grass beside this stream, you feel a warm breeze gently moving through your hair. Inhale deeply and experience how fresh and clean this air is. Inhale again and exhale. Listen carefully as the stream flows beside you. A quiet whoosh noise, filling your ears and relaxing you even further.

It is becoming less and less important for you to listen to me. Your subconscious mind takes hold and listens to everything I am saying. All you need to do is to enjoy the beautiful nature around you. The sunlight shines through the trees and kisses your skin gently. The birds begin to sing a happy tune. You smile, feeling yourself become one with nature.

Each time you exhale, I want to imagine your whole body relaxing more. You are becoming more at ease. As you do this, I want you to begin to use your imagination. You are lying on the grass. It is located in a green meadow with the sun shining down on you. The sun is not hot, but a comfortable warm.

Imagine that there are beautiful flowers blooming everywhere around you. Watch as the flowers move gently in the breeze. Their scents waft toward your nose as you inhale deeply and exhale.

When you are ready, I want you to imagine that you begin to stand up. As you do this, you look over your left shoulder gently, and you see a mountain near the edge of the beautiful meadow. You decide that you would like to take a trip up to the top of the mountain to see this beautiful view from a different angle.

As you begin to walk, you follow the stream. Imagine gently bending over and placing your hand, not the cool, rushing water. As you look upon the water, imagine how clean and cool this water is. The stream flows gently across your fingers, and it relaxes you.

When you are ready, we will head toward the mountain again. As you grow closer to the mountain, the birds begin to chirp. Inhale deep and imagine how the pine trees smell around you. Soon, you begin to climb the mountain at a comfortable pace.

You are enjoying the trip. It is wonderful to be outside with this beautiful nature, taking in all the sights and sounds. Now, you are already halfway up the mountain.

The meadow grows smaller as you climb higher, but you are not afraid. The scene is beautiful from up here, and you are happy at this moment.

As you reach the top, take a deep breath and give yourself a pat on the back for your accomplishment. Take a look down on the meadow and see how small the trees look.

The breeze is blowing your hair around gently, and the sun continues to shine down on the top of your head. Imagine that you are taking a seat at the very top of the mountain. You close your eyes in your mind's eye and take a few moments to appreciate this nature. You wish you could always be this relaxed.

When you take your life into your own hands, you will be able to. This is why we are here. Of course, you may be here because you want to sleep, but you can't do that unless you truly learn how to let go of your stress. Through guided meditation and exercises within this audio, you will learn how to become a better version of yourself. I am here to help you every step of the way.

Soon, we will work on deepening your trance. You are beginning to relax further into the meditation and are opening your heart and soul to the practice. Remember that you are safe, and you are happy to be here.

How Hypnosis Can Help Control Food Addiction

The national holidays in Chile begin with the temptations of tasty choripanes, roasts, empanadas, terremotos, and a host of other foods, a situation that becomes a real challenge for those who suffer from problems to control their weight and eating disorders.

A few days before the national holidays begin, there are several who are already preparing to enjoy a weekend of celebrations, a situation that becomes a real challenge for those who have problems controlling their weight. Empanadas, choripanes, anticuchos, and terremotos are the temptations and true enemies of those who suffer from eating disorders or true food addiction.

However, the good news is that, like other uncontrollable desires, appetite can also be controlled through psychological therapies or hypnotherapies with great effectiveness, which would help you enjoy a "Dieciocho" with no excesses.

Hypnosis points out, eating disorders or the inability to control food consumption have various causes. "Some factors that could contribute to these eating disorders are low self-esteem, lack of control of life, depression, anxiety, anger, loneliness, and personal psychological factors.

There are others that are more interpersonal, and that can help people to lose control of their diet at an unconscious level, such as family problems, difficulty expressing their feelings and with hypnosis, you can go to the source of the problem, in this case, food "

Eat portions in smaller plates and have measures to eat, for example, half of the bread, half of the vegetables, of soups, either at home or in a restaurant. Fad diets usually cause rebound; therefore, it is recommended to eat four times a day, and only when you are hungry. This can work through hypnosis.

Through hypnosis, you can visualize and consume food more slowly. Be clear that in the national holidays the food does not end," advised the professional.

Regarding treatment with hypnosis to maintain a nutritional balance, the expert explained that "it consists of two stages. First, educate the patient, explain what it is and what the scope of hypnotic therapy is. Second, explain that there is a job on their part.

As for weight control, it has to do with generating the patient a cognitive modification of their brain through hypnosis that allows them to visualize differences in physical and psychological terms and also change the eating habit in terms of the amount of food eaten.

For this, we work with reinforcements, which is where the patient takes audio recorded by the Center for Clinical Hypnosis, where there are three levels and thus gradually move towards a new vision regarding what it is and what we eat. "

Unlike other methods, the specialist stressed that "does not generate rebound effect, it is so powerful when people do the work they decide to do what they are taught, such as generating behavioral change, hypnotic work with reinforcement at home, that It is a natural way to understand again what food is.

The rebound effect is generated in other instances. With hypnosis, a profound change is generated in the person's behavior and perception of what they really eat for."

On the other hand, it is difficult not to gain weight is this holiday season, since "at least on average we gain four kilos, depending on the holidays."

Anyway, he gave some tips that can help not to overdo the diet and control weight, for example, "don't drink anything with sugar change it for one without sugar, do not use dressings such as mayonnaise or others, consume roast but with salads and not with potatoes or rice, ideally green salads that have fewer calories, or one day eat empanadas and another day roasted.

The important thing is not to mix everything on the same day and avoid canned fruit. If you are going to drink alcohol, try it with a light or zero soda, and thus decrease the caloric intake.

How to Stop Overeating?

Overeating is a disorder characterized by a compulsive diet that prevents people from losing control and being unable to stop eating.

Extreme episodes last 30 minutes or work intermittently throughout the day.

An excess dining room will eat without stopping or paying attention to what you eat, even if you are already bored.

 Overeating can make you feel sick, guilty, and out of control.

If you want to know how to stop overeating, follow these steps:

Procedure

- ## Maintaining Mental Strength

Stress managing stress is the most frequent cause of overeating. Regardless of whether you are aware or not, the chance is to make a fuss because you are worried about other aspects of your life, such as work, personal relationships, and the health of loved ones.

The easiest way to reduce compulsive intake is to manage life stress. This is a solution that cannot be achieved with a tip bag that can help with stressful situations.

Think about: are there some factors that are stressing your life? How can these factors be minimized? For example, if you are living with an unbearable roommate, that is one of the main causes of stress in your life. Activities such as yoga, meditation, long walks, listening to jazz and classical music can be enjoyed comfortably.

Do what you have to do to feel that you are in control of your life. Try to go to bed at the same time every day and get enough rest. If you are well-rested, you will be better able to cope with stressful situations.

- ## Connect Your Mind and Body over Time

You can get more out of your feelings by writing a diary that lets you write what you have come up with, talk about your desires, and look back after an overwhelming episode.

Taking a little time a day to think about your actions and feelings can have a huge impact on how you approach your life.

Be honest with yourself. Write about how you feel about every aspect of life and your relationship with food.

You can surprise yourself too. You can keep a record of the food you eat unless you are obsessed with every little thing you eat. Sometimes you can escape temptation if you know that you have to write everything you eat.

- **Take Time to Listen to the Body and Connect the Mind and Body**

If you know what your body really is telling you, it will be easier for you to understand what will bring you to your anger and manage your diet. Listen to your body throughout the day and give it time to have a better idea about what it really needs or wants.

Follow the 10-minute rule before eating a snack. If you have a desire, do not grant yourself immediately, wait 10 minutes, and look back at what is actually happening. Ask yourself whether you are hungry or craving. If you are hungry, you have to eat something before your desire grows.

If you have a strong desire but are tired, you must find a way to deal with that feeling. For example, take a walk or do something else to distract from your desires. Ask yourself whether you are eating just because you are bored.

Are you looking in the fridge just because you are looking for something? In that case, find a way to keep yourself active by drinking a glass of water. Please have fun from time to time.

If you have the all-purpose desire to eat peanut butter, eat a spoonful of butter with a banana. This will allow you to reach the breakpoint after five days and not eat the entire peanut butter jar.

Maintain healthy habits Eat healthy meals three times a day. This is the easiest way to avoid overeating. If you haven't eaten for half a day, you'll enjoy the fuss. The important thing is to find a way to eat the healthy food you like. So instead of eating what you really want, you feel that you are fulfilling your duty through a dull and tasteless meal. Your meal should be nutritious and delicious.

The method is as follows.

Always eat in the kitchen or other designated location. Do not even eat in front of a TV or computer or even when you are on the phone. There is less opportunity to enjoy without concentrating on what you eat. Eat at least 20-25 minutes with each meal.

This may seem like a long time, but it prevents you from feeling when your body is really full. There is a gap between the moment your body is really full and the moment you feel full, so if you bite a bit more time, you will be more aware of how much you eat.

Each meal needs a beginning and an end. Do not bob for 20 minutes while you cook dinner. Also, do not eat snacks while making healthy snacks. You need to eat three types of food, but you should avoid snacking between meals, avoiding healthy options such as fruits, nuts, and vegetables.

Eat meals and snacks in small dishes using small forks and spoons. Small dishes and bowls make you feel as if you are eating more food, and small forks and spoons give you more time to digest the food.

- **Managing Social Meals**

When eating out, it is natural to increase the tendency to release because you feel less controlled than the environment and normal diet options. However, being outside should not be an excuse to enjoy overeating.

You must also find ways to avoid them, even if you are in a social environment or surrounded by delicious food. The method is as follows.

Snack before departure. By eating half of the fruit and soup, you can reduce your appetite when surrounded by food. If you are in an area with unlimited snacks, close your hands. Hold a cup or a small plate of vegetables to avoid eating other foods. If you are in a restaurant, check the menu for healthier options. Try not to be influenced by your friends. Also, if you have a big problem with bread consumption, learn to say "Don't add bread" or smoke peppermint candy until you have a meal.

- **Avoid Temptation**

Another way to avoid overeating is to stay away that can lead to committing them.

Taking steps to avoid overeating when you leave home has a significant impact on how you handle the high-risk situation and creating a plan to avoid it. This is what you should do:

Try to spend more time on social activities that do not eat food. Take a walk or walk with friends, or meet friends at a bar that you know is not serving meals. If you are going to a family party that you know will be full of delicious food and desserts, choose a low calorie or healthy options.

Try to escape from unhealthy food when you are at a party. Modify the routine as needed.

Eliminate or save a little bit of unhealthy food at home. I don't want to remove all unhealthy snacks from home and go to the stores they sell at midnight.

Positive Affirmations for Weight Loss

An affirmation is something that you assert. It is a phrase that is stated in a factual manner, making sure that it is knowledge to be known. We often say affirmations to ourselves without even thinking about it.

You might consistently say to yourself, "I hate my job." You might think it over and over again, and before you know it, you're miserable and hate your job because the thought affirmed that in your head on a daily basis. We need to flip affirmations around and use them to our advantage. Instead of consistently repeating negative things in your mind, you should aim to repeat positive phrases.

We will discuss ways to include affirmations in your daily lives. It takes minimal effort to say these sentences, so you should start to implement these methods into your life ASAP. The more you say these things, the truer they will feel, and the easier it will be to follow through with your weight loss goals. Saying these things will start to come naturally to you.

We think about symbolism a lot when it comes to our pattern of thought. If you're hungry, you think, "I am starving," "I am sick," "I am not myself." These are dramatic statements, but they are themes that pop into our heads because that's how our brains are wired. You might fail once in a diet and think, "I can't do this." We create these assumptions because that's how our brains come up with a solution.

We need to turn that thinking around and, instead, wire our brains to think positively. To create your own affirmations, speak in "I can," "I am," "I will," "I have." statements. Use "I" in every affirmation you do, because this is all about increasing your positivity and creative thinking, not doing so for another person.

After you use the "I" phrases, next move onto making a positive statement, never describe what you lack, and try to avoid pointing out your flaws, even if you are doing it positively. Speak in strong absolutes. Whichever area you struggle with the most is the one you should include the most affirmations from.

Affirmations

I can easily divert myself from restaurants and establishments that can serve as a temptation to practice unhealthy eating habits.

1. I can easily resist processed food, refined sugars, and salty snacks.

2. I have developed a new healthy eating habit.

3. I keep myself hydrated to aid in my weight loss.

4. I have embraced a life of clean and healthy living.

5. Eating healthy foods helps my body get all of the nutrients it needs to be in the best shape.

6. I celebrate my power to make good and healthy choices around food.

7. I eat healthy meals.

8. When I exercise, I feel powerful and alive.

9. I am burning calories every day.

10. I love exercising. I love working out. I love eating natural foods.

11. It is easy for me to control my weight.

12. I love the taste of healthy food.

13. It's exciting to discover my unique food and exercise system for my ideal weight.

14. Everything I eat heals, nourishes my body, and helps me reach my ideal weight.

15. I have a strong urge to eat only healthy foods and to let go of any processed foods.

16. I only eat nutritious foods, and I can easily resist temptations.

17. I am so grateful now that I have healthy eating habits.

18. Eating healthy comes naturally to me.

19. Healthy, nutritious food is what I eat every day.

20. My body benefits from the healthy food that I eat.

21. I eat fruits and vegetables daily.

22. I easily manage my weight through exercising and through healthy eating.

23. I work out and see the results right away in my energy, stamina, and strength.

24. I'm becoming lighter and stronger every day.

25. I burn calories easily and frequently.

26. I'm dedicating myself to staying in shape.

27. I eat foods that make me feel and look good.

28. I have a good pattern of behavior around food.

29. My desire for fat-rich foods is dissolving.

30. My body digests food well and takes out the nutrients I need.

31. I eat in proper portions.

32. Food is my fuel, so I give my body clean, healthy fuel.

33. My relationship with food is positive and healthy.

34. I maintain my body with optimal health.

35. My health is improving more and more every day, and so is my body.

36. I'm creating healthy habits.

37. The energy of my relationship with food is healthy, loving, and flowing.

38. I am now experiencing my ideal weight.

39. Following a healthy food the plan is natural to me.

40. Eating healthy foods helps my body get all of the nutrients it needs to be in the best shape.

41. I attentively take care of my body every day by eating only healthy foods that heal and nourish me.

42. Everything I eat nourishes and strengthens my body and mind.

43. I make wise food choices.

44. I eat food that energizes me and makes me feel good.

45. I give my body only the food that is best for it.

46. My body gets the maximum benefits from its food intake.

47. My metabolism rate is at its maximum level, and I am reaching my ideal body weight.

48. I am increasingly reaching my ideal weight with each passing day.

49. I only eat nutritious foods, and my body retains all the nutrients.

50. I eat controlled portions of food.

51. I enjoy doing the exercises. They make me feel really good and healthy.

52. I am happily exercising every day.

53. I eat fruits and vegetables daily.

54. I am attaining and maintaining my desired weight.

55. Every cell in my being is perfect and healthy.

56. I exercise, and I enjoy a strong, toned body.

57. Exercising comes naturally to me.

58. I easily take control of my weight by eating well and by exercising.

59. I enjoy eating nutritious, balanced, and healthy meals.

What Are Positive Affirmations?

Positive affirmations are positive statements describing a desired outcome, routine, or goal you wish to achieve. Repeating these positive statements often affects the subconscious mind deeply and stimulates it into action, bringing into real life what you are parroting.

The act of mentally or loudly repeating the affirmations motivates the individual to repeat them, enhances confidence and inspiration, and creates incentives for change and success.

This act also programs the mind to act in accordance with repeated words, sparking the subconscious mind to work on one's behalf, making the factual claims come to fruition.

• Affirmations are really helpful in creating healthy routines, achieving meaningful improvements in one's life, and attaining goals.

• The affirmations help to lose weight, to become more centered, to learn more, to improve behaviors, and to fulfill the goals.

• They may be useful in athletics, industry, health-enhancing, bodybuilding, and many other fields.

• These positive statements affect the body, the mind and one's feelings in a favorable way

It is very normal to repeat affirmations, but most individuals are not conscious of this. People often echo pessimistic, not constructive proclamations. This is known as negative self-talk.

When you tell yourself how miserable you are, how inadequate to learn, have not enough resources, or how tough life is, you reinforced pessimistic affirmations.

In this way, you generate more difficulties and many more issues because you focus on the troubles, and therefore increase them, rather than concentrating on the solutions.

Most people repeat negative words and statements in their minds about the unpleasant experiences and situations in life and thus create more unwanted situations. Words work to build or demolish in both ways. It is the manner we utilize them that decides how they can produce positive or negative outcomes.

Do Affirmation Work?

There might be skeptical about this topic, especially since motivational phrases are often provided as wondrous but under a more diviner light, in which we are probably not identifying ourselves.

Reiterating the same sentences multiple times can not appear to be the most exciting thing to do, and might even sound tedious.

But are you risking something if you attempt it? You are the only one who has direct exposure to the inside of your head, and no one else knows what happens inside it if you either repeat some positive affirmations or if your parts of the brain have chosen to go to the beach.

Positive affirmations which work, but don't make miracles

Compelling affirmations don't perform magic, and they don't add miracles to our lives just by attempting to read them for several days. However, they can be quite advantageous if used to accomplish our changes/goals in accordance with the approved behavior chosen.

For instance, if you reiterate to yourself that the only meal I want is nutritious food, my behavior will have to go along, that is, I will try whatever I can to stop taking some fast food home and simply avoid purchasing it.

Another reason is that if we say many times per day that we are indeed a good individual, then stick on the same behaviors as normal, it would be really unlikely for us to lose weight, gain strength or grow stronger.

A Daily Practice

- Choose from a list of two or three affirmations. Adjust them to fit you better, or create your own.

- Say your statements three to five times, or more, all day long.

- Write them on 35 cards to take with you, apply them to the backdrop of your screen, or write them on post-it notes located in noticeable places such as your bathroom mirror or vehicle.

- Create a quiet time during the day when you can sit back and repeat them peacefully.

- Say your affirmations with a profound feeling, as when you already acquire the qualities that you assert.

- Positive statements are worthless in the absence of practice.

- Using inspirational affirmations will also encourage us to hold our target current, to reassure us that we will achieve what we desire and sustain a good outlook, but we must bear in mind that we do need to put some effort into it.

CHAPTER 2:

Reasons Why We Overweight

Aside from hormonal and genetic factors, weight gain has a direct correlation to our negative emotions. Overindulgence and overeating seem to be connected in our brains with specific events, relationships, feelings, and our thoughts have ascertained that in some cases, the food is serving a crucial reason, i.e., the usage of food inf comforting stress.

It appears everybody nowadays is attempting to lose weight. We are modified by our condition to look, dress, and even act in a specific way.

Each time you get a magazine, turn on the TV or check out yourself, you are reminded of it. You start to hate your body losing control, disappointed, focused on, apprehensive, and now and again even discouraged.

If losing weight is tied in with eating fewer calories than your body needs and doing some activity to support your digestion, at that point, why are such a significant number of individuals as yet attempting to lose weight?

Losing weight has to do with your considerations and convictions as much as it has to do with what you eat. Give me a chance to give you a model. You are staring at the TV, and an advertisement is shown demonstrating a chocolate, cheddar cake that you can make utilizing just three fixings. However, since you have seen that cheddar cake, you might feel denied, and you need to eat. Your feelings are revealing to you that you have to eat, although your stomach isn't disclosing to you that you are hungry.

This is called emotional. It is our feelings that trigger our practices.

You may find that when you are feeling focused or depressed, you have this need to eat something since it solaces you somehow or another. The issue is that generally, it isn't healthy that you get for, and once you have done this a couple of times, it turns into a passionate stay, so every time that you experience pressure or grief, it triggers you to eat something.

Grapples keep you attached to convictions that you have about your life and yourself that prevent you from pushing ahead. You regularly compensate yourself with things that prevent you from losing weight. When you're utilizing nourishment to reward or repay yourself, you are managing stays.

Although the grapples that I am alluding to around passionate eating are not healthy ones, they can likewise be utilized intentionally to get a specific outcome. Enthusiastic eating doesn't happen because you are physically hungry. It occurs because something triggers a craving for nourishment. You are either intuitively or deliberately covering a hidden, enthusiastic need.

Food has become the unconscious reflex when one is stressing out. Habits of the mind like this are exactly the reason for losing weight can be challenging a lot for people.

Far down our unconscious minds, we have built rigid thoughts about behaviors that are not healthy. As a matter of fact, as time goes by, one might have developed the mind into believing that these behaviors that are not healthy are crucial, i.e., they are important for sustaining our good health. Suppose the mind is convinced these behaviors are much needed, change that is for the long runs is difficult. Emotional eating or stress eating is just one instance out of several. There many unhealthy companies and associations we build that negatively influence our choice of food. Some usual associations that hinder weight loss involve:

- Consuming food is a convenient blanket, used for comforting one's self in times of depression or despair.

- When we eat, it brings a great distraction to us from feeling sad, worry, or angry.

- Excessive intake of sugary, fatty, or unhealthy foods is connected with party celebrations and other great times.

- Foods full of sugar or ones are a sort of reward or compensation.

- Overeating makes you reduce the fear that you won't be able to achieve losing weight.

- Food can give one entertainment when one is feeling bored.

The fear of eating can assume control over your life. It expends your musings, depleting you of your vitality and self-discipline, making you separate and gorge. This will create more fear and make matters more regrettable. So how might you conquer your fear and different feelings around eating? You can transform the majority of your feelings around eating into another more beneficial relationship.

In all actuality, you have a soul. You should find it. It is that spot inside of you that is continually cherishing, forgiving and tranquil. It's a spot that speaks to your higher self, the genuine you, the sheltered, loved, and entire you. When you find this, the resentment, dissatisfaction, and stress that you are feeling about your weight will vanish.

Things never appear to happen as fast as we might want them to... perhaps your body isn't changing as quickly as you need. This may demoralize you giving you further reason to indulge. Comprehend that your body is a gift, and afterward, you will begin to contemplate it.

Quit harping on your stomach fat, your fat arms and butt, your enormous thighs that you hate, and every one of the calories that you're taking in, and see all that your body is, all that your body can do, and all that your body is doing right now. This new mindfulness will make love and acknowledgment for your body, such that you never had. You start to treasure it like the astounding gift that it is and center around, giving it wellbeing every day in each moment with each breath.

Begin concentrating on picking up wellbeing as opposed to losing weight, and you will be progressively happy, alive, and thankful. Find the delight of carrying on with a healthy life and feeding your soul consistently. Develop more love increasingly with your body and yourself, and this love will move and transform you from the inside out.

When you tap into an option that is greater than you, you have the constant motivation, which is far more dominant than any battle of the mind or feelings. Tolerating and adoring your body precisely as it is correct presently is the thing that sends the mending vibrations that will quiet your mind and transform your body from the inside out.

When you find out how to love and acknowledge your body, you are in an arrangement with your higher self, that adoring and inviting self.

Grasp what your identity is and not who you think you are or ought to be. Understand the endeavors that you make are seeds. Try not to see the majority of your efforts to lose weight as disappointments. Consider them to be seeds you are planting towards progress.

Pardon yourself. Try not to thrash yourself, regardless of how frequently you think you've fizzled, irrespective of what you resemble at this moment, and irrespective of how often you need that new beginning. Pardon yourself!

CHAPTER 3:

How Does the Mind Works?

D o you want to lose weight? If you are reading this book, your conscious response is probably 'yes.' But what is the answer to your subconscious? If you experience weight loss, it is because your subconscious collaborates well with your inner self. In case of a negative reply, you would doubt whether every part of you wants to go in the same direction. It often happens that the conscious and subconscious mind doesn't speak the same language. For this reason, it is essential to harmonize all parts of your brain and give them the same command. How can you do it?

Imagine writing a manual for a car that deals eloquently with the body, comfort level, style, color, safety, and acceleration features of the car, without saying a word about how its internal engine operates. Could you repair your vehicle if something breaks down while relying on such a description? Clearly not, in the case of machines, we are lucky because we can take the car to a workshop where somebody does comprehend the functions of the engines and can repair it. But what to do when it comes to fixing our minds? We can go to a psychologist for advice, but it is eventually our duty to get our minds right. All our behaviors, constructive or destructive, can be modified by our thoughts. If we learn the nature of our thought system, we find the very secrets of human psychology. The gate to our freedom opens before us as soon as we expose ourselves to the sunlight of purity and wisdom with the right knowledge and comprehension of the functions of our minds. The very first step is to understand how the brain and human consciousness work in general.

How Does Our Inner Consciousness Work?

We traditionally divide the human mind into two parts: The conscious and the subconscious mind. Conscious functions include analytical thinking, logic, reflection, reasoning and judgmental abilities, short-term memory. The subconscious commands our biological systems, handles the response, emotions, and long-term memory. While the conscious mind's terrain is only 10%, the subconscious mind occupies 90% of our brain. Therefore, you should keep in mind that the only way to change your life is to learn to command your account at a subconscious level.

What Should We Know About the Subconscious Mind?

The subconscious mind always follows our instructions. What does this mean? It means we are in trouble if we do not program it in our favor, and we can reap the rewards if we give the right commands. It will receive the inputs and realize what is reinforced by our emotions. The subconscious mind is an excellent servant but a terrible master. Everything, whether wanted or not, is accomplished once we have accepted the related emotions. The stronger the feelings we recognize, the more effectively and promptly, we can achieve a goal. How does it work? We create a thought, the thought creates an image, an image creates emotion, and the feeling creates a reality. We process first through our creative manager in order for the conscious mind to create a thought. It means that we have the keys to open the gate to the subconscious mind, the executive manager. So, we can learn how to control our thoughts in order to manage our emotions (Tracy, n. d.).

Sadly, beginning from our childhood, it is inculcated into us that we have to listen to, say, and even think, what we do not want, instead of concentrating on what we do want. When you aren't feeling well, what do you usually think, "I do not want to be sick" or "I want to be healthy"? Unfortunately, we very often tend to bring the first sentence into our mind; however, in this case, we put the focus on sickness and not fitness. As you pronounce or think of a word, it already forms a picture in your head. And we know that mental images generate emotions, even strong emotions in us. Let's do a mini exercise. For this, I will ask you not to imagine a specific object! Are you in? OK! So, don't believe a blue apple. What did your mind do immediately? It imagined precisely that: a blue crab. Why? Because as soon as you say the word, the image appears immediately, as the mind does not understand the negations. The negative name cannot be displayed in a picture. Thirdly, if you want to program something in your brain, pay attention to imagining the related scene in the present or in the past, because if your picture takes place in the future, your subconscious mind will think it is only a future project; therefore it wants to realize it only someday in the future. If your subconscious feels the urgency of a project, the realization process will be shorter.

Therefore, we have to convince our creative manager to give the right command to the executive manager. To accomplish this task, we need to understand what to focus on with our thoughts simply because we acquire what our thoughts are directed to. It is fundamental to comprehend this simple equation. What you pay attention to now will return to you in the future. The only thing you need to do is to preserve and nurture it because these thoughts are the creators of your future. If you center on what bothers you, even if you don't want it to be realized, you will have to meet it in the future. Have you ever happened to face the difficulty that you were afraid of? I am sure your answer is affirmative. This is because many times, we experience the fate we want to avoid.

CHAPTER 4:

Hypnosis in Our Subconscious Mind

They say we only use about 10% of our brains. That may be real, but I'd instead look at it differently. Consider 10 percent of your conscious mind. In other words, that part generates what you want, the part that thinks about you, analyzes what's going on, makes decisions, and is your will power. So, it's a powerful mind pair.

But where's the mind's other 90%? Imagine the subconscious part. It's different from the conscious component. It doesn't think so. This holds all of your ideals, convictions, behaviors, history, and much more. That's the mental part that regulates you.

Once you've learned to ride a bike and balanced, you'll never forget. If you haven't been on for a while, you may be out of practice, but once you get on your subconscious, you get into gear, and you're able to balance and ride quickly.

The subconscious is computer-like. When you've programmed it, you'll get what you put in it. When your subconscious mind is full of trash and things you don't like, then that's what it's going to give you. It doesn't think eating when you're full is evil. It's just because, in the past, you designed it that way.

If the subconscious is about 90% of the mind and, therefore, stronger, why does it not respond to what the imaginative analytical conscious mind says? It's all about what you know and says it. Imagine a 7-year-old girl. She can be supportive, dig her heels down, not do what you want, and ignore you. When she's supportive, your mind's open to new ideas and improvement. Yet when she's unhelpful, avoiding the negative situation, that's different. When you try to tell her what you want, she'll probably forget you. When you try to push her to listen, it won't work either. And how can you make changes to the subconscious? I use self-hypnosis myself, but if you haven't mastered it yet, you can use an affirmation instead. An affirmation is a constructive message you like. When you repeat an affirmation several times out loud and yourself, then the subconscious can note and take in what you affirm.

To make the affirmation function better and improve your mind's strength, you should do two things:

- Make sure the affirmation has some value for you. When you have eating disorders, and you make an affirmation, "I'm in control of my weight," the subconscious will forget the affirmation because it's not real. However, if you said, "I get more control of my eating habits every day," then work is more likely.

- Put as an issue. If you seek confirmation, the mind must first take it and find out what it means before it's real. It already starts after the affirmation and is practical for you.

Conscious Mind and Subconscious Mind

Conscious Mind

The conscious mind can be compared to a word processor. It is the decision-maker for our day to day chores. This "processor" sends programs to the subconscious mind to perform specific tasks, observes how subconscious programs perform them, and then decides what else needs to be done.

The conscious mind is estimated to be only 12% of our minds. What it perceives as a belief is not exactly what our subconscious beliefs. You may think that there is no limitation in the subconscious for an issue, but they may still be there.

A unique quality of the conscious mind is that it can quickly judge what is right and what is wrong, which the subconscious does not do. The aware decide which information should be kept in the brain and which should not.

Subconscious Mind

The subconscious mind is like a computer's hard drive. It contains memories, habits, beliefs, self-image, and controls autonomous bodily functions. It is both the deposit of information and the executors of the tasks. It also contains "pre-defined instructions" that we don't have to think about consciously, such as keeping our heart beating, breathing, digestion...

The subconscious is estimated to be 88% of the mind. This means that when we recognize that one of our beliefs is negative, 12% of our mind wants to change the other 88%. Any decision to change is formed mainly in our conscious mind. This decision will, in some way, conflict with existing beliefs.

The subconscious mind's strength is incredible. By knowing the power of the inner mind, people can alter their unhappy life aspects. The subconscious mind occupies nearly all minds by about 88 percent. If people learn how to manage this subconscious mind properly, they can do everything in life. Your subconscious mind component represents personal patterns, temperament, and memory. And if you're looking for a positive shift of attitudes, actions, or consciousness, you have to focus on the subconscious mind.

The mind is closely associated with our experience, and it can show in the form of mental or physical disorder if we feed negative thoughts. Not letting negative thoughts spread in the subconscious mind. The future relies on people's views and beliefs. If a person wants to win, they must have a winning attitude. Only then will they accomplish other things in life. It also gives positive inputs for positive output. Ignore negative thoughts because your subconscious mind cannot distinguish the difference between good or bad. So, thrive with excellent views to increase the mind's healing power. Meditation and relaxation can effectively regulate the body.

Individuals can connect quickly with their subconscious mind using powerful affirmations. Affirmation is just constant reinforcement of optimistic thoughts. And it's essential to direct the functional aspects. Through adding the strength of affirmations, people will strengthen their subconscious influence and boost enormous quantities of ability they never knew they had. And whatever the mind thinks it can do. Therefore, hitting the part of the subconscious mind may be a better way to expose the latent ability of the mind. So, if people keep saying good thoughts always and holding faith in subconscious forces, they efficiently resolve their pain and hard times and pull circumstances that will make this conviction come true. Subconscious mind strength is always misunderstood because people do not recognize their virtues. The part of the subconscious mind is the storage bank of all reinforcement (good or bad) we obtain in our surroundings. In adolescence, this affirmation directly affects one's behaviors. These same patterns decide our personality. To enhance our minds' capacity, feeding the right affirmation (repeatedly) into the subconscious is necessary. This is possible with subliminal contact. People may write a tailor-made text message denoting positive affirmation. The encouragement is directed at the subconscious mind to develop a new habit. With age, developing new habits is extremely difficult for an aged person. Subliminal messaging can frame new habits. All of these allow for versatility to adapt to new behaviors. If properly used, the subconscious mind has forces far beyond human understanding. Uncover subconscious mind control by subliminal messaging.

CHAPTER 5:

Guided Meditation

There are seven meridians located along your spine. They include your: root, sacral, solar plexus, heart, throat, third eye, and crown chakras. Each chakra represents a certain part of your mental, emotional, physical, and spiritual wellbeing. Ideally, when all of your chakras have been nurtured and balanced, you will find yourself experiencing complete health within your mind, emotions, body, and soul. This means that in addition to feeling grounded and balanced, you will also notice that your physical body actually begins to operate in optimal health. This includes anything and everything relating to your ability to lose weight and create and maintain a healthy and fit body that serves you.

Many cultures and healers, such as hypnosis masters, will tell you that if you focus on the wellbeing of each of your seven chakras, you will have a complete and structured guide for maintaining your wellness overall. They also insist that if you truly want to lose weight and have your healthiest body possible, educating you on and taking care of your chakras are crucial to your wellbeing. This is because your chakras are tangible points within your body, but they are also points that represent a bigger picture in your general wellbeing, and in all ways. For weight loss specifically, having healthy chakras means that you are not holding onto anything emotionally, mentally, physically, or spiritually that may be preventing you from having a healthier body. This means that you will release any traumas, negative thoughts, energies, and unhelpful habits or behaviors that may be negatively interrupting your physical wellbeing.

In order to better understand each of your chakras and how they contribute to weight loss and general wellbeing, let's take a brief look at each of your seven chakras.

- **Root Chakra**: Your first chakra is your root chakra, located by the base of your tail bone and represented by the color red. This chakra reflects your physical stability, survival, and instincts. When it is imbalanced, you may retain weight as a way to "guarantee" your survival, sort of like a bear carrying weight to preserve his survival through the winter.

- **Sacral Chakra**: Your second chakra is your sacral chakra, and it is located three finger-widths below your navel. Carrying some extra weight around your sacral chakra is natural for women of childbearing years; however, having too much weight can be unhealthy. Extra weight in this area is often linked to sexual health or sexual trauma.

- **Solar Plexus Chakra**: Your third chakra is your solar plexus chakra, and it is located about three inches above your navel and below your rib cage. It is represented by the color yellow. This chakra represents your feelings of personal power and personal strength. If you have repeatedly had your personal power taken from you or threatened, you may carry extra weight on your body as a way to protect yourself from those who have hurt you in the past. This is often seen as a "barrier" that protects you from the abuse of others. An imbalanced solar plexus chakra does not necessarily mean that you will carry more weight around your mid as this weight may be distributed anywhere across your body.

- **Heart Chakra**: Your fourth chakra is your heart chakra, it is located in the middle of your chest, and it is represented by the color green. Your heart chakra represents your feelings and your emotions. If you are carrying weight due to lethargic heart chakra, this means that you are carrying emotional burdens that are "too heavy" for you and that need to be released so that you can let go of the extra weight of these burdens.

- **Throat Chakra**: Your fifth chakra is your throat chakra, and it is located at the base of your throat, in that indented space where your throat meets your chest. Your throat chakra is represented by the color blue. Your throat chakra reflects your ability to communicate, including your ability to speak and your ability to hear what others have been saying to you. Your throat chakra may become imbalanced if you are regularly saying unkind things, or if you are regularly hearing unkind things, both of which can lead to you wanting to protect yourself with extra weight to "block" the pain.

- Rarely an imbalanced **Third Eye Chakra** lead to weight gain, although an imbalanced third eye can indicate that you are experiencing imbalance elsewhere in your body. Symptoms of imbalance include nightmares, headaches, and struggling to see the entire truth of your life. One way this may translate to wellness could be in your inability to see your own beauty and the reality that you are more than just your body, particularly if you are struggling with body image issues and self-esteem.

- **Crown Chakra**: Located at the crown of your head, directly over your spine, is your seventh chakra. An imbalanced crown chakra means that you are not connected to the divine, which may lead to feelings of loneliness, isolation, or depression, all of which can encourage people to engage in unhealthy behaviors surrounding their wellness.

By balancing each of your seven chakras, you increase your likelihood of being able to effortlessly lose weight in a way that looks and feels good. Through this, you are not only going to create the body image that you want, but you are also going to be able to create the wellness that you desire so that you can genuinely feel happy and healthy in your life. This is imperative when losing weight, as many people do not realize that happiness is not inherently attached to weight loss, but instead to a willingness to accept yourself and respect and support yourself in all ways.

How Integrating Chakra Work Will Help You Lose Weight

Many people find that in choosing to work with their chakras, they discover a healthy and effective structure for how they can approach their wellness as a whole. In order to introduce you to this structure and give you some ideas for how you can integrate your chakras into your wellness and weight loss, let's explore each chakra individually and what you can do to create your desires through that chakra itself.

Your Root chakra represents survival and instincts, which means that it connects with your primal subconscious in the deepest way possible. Learning to heal your fears around survival and wellbeing is a great way to allow your instincts to stop instinctively harboring extra weight on your body. This particular symptom often arises when people have grown up in poverty, or in a way that meant they struggled to have access to food or other necessities of survival. Creating a life where you can safely and consistently access healthy food and trusting that your food supply will not run out is a great way to start letting go of habits related to food hoarding and excess eating caused by a fear of survival.

Your Sacral Chakra represents your sexual urges and energy, as well as your cravings and desires. In order to integrate sacral chakra work into energy loss, you need to balance this chakra so that you can learn how to delay pleasure and desire. This way, you will be less likely to excessively indulge in cravings in order to meet your desires, and when you do choose to mindfully indulge, you will derive far more pleasure from your indulgence. Creating this balance will also help you release any fears you may have around "having enough" and "being enough" so that you can feel more at peace with yourself, your desires, and your desirability.

Your Solar Plexus Chakra represents your personal power and confidence, which is something that many people who are unhappy with their bodies tend to struggle with. Learning to integrate your solar plexus chakra work by becoming more confident in yourself and more certain in your worthiness is a great way to release any weight or blocked energy that you may be carrying in your solar plexus chakra. As you create this balance, you will find yourself naturally building a body and a life that you feel more comfortable in and confident about.

Your Heart Chakra represents your emotions, which are something that many people struggle with. Becoming more attuned with your emotions and healing any emotional trauma or pain that you may be carrying is a good way for you to release anything that may be causing you to hold onto weight through your emotions. You will likely find that as you heal, your emotions, energy, and motivation come far more naturally and effortlessly for you.

Your Throat Chakra represents your ability to communicate and can have a negative impact on your weight when you have repeatedly been telling unkind things about yourself, or you have said unkind things about yourself or others on a consistent basis. Remember: your mind is the foundation of your entire reality and identity. Healing your communication abilities and habits will help you lay the foundation for healthier communication, a healthier identity, and a healthier reality. You can do this both by changing the way you speak about yourself and others and setting boundaries around how you are willing to allow others to speak about you.

Your Third Eye Chakra can reflect your ability to see the truth and to see the bigger picture. If you want to use your third eye chakra to help you lose weight, you need to be willing to see the truth about yourself and your reality, rather than seeing the narrow view that you may have become obsessed with. Learn how to see the truth in your bigger picture, and how to keep your focus on the end goal. The more you can maintain this focus and vision, the more you will find yourself having better health in your body, mind, emotions, and spirit.

Your Crown Chakra reflects your ability to remain connected to the divine and to your own divine energy. This divine connection helps you remember that you are not alone, that you are supported, and that you are a valuable and worthy individual. When it comes to weight loss, healing this chakra can help facilitate healing in your lower chakras, such as healing surrounding your survival, desire, cravings, emotions, confidence, and more.

Healing each of your chakras is going to help you clear up any discomfort or dysfunction in your life and spiritual energy that may be leading to you having a difficult time releasing excess weight that you have been carrying. Furthermore, it is going to help you experience more thorough vitality and wellness in your life, making your weight loss about so much more than just weight loss, but also about the creation and integration of a healthier, happier, and more authentic you.

CHAPTER 6:

Program Your Mind

Your mind holds the key to the daily life of yours. You are able to either let your mind drive you to malcontent or perhaps happiness. The best part is you are able to reprogram your subconscious mind to lead the life you wish. When you were younger, your brain was a blank slate; it didn't have any existing interpretation, beliefs, or ideas of events. Every time someone said something to you, the subconscious absorbed it and stored it away for reference. For instance, in case you had been called fat, embarrassing, ugly, worthless, all that negative info was stored away because the brain is always listening and always impartial.

Now you're older and know better; you feel it's merely a case of getting rid of the false notions that your subconscious took hold of in your youth and childhood. It's easier said than done because the subconscious doesn't react to the conscious mind. This's since your programming can make decisions for you. To reprogram your brain successfully, you must:

Make a Decision

Determine the exact outcome you wish for yourself. With clarity comes the power to shape the subconscious of yours in the new paths to follow. When you've settled on what you would like for yourself and in the future, you're offering your mind resources toward the fulfillment of the goals of yours.

Write It Down

Let's say you want to be 17-pounds lighter by summer three months away. That is a clear-cut objective which you have set for yourself. Put it down clearly on paper, place it within sight so you can see it as often as possible. Therefore, when "external" forces try to sway you into say, indulging, or binge eating, you remember that you have set a goal. You have decided to shed seventeen pounds in three months. All of your mental power is aligned to help you accomplish this task.

Commit

Once you have made a clear decision, commit to sticking by it. Commitment means allowing the decision to inform your choices. You may, however, expect to encounter fear. Fear is the biggest threat to success. The fear of failure drives people into giving up on their dreams-not failure itself.

Fear can lead to procrastination of your goals, which in turn feed the fear with negative thoughts such as, "I am better off not trying" or "Why should I risk disappointment in case I fail?" These thoughts cause you to feel even worse than you did before. The best solution for fear is facing it.

Failure is not the end of everything; it is a lesson in itself. Access the first trial, everything you did and how you did it. Examine if there is a way to modify the exercise to alter the result. Therefore, fear should not hold you back from your goals. Your efforts should be coupled with a commitment to a healthier lifestyle, devotion to overcoming the negative thoughts, and commitment to yourself.

Modify Progress

Allow flexibility in your mental capacity. When you have committed to your decision, check the progress to see what is working and what can be amended. Striking a balance between alteration and overhaul can be difficult if you do not have a guide- be it a plan or a mentor or sponsor.

Do not limit yourself to "It's my way or the highway" mentality. Having a peripheral vision can direct you to alternative possibilities and opportunities in case problems arise during your course. Adjusting your programming to cater to these speed bumps builds your resilience to the challenges.

Your subconscious develops a winning attitude where failures become lessons, hurdles become catapults, and change becomes inevitable.

Overcoming Limitations

To overcome limiting beliefs, you must first acknowledge them and accept them for what they are and their role in your life to this crucial point. It is of significant importance to accept them because you cannot change what does not exist. These beliefs are repeated to us by society, causing us to relate negatively with ourselves, food, money, and others. When you realize that these beliefs do not define your worth, you will start to see your true potential and develop self-confidence in your abilities. You will feel free to win at everything in which you set your mind.

Note Down Your Personal Limiting Beliefs

While getting rid of all your limitations, write down the beliefs that you have had from childhood that simply do not serve your purpose anymore. For example, "I am overweight" or "I do not look as good as my petite friends." Such beliefs have likely caused you to look upon yourself with disdain. The negative "I am" thoughts are not honestly what you think of yourself unless someone said them to you.

Understand Causality

The circumstances you find yourself in are not the cause of your limiting beliefs but the effect. Let us take an example of struggling with weight; the reason you are "struggling" is your limiting beliefs about food and yourself. Knowing this, you can alter your mentality about your limitations and flip them to work for you instead of against you. Along with learning how to reprogram our mind, it is essential to note that the subconscious is still taking in new information and using it for reference for future decisions. There are several ways to reprogram your mind successfully.

Environment

The environment that surrounds us impresses significantly on our minds. Imagine if you always have people talking down at you at work or school. That kind of negativity can lead to a host of psychological problems, including depression.

Remove yourself from toxic environments; the instance you start to notice a pattern of ill-intentioned thoughts. Immerse yourself into an environment that fosters loving and positive thoughts. This way, your mind will absorb all the kind thoughts and gradually begin to reprogram your thought pattern. Support groups are an excellent environment to immerse yourself into because these people are working with the same set of circumstances, but some have also succeeded in daily progress. They know how rough it can be; therefore, they are the best reference for guidance and support.

Visualization

Visualization is a powerful reprogramming tool. Try to envision your transformed self in day-to-day activities. Envision your perfect romantic life, professional life, family relationships, financial relationships, and how you relate to yourself. See yourself as you would like to lead your life and feel fulfilled in these visions. When these images are accompanied by emotions of accomplishment, gratitude, and joy, they will more effectively redraw on your images. Your subconscious will see these images as the truth and guide your decisions based on the repetitive visualization of the images, as mentioned earlier. For creative visualization to work, you must first change the underlying negative beliefs. This is because the subconscious, being the autopilot, corrects the shift in course whenever you seem to deviate from the norm. Ignoring the limiting beliefs can, by all means, curtail your efforts at reaching your objectives. Address the underlying cause first or use the mental by- product focus method to attaining what you want. This method allows you to focus on something that you do not have negative thoughts about, and therefore, by association, helps you achieve what you desire. For example, you may want to travel abroad for summer vacation. You have been saving up for this trip, and you are looking forward to it. By visualizing your perfect self in your ideal trip will enable you to take the necessary steps to shred the undesired 17-pounds.

Affirmations

Affirmations are necessary when you want to focus on another thought pattern. During affirmations, you phrase your statements positively, attach personal meaning to them, and repeat them to yourself multiple times throughout the day. Corresponding emotion helps the subconscious to understand the statements and believe them as the new status quo.

At first, getting your conscious mind on board with affirmations that may seem far-fetched can be difficult. As time goes on, however, the power of these affirmations has taken root into your subconscious, and you start to believe them to be true even with your rational mind.

Act as If

This method builds your confidence. It really works in the same manner as affirmations, but uses actions rather than words and thoughts. It's the equivalent of the "fake it till you make it" mode of thinking. While the conscious brain of yours is actually busy judging you about your deceiving mannerisms, your subconscious is loyally picking up on all of the subtle differences in sensation and thought as you fake the way of yours to your desired objective.

Actively changing your behaviors causes a change in habits, and later or sooner, the entire narrative of yours will change.

Hypnosis

Hypnosis is another tool used to reprogram the mind where the hypnotherapist puts you in a state of complete relaxation and reaches into the subconscious mind. Afterward, messages of empowerment and self-reliance are delivered repetitively to the listener. Hypnosis is used to reprogram the self-defeating habits and thoughts that keep you from achieving your goals.

This technique uses creative metaphors, illustrations, and suggestions to rewire the brain. In the wake of hypnosis weight loss studies, women who participated in hypnosis lost twice as much weight as the women who merely watched what they ate. The research, however, is not enough to be conclusive.

The best way to effect hypnosis is to play the messages when you are retiring for the day. As you are about to fall asleep, play the hypnosis tape, and let it carry your mind forward. Doing this in your sleep is more effective because there are limited to no distractions of the conscious mind chatter. The subconscious, being the sponge, absorbs the new thought patterns and rewrites the societal limitations held.

All these modes of rewiring your mind are dominant, but how exactly do you know what to expect? What signs do you look for to show improvement before you start discouraging yourself with negative thoughts? In short, when a paradigm shift takes place in your subconscious, you begin to feel a sense of change in your inner and outer self,

- You begin to feel more confident.

- You begin to feel happier.

- Your anxiety dissipates, meaning that your objectives do not scare you anymore.

- You begin to take more risks and assume the courage to face more challenges.

You find the ability to recognize all the opportunities coming your way. Once you have selected a method to apply in reprogramming your mind, it is essential to stay consistent with it before moving on to another plan.

Repetition is crucial in creating new neural paths. It is also good to remember that:

- In this world of instant gratification, reprogramming your mind can take thirty to forty days, so you must cultivate patience.

- Results are directly proportional to the work, so you must put in the work.

- Start now! The longer you put off the work, the more you will doubt your ability to succeed.

- The solution lies within

Training your mind is much more efficient than using mere willpower to weight loss. Only by repetitive insertion of positivity into the subconscious can new thoughts and habits become ingrained and manifest in the conscious level. To program your mind to become slimmer is not only about combating the eating habits, but a general lifestyle approach that focuses on a healthier life that traverses beyond weight.

CHAPTER 7:

How to Prepare Yourself for Hypnosis

S elf-hypnosis is merely creating this trance state within yourself and giving affirmations to your mind. There is nothing to be afraid of; you are still aware of yourself and in total control during self-hypnosis.

How Do You Hypnotize Yourself?

1-Remain relaxed

Find a convenient place to sit and lie down. Don't cross your arms or legs unless you frequently practice yoga in this position-maintain a relaxed posture that is easy to remain in for the next 20 minutes. Take a deep breath a few times and know for at least the next 20 minutes that you can forget about anything that happens in your life and just let the world take care of itself. Let your eyes naturally close and let your mind relax.

2-Unleashes every tension

Reflect on removing any physical stress in your whole body. Start at your toes, and then imagine each muscle relaxing in turn. It should feel like a moist, welcoming feeling. Remove each muscle group slowly, and work your way up to your legs and backward. Spend more time on your elbows and your upper back, which appears to hold up a lot of stress. Visualizing your body filling up slowly with bright, glowing light can help loosen up your muscles.

3-Link with the subconscious

Roll your eyes slowly back into your head (this is their preferred calming position) and imagine yourself at the top of a staircase. That staircase reflects your consciousness. Now you'll transfer your concentration from your conscious awareness at the top of the stairs into the bottom of your subconscious.

Start descending slowly down the stairs, taking each step one at a time. Take a slow, deep breath with each staircase and let yourself feel even more relaxed, drifting further and further into your relaxing trance state. Starting at ten counts, you go down every step until you get to 1 at the bottom of the staircase.

4-Place your claims in your subconscious

Once you hit the bottom of the stairway, you are ready to implant your subconscious with hypnotic suggestions. Repeat one or more of the following sentences gently in your mind (choose whichever you feel is right):

- "I'm calm and laid back."

- "I am confident and solid."

- "My future is in my hands."

- "I can get everything I want."

- "I am healthy and full of energy."

- "I memorize my dreams."

- "My dreams can be lucid."

You can, of course, make up any sentence you want. Only remember to make any sentence positive and tense to the present.

5-Wake up cautiously

Repeat as many times as you wish your desired confirmation. Take the time to experience the sensation of deep relaxation. Prepare yourself to wake up from your trance state when you are ready. Tell yourself that you will be counting up to 10, and you will gradually return to full awareness with each step. Now start at one count up to 10 as you ascend the steps in your mind backward. (Exactly the opposite of what you did in Stage 3 trance induction).

Upon hitting the top, take a deep breath, then open your eyes if you like to sit for a moment and remember to get up slowly.

Why Self-Hypnosis Works for Weight Loss

Now put that together for weight loss; you decide to lose weight first. Mentally, you might have a specific gravity in the numbers you'd like to be, or a size dress you'd like to fit in. At this point, it would be somewhat necessary to use self-hypnosis for weight loss. To increase your desire to lose weight, using self-hypnosis, you can imagine your life at your desired weight, while in a self-induced hypnotic trance. Imagine putting on that particular size of the dress. Begin to imagine all the benefits that come with wearing that dress, how it feels, how you look in the mirror, how people respond to you, and so on. What you want to do is stimulate all the positive feelings that will make you want to lose weight even more. Utilizing your mind to rehearse behavior makes you comfortable.

So is self-hypnosis a fraud regarding weight loss? If you think you're putting yourself in a trance and telling yourself that fat will automatically melt away from you without changing any of your actions, then you're stupid. And if someone said to you that they would do that using their product, I'd say you're probably being deceived. With that said, when you change your mind, mentality, and drive, it can seem like you're only doing what you do every day, of course, but you've changed your habits enough that weight appears to melt away from you magically.

Because self-hypnosis isn't going to make fat melt away from you magically, you know there are specific actions that are needed to lose weight. These actions typically involve eating less and getting more exercise or activity in your life. Then, the next move will be to use the trance of self-hypnosis to visualize doing whatever action you have wanted to do to help you lose weight. And if you're going to eat less food, you can use your imagination to imagine that you eat less, leave food on your plate, take smaller quantities, eat less often, etc. And every time you use your imagination to behave this way, you add to the emotional feeling of accomplishment, joy, and all of the emotions felt to enhance your appetite for weight loss.

What you're doing is connecting habits to good emotions that will help you in your weight loss plan to remain on track. If you believed that weight loss self-hypnosis meant that you would magically melt fat off your body without any improvement in your habits, then you underestimated what weight loss self-hypnosis was all about. Weight loss self-hypnosis is an effective way to make changes happen by programming your mind for what you really want rather than what you're accustomed to.

Kind of Self-Hypnosis Used in Losing Weight

People have tried many ways down through history to lose weight. You may feel you've explored all of your choices, but you certainly didn't think about "self-hypnosis." Even though this works for many people, it doesn't work for everyone. The success rate is high enough to make self-hypnosis a practical technique for weight loss. This technique has drawbacks, as well as benefits, as follows:

Merits

No special gear is required. You don't need a hypnotist either; you can do this yourself!! Initially, you may want to meet a hypnotist to ask questions to understand what that kind of system entails. Consulting a doctor and a nutritionist to come up with a healthy eating and exercise plan is worth the time and money, especially if you are unfamiliar or used to dieting and exercising. Those acts will help you slim down. Self-hypnosis is one established self-help mechanism. Hypnosis was used for a variety of things, from quitting smoking to recovering memories lost. Many people are still skeptical about its merits; however, many people stand by it. Hypnosis has helped lift weight for many men. If you're talking to someone who's used self-hypnosis to lose weight, they're not going to know the exact mechanisms that are being used, but they're going to tell you that when nothing else has worked for them.

Demerits

That's not scientifically verified. There was no apparent connection between hypnosis and weight loss. It is believed that, during medical trials, many patients experience different results. People who think it will yield results will usually see results, though it has been found that hypnosis has no real benefits. The main thing is that a lot of people contribute to self-hypnosis with their weight loss. Since they have unsuccessfully tried other methods, they highly recommend this procedure. Hypnosis is a great one for those individuals! The principle of belief is a significant aspect of the Law of Attraction. Also known as the mystery. Followers of this method believe that if you think it is something that will eventually become real. You're going to become rich; if you think you're going to become wealthy and make suitable investments. In terms of weight, the same holds; if you believe that you will lose weight and make wise dietary choices, you will lose weight.

For everyone, hypnosis is not. For one reason or another, some people just can't be hypnotized. If you are having trouble being hypnotized, try relaxing and engaging in some form of exercise visualization. Yoga is one activity where visualization can help. Once you've learned to control breathing, clear your mind, and focus through yoga on a goal, maybe self-hypnosis isn't far behind! Look for a detailed tutorial online to help you get started if you're serious about using self-hypnosis. You may want to check out a self-hypnosis guide on a book store or library. This guide will take you through the hypnosis process, step by step. You may want to try self-hypnosis to lose weight; if you have tried other weight loss methods without success, it may function for you.

CHAPTER 8:

What is Meditation?

S ome people's lives come to a grinding halt because of this menace, and it continues to do so on a daily basis. It also gives light (although not expounded) about some techniques that can come in handy when battling anxiety. Meditation, although not mentioned, happens to be one of these handy techniques.

To many people, the technique appears as somewhat vague and difficult to grasp without giving it a bit of time to see the results. To some, the battle with the fleeting mind only discourages them from taking a step further to calm the mind. To others, religious dogma stands in their way. Some folks have chosen to embrace the practice and report numerous benefits, some even taking up journeys to go and meditate in every known meditation center. It is completely okay to belong to any of these groups because the practice in itself requires a lot of dedication and open-mindedness, without which the practice may appear boring or unfruitful. It is a practice for a reason!

Yet, what is this phenomenon called "meditation"? Meditation is a practice that involves the application of various techniques such as breathing and mindfulness in order to achieve a calm mental state and train focus and attention. The main purpose of the practice is to help you observe your feelings and emotions without judgment, with the benefit that you will get to understand them well. Therefore, meditation does not make you a holy person or a different person, but it has the potential to if you wish to take the path.

What is not meditation? Meditation is not a practice meant to make you high or zone out or even have bizarre experiences. Many people carry this notion around with them. It would be a good idea to dispel some of these thoughts before getting yourself to start the practice lest you feel deceived. Meditation is an avenue to train your mind in awareness.

Guided Meditations for Weight Loss

Before you can begin using meditations to do things such as help you burn fat, you need to make sure that you set yourself up correctly for your meditation sessions. Each meditation is going to consist of you entering a deep state of relaxation, following guided hypnosis, and then awakening yourself out of this state of relaxation. If done correctly, you will find yourself experiencing the stages of changed mindset and changed behavior that follows the session.

To properly set yourself up for a meditation experience, you need to make sure that you have a quiet space where you can engage in your meditation. You want to be as uninterrupted as possible so that you do not stir awake from your meditation session. Aside from having a quiet space, you should also make sure that you are comfortable in the area that you will be in. For some of the meditations I will share, you can be lying down or doing this meditation before bed so that the information sinks in as you sleep. For others, you are going to want to be sitting upright, ideally with your legs crossed on the floor, or with your feet planted on the floor as you sit in a chair. Staying in a sitting position, especially during morning meditations, will help you stay awake and increase your motivation. Laying down during these meditations earlier in the day may result in you draining your energy and feeling completely exhausted, rather than motivated. As a result, you may work against what you are trying to achieve.

Each of these meditations is going to involve a visualization practice; however, if you find that visualization is generally difficult for you, you can listen. The key here is to make sure that you keep as open of a mind as possible so that you can stay receptive to the information coming through these guided meditations.

Aside from all of the above, listening to low music, using a pillow or a small blanket, and dressing in comfortable loose clothing will all help you have better meditations. You want to make sure that you make these experiences the best possible so that you look forward to them and regularly engage in them. As well, the more relaxed and comfortable you are, the more receptive you will be to the information being provided to you within each meditation.

A Simple Daily Weight Loss Meditation

This meditation is an excellent simple meditation for you to use daily. It is a short meditation that will not take more than about 15 minutes to complete, and it will provide you with excellent motivation to stick to your weight loss regimen every single day. You should schedule time in your morning routine to engage in this simple daily weight loss meditation every single day. You can also complete it periodically throughout the day if you find your motivation dwindling or your mindset regressing. Over time, you should find that using it just once per day is plenty.

Because you are using this medication in the morning, make sure that you are sitting upright with a straight spine so that you can stay engaged and awake throughout the entire meditation. Laying down or getting too comfortable may result in you feeling more tired, rather than more awake, from your meditation. Ideally, this meditation should lead to boosted energy as well as improved fat burning abilities within your body.

The Meditation

Disclaimer: when listening to meditation recordings, do so in a safe place, preferably where you will not be disturbed for the duration of your recording. Please use your headphones. Never listen to recordings or practice meditation while driving in a car, operating machinery, or doing anything else that requires your attention for safety reasons.

Start by gently closing your eyes and drawing your attention to your breath. As you do, I want you to track the next five breaths, gently and intentionally lengthening them to help you relax as deeply as possible. With each breath, breathe in to the count of five and out to the count of seven. Starting with your next breath in, 1, 2, 3, 4, 5, and out, 1, 2, 3, 4, 5, 6, and 7. Again, 1, 2, 3, 4, 5, and out, 1, 2, 3, 4, 5, 6, 7. Breathe in, 1, 2, 3, 4, 5, and breathe out, 1, 2, 3, 4, 5, 6, and 7. Again, breathe in, 1, 2, 3, 4, 5, and breathe out, 1, 2, 3, 4, 5, 6, and 7. One more time, breathe in, 1, 2, 3, 4, 5, and breathe out, 1, 2, 3, 4, 5, 6, and 7.

Now that you are starting to feel more relaxed, I want you to draw your awareness into your body. First, become aware of your feet. Feel your feet relaxing deeply, as you visualize any stress or worry melting away from your feet. Now, become aware of your legs. Feel any stress or worry melting away from your legs as they begin to relax completely. Next, become aware of your glutes and pelvis, allowing any stress or worry to fade away as they completely relax. Now, relax your entire torso, allowing any stress or anxiety to melt away from your body as it relaxes completely. Next, become aware of your shoulders, arms, hands, and fingers. Allow the stress and worry to melt away from your shoulders, arms, hands, and fingers as they relax entirely. Now, let the stress and fear melt away from your neck, head, and face. Feel your neck, head, and face relaxing as any stress or anxiety melts away completely.

As you deepen into this state of relaxation, I want you to take a moment to visualize the space in front of you. Imagine that in front of you, you are standing there looking back at yourself. See every inch of your body as it is right now standing before you, casually, as you observe yourself. While you do, see what parts of your body you want to reduce fat in so that you can create a healthier, more muscular body for yourself. Visualize the fat in these areas of your body, slowly fading away as you begin to carve out a more robust, leaner, and more muscular body underneath. Notice how effortlessly this extra fat melts away as you continue to visualize yourself becoming a healthier and more animated version of yourself.

Now, I want you to visualize what this healthier, leaner version of yourself would be doing. Visualize yourself going through your typical daily routine, except the perspective of your healthier self. What would you be eating? When and how would you be exercising? What would you spend your time doing? How do you feel about yourself? How different do you feel when you interact with the people around you, such as your family and your co-workers? What does life feel like when you are a healthier, leaner version of you?

Spend several minutes visualizing how different your life is now that your fat has melted away. Feel how natural it is for you to enjoy these healthier foods, and how easy it is for you to moderate your cravings and indulgences when you choose to treat yourself. Notice how easy it is for you to engage in exercise and how exercise feels enjoyable and like a beautiful hobby, rather than a chore that you have to force yourself to commit to every single day. Feel yourself genuinely enjoying life far more, all because the unhealthy fats that were weighing you down and disrupting your health have faded away. Notice how easy it was for you to get here, and how easy it is for you to continue to maintain your health and wellness as you continue to choose better and better choices for you and your body.

Feel how much you respect your body when you make these healthier choices, and how much you genuinely care about yourself. Notice how each meal and each exercise feels like an act of self-care, rather than a chore you are forcing yourself to engage in. Feel how good it feels to do something for you and your wellbeing.

When you are ready, take that visualization of yourself and send the image out far, watching it become nothing more than a spec in your field of awareness. Then, send it out into the ether, trusting that your subconscious mind will hold onto this vision of yourself and work daily on bringing this version of you into your current reality.

Now, awaken back into your body where you sit right now. Feel yourself feeling more motivated, more energized, and more excited about engaging in the activities that are going to improve your health and help you burn your fat. As you prepare to go about your day, hold onto that visualization and those feelings that you had of yourself, and trust that you can have this enjoyable experience in your life. You can do it!

CHAPTER 9:

Meditation for Weight Loss

S o far, we have learned a lot about what meditation is about? How meditation can change our mind and how it is useful in the efforts for weight loss. Building on that conviction, here we would elaborate on the several exercises one can undertake to bring about those changes.

Opening yourself for change

- Inhale by taking deep breaths

- Center yourself

- Just focus on one thing—yourself

- Feel all the peace that is around you

- Feel all the happiness that is around you

- Take these feelings now to infinity large amount that cannot be measured, immeasurable peace and immeasurable happiness

- Take a step into this outer space you are visualizing filled with all the peace and happiness

- Visualize yourself merging with this happiness

- Take it a step further and imagine merging your consciousness as well with the objects around you

- See everything is connected

- Also, see everything as one

- Once you have reached this state, let it be like this for some time

- Enjoy this moment with a gentle smile.

Mindfulness Meditation

Mindfulness is one of the most effective ways of meditation. Practicing mindfulness can prove beneficial both for finding your calm and also for meeting your goal of weight loss.

Mindfulness is defined as being aware of self, every tiny detail your existence has, and you are experiencing inside within self or outside in the surrounding. The practice of mindfulness is centered on focusing on the smallest of detail and not overlooking anything tagging it as trivial or not important. Also, what makes this practice very useful that it can practices any time, throughout the day, one can practice mindfulness while doing the chores, while at work, etc. It can be incorporated with even mundane work or work that excites you. Also, mindfulness aims to pay attention to everything, be mindful of everything under a positive light. Practicing mindfulness is not just about allocating 5 to 10 min in a day, but slowly be more aware and extend mindfulness in your way of living, slowly reprogramming our brain to have interest in each moment of your day. A few of the critical factors of the mindfulness practice are as below:

Do not leave or give-up and maintain a routine with the practice.

Mindfulness is an apt choice of meditation for people with hectic schedules and lives. Every day we come across so much information, variation, and changes that at a certain point, it stops making sense— the time when we say my head is jammed, I am not able to grasp the information. Mindfulness can help you find your calm. The ideal approach is to allocate some specific time every day and do it in a place where there is less disturbance. It is best not to do it on your bed or sofa as you may doze off while meditation requires you to be very much awake.

You can take a yoga mat to find a calm spot, with a reassuring ambiance with softer lights. You can also visit a park, or sit in your backyard, in the open listening to your surroundings, feeling the breeze, the aroma around you.

However, even if you do not have provisions for doing the practice outside, it should not stop you from doing it inside. The exercises should be done daily and recommended at the same hour to make your mind learn and become habituated to practice mindfulness.

Do not restrain your mind and let it wander and wonder.

One of the challenges with the practice is the very nature of the mind, its fragile nature. The moment you try to focus on something, it runs away. So it becomes essential to understand this and keep trying, no matter if you fail, again and again, no matter how many times you drift back and again.

One of the ways to find control over your mind is to let it fall in place naturally. This can be achieved by allowing your mind to wander, let it be free and observe where it all can go, what situations it can walk to. And, once you realize it has seen enough, gently pull it back. Be gentle on yourself, and keep trying. Do not be too restrictive, and do not lose the smile while doing it.

Do not bring judgment in practice.

People who are new to meditation practices often find it challenging to cope up with the influx of thoughts and memories. However, this is what the practice of meditation teaches us to bear whatever is rolled in our way. It is about seeing those thoughts, but now giving power to it. You must practice this and let your dreams come and go.

This is a cornerstone of your weight loss practices as well. If you are able to cope up with the influx of thoughts and flurry of emotions, you will not naturally resort to food and binge eating. However, this is difficult to gain but not impossible. So, for people who want instant results often takes it a step further and try hypnosis.

Come back sooner than later

The idea of meditation is not to sit with a stiff body and heavy heart, but with an open mind and to find new limits. Naturally, our brain will lose focus, and the more we try to tame it, the more berserk it will go. One of the simple and effective ways is to connect your breathing with your thoughts. The moment you realize that the mind is at places beyond, bring it back with a simple, deep inhalation and get on with the meditation.

We have seen something in the practice of dissociation hypnosis. There we have a control mechanism guided by the hypnotherapist to ensure that our mind does not become unhinged or strangled in an alternate reality, which is not a risk; however, it is worth mentioning that people with some mental conditions, cautionary measures will not hurt.

For weight loss, this becomes a valuable tool as well, dissociating yourself from the feeling and eventually the need to binge eat.

Guided meditation

Guided meditation is recommended for people who have not tried meditation and new to this practice. This method is both accessible and easy to grasp. Here you have help from the field experts who will teach you—How to begin? How to relax? How to keep up with your mind? How to navigate through your account, through all the anxiety and unnecessary information? How to be in peace with your mind?

Guided mediation is done with the help of a professional or expert. The practice requires you mainly to focus on the voice, only one view of the speaker, and do as the voice asks you to do so. Even with voice guidance, you would lose track. However, with practice, this will become better. The duration of the training is up to you. You can start small and slowly aim big.

You can enroll in classes for guided mediation. You can also choose to do it from the place you like. There is an online self-help guided meditation, which will provide you the instructions to set-up the ambiance and even the session instructions in the form of recordings, podcast sessions, or live classes. Whichever way you choose; it is beneficial to follow the below pointers:

- Sticking to a schedule helps.

- It is recommended that you choose a specific time for the practice of guided meditation and also make a conscious effort to try to come back to it every day. Selecting the same time window also helps to reprogram your mind into being habituated with the practice.

- Even if you are not able to meet the timing, sometimes it is alright to be a little flexible and do it whenever it suits you best.

- Repetition is the key. To reap the benefits, you must do it regularly and also with a smile

- For beginners, you can choose alternate days or thrice a week. If every day works fine, then it is better, and you can grow faster into this practice.

- Setting up the right ambiance is essential. The place should be calm, without disturbance, and with ample lighting. Do not sit in an area that is too bright or entirely dark.

Breath meditation

Breath meditation is an effective and popular meditation technique. It could be simple inhalation and exhalation, slow and deep inhalation and exhalation, rhythmic inhalation and exhalation, etc. When you follow the breath consciously and also feel the relaxation, thoughts, things happening around you are attaching inspiration to the practice of meditation.

This exercise can be done anywhere and known to calm a person down, reduce anxiety, and also several health benefits. Even modern science is acknowledging the power of meditation and several breathing techniques it involves.

- Sit in an upright posture, loosening your shoulder and place your eyes comfortably gazing at a safe distance or shut gently closed.

- It is recommended to use a yoga mat on the floor or raised platform.

- Focus on your breath and breath only

- Start by taking a deep, slow breath and listen to the sound of air entering and leaving, feel the air fill your lungs and expanding as you inhale, and also it returning to normal when you exhale.

- Observe the rhythm.

- Observe the thoughts—are there any thoughts and ideas which is coming and going

- You can also choose a specific yoga posture—known as 'Mudras.' In the defined 'Mudras,' you would be required to sit in a particular way and perform the meditation is a specific direction. It is best of lookup or checks with a professional for particular guidance on Yoga Mudras. These Mudras have an impact on the quality of meditation.

- Choose your breathing technique—The techniques of deep breathing, rhythmic breathing, switching of nostrils, etc.

Breathing form of meditation is quite useful when it comes to rapid weight loss. The simplicity of the technique makes it practical and possible to be done even by beginners. So, whenever there is a significant flux of anxiety that may lead to binger eating, practicing the breathing meditation for a few minutes can save you from regret.

CHAPTER 10:

Your Daily Meditations

Day 1. TAKE TIME TO PREPARE A HEALTHY MEAL

Home cooking has many advantages because it's a form of mindfulness. You personally choose high quality and nutritious ingredients. Keep in mind that grocery stores are based on cheap fats and cheap carbohydrates, not your nutritional value. You are controlling where your calories come from: they come from trans fats, additional sugars, well!

They ensure that there are no flavor enhancers like MSG or other brain-disrupting substances. As mentioned earlier, the net effect of these addictive substances is that you eat more. Creating a healthy diet is expressing your love for yourself and your family. It's a creative achievement. Save money with this exciting vacation-like activity in Tahiti, Paris, and the Galapagos Islands. You can spend as much time as you want. You can come up with several tricks and shortcuts to save time in the kitchen. It is honest and to recover your cooking skills. It only takes a few hours to revive the master chef inside.

In comparison, to go somewhere to pick up food. Clarify the facts, go there, park, get food, eat there, or take it home. According to the Center for Disease Control (CDC), cases of more than 76,000,000 people who suffered from food poisoning annually due to bacteria, viruses, and parasites that lead to food contamination. Think about it; you have to eat carefully. The only area that affects 95% of this possibility is the quality of the food you eat. If you don't know who cooks or exactly what ingredients they use, are they cheap trans-fat oils, lots of extra sodium, extra sugar? How can you manage yourself?

Sitting In Beauty

Establish a simple and beautiful environment, especially if you eat alone. Even if you're hungry, it can take a few minutes to reach an attractive setting. If you don't have the time, are in a hurry, and want to eat directly from the fridge, this is a big sign that you're usually absorbed in foods that are perceived as high levels of anxiety. This may feel irresistible while restoring a naturally lean female neural network. This heals the "hungry brain," so it is important to calm before eating. There are several ways to reduce high levels of anxiety, deep breathing, meditation, journaling, active jogging, and anything else that seems personally effective in reaching a place of peace. Remember to measure your progress. Can you set up the table without fear? If not, could you be wise to identify the cause of anxiety and address it?

Eating Experience

In a culture that emphasizes multitasking, eating is a secondary activity. We do not combine food with the nutrition of our bodies. Eating is what we do without attention while doing more meaningful work.

Have you automatically turned off your car radio while looking for a new address? I instinctively know that removing a voice stimulus increases your ability to focus on finding its address. Silence also allows us to pay attention only to food and to be fully present for a dining experience. Watching TV, interacting with computers, talking on the phone, reading books, and doing other activities is not a supplement to a careful diet. Mindful meals require indiscriminate attention, so it's a great way to overeat.

If you have resistance to silent hoods, rewiring can help you recognize that you ate for the first time when you had another activity. It is a custom that has been cultivated for many years. You rarely eat the main focus.

When you sit quietly and eat, you can hear inner conversations such as how to enjoy the meal and subtle messages from the body when you are satisfied. If turning off competing stimuli creates fear, inhale, and note the cause of the anxiety.

If you are dining with your family, invite them to participate in the careful process of eating. Trying to turn off as many distractions as you can during your meal is better than overeating during multitasking. Discuss your senses and taste of food. Slow food does not have to be extreme. Nevertheless, it is a good idea to remind the family that eating is not a race. Encourage the family to chew on every slice of food, examining the taste, texture, and odor in detail. Ask them about their feelings, thank them for collecting brownie points, and thank them for their blessings and share their meals with their families.

Remember to measure your progress: how do you feel in silence after a meal? Can you eliminate all distractions and eat quietly without fear? Is practicing this property easier to eat silently?

Enjoy Your Meal

Of course, the thin women have an internal dialogue of appreciation and appreciation and joy: "This is delicious. And it saturates. Shoveling food not only misses every bite of taste, but the entertainment center is in place. You'll need more food to meet gourmet merchants because you're not inspired by it.

We acknowledge that this resistance to internal dialogue is the current practice of not attending for the pleasure of eating. Usually, our conversation feeds on something other than our body, so it's more relevant to issues, concerns, and current to-do lists.

If you pay 100% attention to eating and enjoy eating carefully, you will find that the restoration of NATURALLY THIN WOMEN'S wiring is approaching. Remember to measure your progress. How do you feel after allowing an internal dialogue about the pleasure of eating? Do you enjoy this conversation without fear? If the answer is no, what are the obstacles to achieving this trait?

Small Bites

If you overeat food, you will burn more calories and experience the same amount of pleasure. We must recognize that we have made significant efforts in the past. The wise action is to eat some meals with a small spoon like a wheel while we learn to take smaller bites. However, once you measure progress in this area, it is essential to make the scoop larger. The reason is that if you take a small bite just because the spoon is low, the neural network won't be restored, and you are entirely dependent on the tool.

Don't forget to check for your progress. How does it feel like after eating the whole meal with just a few bites? How was your fear? Did you experience the fun with such a small morsel? Did you have to hit the kitchen and get a more oversized spoon? Or did you just start eating with your fingers?

Fork Down

Whatever your fork or tableware is placed in a bite, you are encouraged to eat wholeheartedly. We are ready to enjoy every bite, every bite, every subtlety, every spice, every texture. Eating is foreplay, not a race. It's a sensual experience. Arashi defeats the purpose.

Remember to measure your progress: how do you feel after eating a complete meal and placing a fork in a bite? What is your fear level? Would you like to enjoy the delicacy of food?

Chew Slowly and Thoroughly

For many obsessive eaters, diet represents a solution for drug users. The faster you can move the shovel, the quicker you can get up. Unfortunately, this behavior leads to total calorie burn and shortens the sensation of pleasure. We try to raise our dopamine levels as soon as possible! We've been doing this for a long time, so biting slowly and slowly can be anxious.

The digestion begins with the first bite, causes the release of saliva, disinfects food, and smooths the way to the stomach. As we bit, the brain releases neurotransmitters that tell the hypothalamus that we are full. Wholly and slowly chewing will remove even the slightest aroma and increase your enjoyment.

Remember to measure your progress. How do you feel after biting slowly? What was your fear? Can you enjoy the slowdown without fear?

Breathing

After swallowing, breathing three times will reconnect with the body. If you prefer, it is a kind of palate wash. Read just for the next bite sensual experience. This is also an opportunity to help us determine if we are full.

Remember to measure your progress. Do you breathe three times during one bite with one meal? Did you notice that your anxiety is growing? Did you enjoy your meal?

Experience Fullness

If you eat it carefully, you'll be full if you lose the taste! By contrast, they are looking for salt, ketchup, mayo, mustard, sugar, or barbecue sauces as overeaters. It's something you can regain a comfortable experience and "enjoy" your food. Additives are an attempt to nullify the intelligence that tells you that you have enough.

I've certainly heard the advice to wait 20 minutes for your brain to catch up with your ecstasy. But when we eat at piranha speed, we consume a lot of food. We don't know how to wait. Until then, everything was invisible. Besides, our brain isn't too slow! By paying attention to when food loses its initial appeal, we can instantly know when it is full.

Note that the beginning of this process feels strange. After all, we are used to consuming everything on the plate. For many of us, throwing away food is very difficult because our conditioning to eat everything on the plate is rooted. A useful tool is to visualize excess food as fat in your favorite body parts. Your taste will tell him that he is good enough, and all overconsumption turns into fat.

Also, understand that we are accustomed to stomach congestion and no food consumption. Initially, this is done mechanically, but if you repeat this a few times, you get the actual saturation. Besides, regaining confidence in the palate signal feels free, as you no longer need to experience the severity of a clogged sensation after a meal. The energy satisfaction after eating, rather than lethargy or immobility, regains your sense of freedom.

Remember to measure your progress. Can you say "it was great" and "I'm full" without having to stuff myself? Can you recognize the abundance?

Day 2. RELEASE OF BAD HABITS

Relax your muscles, close your eyes. Breathe in and breathe out. Do not cross your feet because this will lock you away from the desired experience. Hold your hands together to connect your logical brain hemisphere with your instinct.

Concentrate on your back now and notice how you feel in the bed or chair you are sitting in. Take a deep breath and let your stress leave your body. Now focus on your neck. Observe how your neck is joined to your shoulders. Lift your shoulders slowly. Breathe in slowly and release it. Feel how your shoulders loosen. Lift your shoulders again a little bit, then let them relax. Observe how your neck muscles are tense and how much pressure it has. Breathe in and breathe out slowly. Release the pressure in your neck and notice how the stress is leaving your body. Repeat the whole exercise from the beginning. Observe your back. Notice all the stress and let it go with a profound breath. Focus on your shoulders and neck again. Lift up your shoulders and hold it for some moments, then release your shoulders again and let all the stress go away. Sense how the stress is going away. Now, focus your attention on your back. Feel how comfortable it is. Focus on your whole body. While breathing in, let relaxation come, and while you are breathing out, let frustration leave your body. Notice how much you are relaxed.

Concentrate on your inner self. Breathe slowly in and release it. Calm your mind. Observe your thoughts. Don't go with them because your aim is to observe them and not to be involved. It's time to let go of your overweight self that you are not feeling good about. It's like your body is wearing a bigger, heavier top at this point in your life. Imagine stepping out of it and laying it on an imaginary chair facing you. Now tell yourself to let go of these old, established eating and behavioral patterns. Imagine that all your old, fixed patterns and all the obstacles that prevent you from achieving your desired weight are exiting your body, soul, and spirit with each breath. Know that your soul is perfect as it is, and all you want is for everything that pulls away to leave. With every breath, let your old beliefs go, as you are creating more and more space for something new. After spending a few minutes with this, imagine that every time you breathe in, you are inhaling prank, the life energy of the universe, shining in gold. In this life force, you will find everything you need and desire: a healthy, muscular body, a self that loves itself in all circumstances, a hand that puts enough nutritious food on the table, a strong voice to say no to sabotaging your diet, a head that can say no to those who are trying to distract you from your ideas and goals. With each breath, you absorb these positive images and emotions.

See in front of you exactly what your life would be like if you got everything you wanted. Release your old self and start becoming your new self. Gradually restore your breathing to regular breathing. Feel the solid ground beneath you, open your eyes, and return to your everyday state of consciousness.

Forgiving Yourself

Sit comfortably. Do not cross your feet because this will lock you away from the desired experience. Hold your hands together to connect your logical brain hemisphere with your instinct. Relax your muscles, close your eyes.

Imagine a staircase in front of you! Descend it, counting down from ten to one.

You reached and found a door at the bottom of the stairs. Open the door. There is a meadow in front of us. Let's see if it has grass. If so, if it has flowers, what color, whether there is a bush or tree, and describe what you see in the distance.

Find the path covered with white stones and start walking on it.

Feel the power of the Earth flowing through your soles, the breeze stroking your skin, the warmth of the sun radiating toward you. Feel the harmony of the elements and your state of well-being.

From the left side, you hear the rattle of the stream. Walk down to the shore. This water of life comes from the throne of God. Take it with your palms and drink three sips and notice how it tastes. If you want, you can wash it. Keep walking. Feel the power of the Earth flowing through your soles, the breeze stroking your skin, the warmth of the sun radiating toward you. Feel the harmony of the elements and your state of well-being. In the distance, you see an ancient tree with many branches. This is the Tree of Life. Take a leaf from it, chew it, and note its taste. You continue walking along the white gravel path. Feel the power of the Earth flowing through your soles, the breeze stroking your skin, the warmth of the sun radiating toward you. Feel the harmony of the elements and your state of well-being. You have arrived at the Lake of Conscience, no one in this lake sinks. Rest on the water and think that all the emotions and thoughts you no longer need (anger, fear, horror, hopelessness, pain, sorrow, anxiety, annoyance, self-blame, superiority, self-pity, and guilt) pass through your skin and you purify them by the magical power of water. And you see that the water around you is full of gray and black globules that are slowly recovering the turquoise-green color of the water. You think once again of all the emotions and thoughts you no longer need (anger, fear, horror, hopelessness, pain, sorrow, anxiety, annoyance, self-blame, superiority, self-pity, guilt), and they pass through your skin, and you purify them by the magical power of water. You see that the water around you is full of gray and black globules that are slowly obscuring the turquoise-green color of the water. And once again, think of all the emotions and thoughts you no longer need (anger, fear, horror, hopelessness, pain, sorrow, anxiety, annoyance, self-blame, superiority, self-pity, guilt) as they pass through your skin, you purify them by the magical power of water. And you once again see that the water around you is full of gray and black globules that are slowly obscuring the turquoise-green color of the water.

You feel the power of the water, the power of the Earth, the breeze on your skin, the radiance of the sun warming you, the harmony of the elements, the feeling of well-being.

You ask your magical horse to come to you. You love your horse, you pamper it, and let it caress you too. You bounce on its back and head to God's Grad. In the air, you fly together, become one being. You have arrived. Ask your horse to wait. You grow wings, and you fly toward the Trinity. You bow your head and apologize for all the sins you have committed against your body. You apologize for all the sins you have committed against your soul. You apologize for all the sins you committed against your spirit. You wait for the angels to give you the gifts that help you. If you can't see yourself receiving one, it means you don't need it yet. If you did it, open it and look inside. Give thanks that you could be here. Get back on your horse and fly back to the meadow. Find the white gravel path and head back down to the door to your stairs. Look at the grass in the meadow. Notice if there are any flowers. If so, describe the colors, any bush or tree, and whatever you see in the distance. Feel the power of the Earth flowing through your soles, the breeze stroking your skin, the warmth of the sun radiating toward you. Feel the harmony of the elements and your state of well-being. You arrive at the door, open it, and head up the stairs. Count from one to ten. You are back, move your fingers slowly, open your eyes.

Weight Loss

Sit comfortably. Relax your muscles, close your eyes. Breathe in and breathe out. Do not cross your feet because this will lock you away from the desired experience. Hold your hands together to connect your logical brain hemisphere with your instinct.

Concentrate on your back now and notice how you feel in the bed or chair you are sitting in. Take a deep breath and let your stress leave your body. Now focus on your neck. Observe how your neck is joined to your shoulders. Lift your shoulders slowly. Breathe in slowly and release it. Feel how your shoulders loosen. Lift your shoulders again a little bit, then let them relax. Observe how your neck muscles are tense and how much pressure it has. Breathe in and breathe out slowly. Release the pressure in your neck and notice how the stress is leaving your body. Repeat the whole exercise from the beginning. Observe your back. Notice all the stress and let it go with a profound breath. Focus on your shoulders and neck again. Lift up your shoulders and hold it for some moments, then release your shoulders again and let all the stress go away. Sense how the stress is going away. Now, place your attention on your back. Feel how comfortable it is. Focus on your whole body. While breathing in, let relaxation come in, and while you are breathing out, let frustration leave your body. Notice how much you are relaxed.

Concentrate on your inner self. Breathe slowly and release it. Calm down your mind. Observe your thoughts. Don't go with them because your aim is to observe them and not to be involved. It's time to let go of your overweight self that you are not feeling good about. Imagine yourself as you are now. See yourself in every detail. Describe your hair, the color of your clothes, your eyes. See your face, your nose, your mouth. Set aside this image for a moment. Now imagine yourself as you would like to be in the future. See yourself in every detail. Describe your hair, the color of your clothes, your eyes. See your face, your nose, your mouth. Imagine that your new self-approaches your present self and pampers it. See that your new self-hugs your present self. Feel the love that is spread in the air. Now see that your present self leaves the scene, and your new self takes its place. See and feel how happy and satisfied you are. You believe that you can become this beautiful new self. You breathe in this image and place it in your soul. This image will always be with you and flow through your whole body. You want to be this new self. You can be this new self.

After spending a few minutes with this, imagine that every time you breathe in, you are inhaling prank, the life energy of the universe, shining in gold. In this life force, you will find everything you need and desire: a healthy, muscular body, a soul that loves itself in all circumstances, a hand that puts enough nutritious food on the table, a strong voice to say no to sabotaging your diet, a head that can say no to those who are trying to distract you from your ideas and goals. With each breath, you absorb these positive images and emotions.

See in front of you exactly what your life would be like if you got everything you wanted. Release your old self and start becoming your new self. Gradually restore your breathing to regular breathing.

Day 3. SHAPING HEALTHIER HABITS

We will focus this meditation on shaping healthier habits. Tune in to this or repeat the content in your own voice and use that to help manage you through the meditation. Locate a comfortable position and start when you are ready. Let these thoughts course through your mind naturally, as if you were telling them. I can feel each breath that enters and leaves my body. My breath comes in through my nose naturally. I don't have to consider it, and my body will breathe all alone. This is a habit that I created before I even left my mother's belly. I breathe faster when I am apprehensive. I breathe faster when I am energized. My breathing will slow as I become relaxed. At the point when I am falling asleep, I can feel my breathing going staggeringly moderate. My breathing will regulate itself. This is a habit that I have, and it reminds me I am human. When my breathing is happening in the winter, I can see it leave my body and make the air white. At the point when I am breathing on a hot sunny day, I can once in a while feel my warm breath on my body, making me feel significantly hotter. As I am breathing now, I see this theme. I perceive that habits are patterns that can come as naturally to me as breathing. Without considering it, there are a few habits that I take part in daily.

In the past, I have taken part in habits that were not healthy, and that is okay. I wasn't always aware of the unhealthy habits that I had shaped. Some things took somewhat longer to realize, and it wasn't something I could always recognize all alone either. I can now perceive the unhealthy things that I have done in the past. These unhealthy habits included things like picking a diet I knew wasn't healthy for my body or choosing not to practice, although I realized I expected to get my body going. I won't rebuff myself because of these unhealthy habits. I am at peace with the decisions I used to make for my body. I will focus just on shaping healthy habits for me. I have to emphasize doing things that will better my body, mind, and soul later on. There is no better ideal opportunity to shape a healthy habit, and then, I realize I have to remember it for my lifestyle. The better I can get at perceiving and adding healthy habits, the easier it will be to change my life. I am aware of the things I have to improve, and it is significantly easier to identify what I shouldn't do. I will always search for new healthy habits to remember in my life. I will recall that I have to keep investigating myself and guarantee that I am making the correct choices for the right reasons. There is nothing amiss with framing habits. Now I have to focus on framing healthier ones that will help me for a more drawn out timeframe. Habits will take time to shape. I won't have the option to frame all the habits I want for the time being. I will make sure I attempt every day to accomplish something healthy. From that point, I will locate the most natural habits to utilize, and the ones I have to alter to fit into my life more readily. I can shape healthy habits, as long as I commit myself to make healthy decisions every day. Some healthy habits will shape all alone. This is natural. Easy habits for certain individuals, maybe even more challenging for me, and that is okay. I will go at my pace, and the principal thing that matters is that I will be committed to adding these healthy habits. The more I focus on framing habits, the easier it will be to follow through with them. Habits will take as much time as it needs to form. It is okay to fall back into old habits; I have to have the solidarity to pull me back out. I will prepare for times when I may fall back into these habits, so I don't let it cause me disappointment. If I anticipate flawlessness all through my habit-framing process, I will just set myself up to feel defeated. Instead, I will prepare with encouraging affirmations and positive intuition to help me through the occasions when I want to give up. Now is the best opportunity for me to enter the current world from this meditation and to get focused on adding healthier habits to my life. I am going to put my mind towards guaranteeing that I include meditation as one of my habits, as this will improve my health. I start to leave this state of mind and come back to a superior, healthier place, situated on making healthy decisions. I can feel my breathing in a cadenced pattern that assists with relaxing my mind, body, and soul. I breathe in again, recollecting how it resembles a pattern, a mood, a habit. I feel the breath leave my body, exhaling the bad habits, inhaling the good. As I exhale the bad habits, I continue recalling how I can start these great habits as soon as my breathing has regulated. The time has come to be either focused or drift asleep at this point. As I count down from ten again, I will be out of this meditative state and back into the world that will assist me with forming healthy habits successfully. Ten, nine, eight, seven, six, five, four, three, two, one.

Mindful eating

This meditation will be focused on eating mindfully. You may even attempt this one (after you have already completed it once) while you are eating as another technique. Tune in to this or repeat the content in your own voice and use that to help manage you through the meditation. Locate a comfortable position and start when you are ready. Let these thoughts course through your mind naturally, as if you were telling them. I can feel each breath that enters and leaves my body. I am aware of my breath. I can tell how much air is entering my body and how much air is leaving. I am focus on only the breath that is coming through my mouth. As I become relaxed, I imagine myself eating. I am sitting behind a plate loaded up with delectable foods that will keep me full. I realize that the ideal way to keep me interested in my meal is to incorporate various parts and food groups. Having whole grains will keep me full more. Veggies will give me fiber and fruits give me that pleasantness I need. These foods keep me happy while I am eating them for the day. They are useful not only for my body but for my mind as well.

I feel each chunk of food as it enters my mouth. I love the mix of the surfaces as I bite into each piece. My teeth are strong and amazing enough to have the option to tear up anything from the meat of an animal to the hardest of apples. I am incredible as I bite into my food, feeling the surfaces in my mouth. It feels great to recharge my body. I appreciate the sustenance I get from these tasty meals. I don't have to eat large pieces of food. Small bites are similarly as powerful. I used to eat larger spoonfuls, filling my mouth as much as I could. I now realize that it's smarter to take smaller bites, so I can focus instead on the flavor and not the amount of food that I'm eating. I'm worried about surface and taste, not eating more to keep me full.

The slower I bite into my food, the less I have to process with my body. This will make it easier to pull the supplements from my food. I can feel this giving me vitality; I am gaining as much as I can from this food. I am taking all the supplements and minerals that it offers. All the parts of my food will assist me with being a stronger and healthier individual. I realize that as I let food enter my mouth, I am putting acceptable supplements into my body. As I eat gradually, I realize that I don't have to eat seconds. I am delighted in the amount that I ate. I take smaller bites so that if I want seconds, I am not eating that much. I also prefer to use smaller plates now because I realize that the food appears to be greater to me. There are so many things that I can do to assist me in focusing my attention on mindful eating rather than the mindless practices I used to do while devouring my food. I am relaxed as I eat, not forcing myself to bite excessively fast. There is no surge. At the point when I am feeling raced to eat, I make sure to eat a snack. I am eating my food in a relaxed state. I make sure I breathe throughout this.

I am appreciating my food and creating a relationship with it that will help me lose weight faster. I love my food, and it adores me. It causes me to become stronger, and this relationship is better than the one I used to fear. I am eating more mindfully than in the past, and it makes me feel amazing. I can feel my breathing in a cadenced pattern that assists with relaxing my mind, body, and soul. As I breathe again, I let myself feel full without having to keep eating. I can take a break and be okay with what I exhausted, feeling it attempting to make my body feel good. I continue breathing in and out, letting the air fill me, similarly as the food has.

The time has come to be either focused or drift asleep at this point. As I count down from ten again, I will be out of this meditative state and back into the world that will assist me with losing weight successfully. Ten, nine, eight, seven, six, five, four, three, two, one.

Day 4. SEEKING FULFILLMENT AND FINDING SATISFACTION

The state of emotional eating is about seeking fulfillment and finding satisfaction. The problem is that the way in which you are choosing to do it won't give you what you truly need. Instead, it will harm your health and create further detachment between you and your true self. The connection that you are trying to create with emotional eating is the connection with your identity. You may see that as a way of looking for spiritual satisfaction using food.

Indeed, with mindful eating and a self-loving attitude, food is a good source of pleasure and fulfillment. However, when the act of eating becomes a way for you to detach from your inner being, the trouble occurs.

Meditation, self-reflection, and mindful eating can become a way for you to overcome emotional eating. This is because, with awareness and mindfulness, you will get to connect with your spiritual self. Your inner self remains unchanged and untouched by the difficulties of life and holds a lot of knowledge and instinctive wisdom (Ross, 2016).

How Your Identity Affects Your Relationship With Food

To better understand the essence of your relationship with food, self-awareness is the right approach. To bring the matter closer to your understanding, you can frame the process of discovering the nature of your relationship with food through self-awareness as the process of connecting with your true identity.

Learning how to be in touch with your true identity means becoming able to access your inner strengths and instinctive wisdom. This way, the struggles of life won't overpower you, and you will be able to center yourself and regulate your feelings once challenges occur. This makes a lot of sense from a scientific viewpoint, too, since your body and mind are constantly working on learning, growing, changing, and self-preserve. What happened to you was that early trauma, in the broad sense of the word, taught you that hearing yourself out and trusting yourself was wrong or dangerous. For this reason, you were willing to disregard all of your knowledge and wonderful human qualities and only look into what you perceive are lacks or flaws;

- You are overeating because you think that you can't handle your feelings, which isn't true;

- You are refusing to hear and acknowledge your most profound fears and insecurities that are a result of misinformation;

- You don't believe your own instincts because you deemed them to be a sign of weakness or selfishness. For that matter, you don't seek love, affection, care, and support either from yourself or from others;

How Early Attachment Affects Your Relationship With Food

From the moment you were born, you've associated food with love. Whether you were breastfed or not, the state of hunger was the most distressing experience for you at the time. Being hungry was an agonizing feeling, and receiving the food was a life-saving experience. There's nothing wrong with having a close connection with food. If you think about it, the lack of it, while you were a baby, caused your body to scream for attention. Can you imagine the level of agony you'd have to feel now, as an adult, to react the same way you did when you were a baby? Your initial relationship with food was that the lack of it meant pain and suffering, and getting it meant that you got attention, love, comfort, and care.

Insecure attachment with primary caregivers may have contributed to forming a dysfunctional relationship with food. As a result, food may become a way for you to replace what you feel is missing from your life and obtain love instead of feeling empty and deprived.

Food could have also become a way for you to cope with boredom, as children are often offered snacks to calm down or to keep them from begging for attention from the overtired, overly busy caregiver.

One of the first steps to find your answer in relation to food is to discover what you are trying to compensate for with eating. You need to understand how food is serving as a replacement for truly satisfying your soul, and how to change emotional eating with a good habit that truly nourishes both your body and spirit. To examine your relationship with food, write down the following observations:

- The times of the day when you turn to food for comfort;

- The exact foods you crave at the time; and

- The way in which the foods you crave for make you feel;

Now, a simple way to solve the mystery is to take the food out of the equation and simply connect the times of the day with what you've perceived you can gain with food. This simple exercise will help you discover the type of fulfillment you are looking for with food. This is what your inner self is craving, and because you lack either knowledge or skill to provide that, you are using food. You could be yearning for anything from joy and fun to companionship and comfort.

How Your Body Image Affects Your Relationship With Food

Repeating the same process will help you discover the background of your body image issues and the way in which habitual eating fits into the equation. Here's how to explore the connection between body image and habitual eating:

- Write down the thoughts about your body;

- Write down the situations that trigger these thoughts;

- Write down the social situations that make you crave food; and

- Write down the feelings and thoughts that these situations cause you;

Are you noticing any patterns? Does your negative body image somehow reflect on what you think when you're with friends and family? Could these thoughts and feelings have something to do with social overeating? If so, what are your observations regarding this connection?

How to Create a Healthy Relationship With Food

To start building a healthy relationship with food, focus on the positive ways in which the food serves you and your body. Next, list all the positive ways you want to feel about your body. This will be the beginning of the shift in the way you look at food. Pay attention to that list, and write down how having the ideal body would make you feel;

- How would you feel about yourself if you looked the way you truly desire?

- What would change in your life?

- What would change for you at work?

- How would your relationships change?

The answers to these questions are your core needs in relation to your body image, and the good things that you will obtain from your transformed relationship with food. It could be a desire to be accepted, loved, cherished, adored, respected that lies behind your emotional eating.

Now, look into the similarities behind using the food to distract yourself from the negative thoughts, and the core needs that will be fulfilled with an ideal body. Most likely, there are similar needs at both ends. There could also be differences.

Detach Self-esteem From Food and Weight

If you're used to associating the way you feel about yourself with your weight and the way you are eating, it is very likely to have a negative effect on both your eating habits and your self-esteem. As a result, you've never built up true self-esteem.

You could have spent extensive amounts of time and money chasing after the ideal body, without realizing that the true problem lies in the lack of self-esteem. With food and dieting, you were looking for a way to feel better about yourself. Even reaching the desired weight and shape can't help self-esteem issues.

You need to realize that your self-esteem is unconditional and that it comes from your identity. It doesn't depend on either your achievements or the way you look. As long as you are thinking about self-esteem as something that is earned or achieved, you will never truly have it.

Only by looking at self-esteem as the inborn right to be honored and respected will you make progress.

You learned why your current relationship with food isn't beneficial and why it came to be in the first place. The main shift that you want to make in order to recover from emotional eating is that of your consciousness. Instead of eating to avoid coping, you want to adopt a relationship with food that focuses on the nourishment of the mind and body.

Day 5. CHOOSING A SPOT

Choosing a spot to meditate daily at the same location is invariably very helpful and important, particularly in reducing distraction potential and straying mind. It may not be necessary to fold your legs up into a lotus posture or to sit on the floor; instead, it is the key to locate an upright sitting position conveniently where you will not be interrupted. Both of this help make a jiffy of time to slowly reach serenity and reflect on what is happening inside of us. You don't need to spend a dime to get you off. What you just need is a place to sit down, a bit of decisive power.

For those who want to work it out on kits, there are cushions, stools, and other accessories fashioned for meditation purposes. But seriously, a convenient chair, possibly a soft rug in a calm angle, is needed.

You can also extend your scope of practice with time by engaging in walking meditation. As soon as you're comfortable with sitting meditation and body scan, it could be a choice to try walking meditation. No theory makes walking meditation come afterward, just that it is very helpful for one to know the basics before engaging in walking and meditation simultaneously.

Another form of meditation on mindfulness is mindful eating. An enlightening exercise to try is mindful eating, rather than consuming anything on the menu list, creating time and space for vital attention to experience. This can be done when eating alone. You can experience eating conscientiously with easy food like an apple. Mindful eating is not only a beneficial (often fun and interesting) activity; it often provides a whole lot of wonderful sensory experiences, while evidence has shown that it can lead to loss of weight. If we pay close attention to what we eat when we get hungry, we eat less often.

Take conscious notice of every eating and your responses to it. Observe your feelings as you settle down for a meal. Are you hungry or your mouth wets? Look critically at the food, how does it look? Take a serious examination of the food, hot or cold? Do you have the sensation of how the bit smells, how about it making a sound when you hold it, anything like that? As you set to take the first bite, evaluate your reactions, any salivating? Is taking the next bite your utmost thought now?

What happens at the drop of the food on your tongue? Observe the chewing feelings and the flow it causes to go down your throat, any feeling in your stomach? Set to take the next bite, right? Take a moment to witness every imaginable feeling, urges, and reactions after each bite. Although meditation on the surface looks easy, it might be interestingly difficult; but this doesn't make you a failure.

We need to understand some basic terms which revolve around weight loss meditation. Such specific processes and activities include meditation, mindful eating, and intuitive feeding. These can help our knowledge of having a healthy food relationship with food and the means to evacuate wrong feelings that involve our eating. Weight loss is a result of this renewed, cultivated relationship, but it is also important that we concentrate rightly and wisely in that when weight loss becomes your primary goal, it restricts us from eating intuitively or mindfully.

Pay attention to enjoying the food, as you eat now because you're hungry, not because you're tired, knockdown emotionally, or frustrated. Practices such as this help you love your body for things that it can offer.

When we discuss meditation for weight loss or eating and building a healthy relationship with food, the terminologies will be well understood.

Stress or emotional eating occurs when people seem to eat excessively because of heavy emotions or feelings, rather than reacting to the inner feeling of hunger that runs through them. This emotion tends to overwhelm our physical feelings of satisfaction and fullness, resulting in overeating from strong emotions in a situation such as food being used as a temporary relief tool. However, admitting that this experience adds up to perpetuating a cycle is crucial and important. The feeling of a stressful emotion can result in overeating, leading to guilt and shame, returning to the feeling of negative emotion or stress (without the ability to manage).

Using a mindful eating system or strategy will help you restructure and restore your food relationship and eating experience. It demands our being present and involving our senses – the taste of the food, how it smells, and, essentially, how it makes our bodies feel. Intuitive eating is incorporated through mindful eating. This helps us to delay and listen to our inner feelings of true hunger signs of satiation, and as such, it can help our emotional eating to decline and even completely stop. Therefore, if our type of food is made based on the result or physical outcome we want, it connotes that we have stopped eating attentively.

The approach to wellness and health is a non-diet, mind-body intuitive eating. It disallows the idea of dieting and instructs us to trust our bodies and listen to our internal physical indications to heal our food relationship. However, eating principles are part of intuitive eating. It spreads the enlarged philosophy hat cut across your body as it is interesting to move and harness information about nutrition without partiality.

It is safe to take a positive attitude towards meditation practices. Staying relaxed and friendly will be helpful as you face certain inevitable incoherence of meditation. When you find that you have been working heinously and downcast, take a minute, take a deep breath, and relax and take it easy. Take note of the fact that the object of meditation is not to have your mind completely controlled or abort all your thoughts, but rather to have you calm, loving, and have a clear approach towards happenings.

Basic mindfulness is simple, but it's not always simple to do because it takes a lot of effort. Ordinary admiration of meditation works or produces no result unless there is an engagement. Thoughts will not disappear during mindfulness meditation. Tough emotions may arise when you begin to meditate, especially very early. Staying fixed may seem unrealistic, but with the time, you tend to become more coordinated with the practice. Choose to try to attain feelings of what the present moment looks like, rather than aim for some exercise outside of the body. The perfect thing is to set aside any judgmental picture and excitement only to observe what is happening.

When we start meditating, how we criticize ourselves is so funny. Sayings like "I'm doing it wrong," "I can't be good at meditating," "I'm never going to be able to make up for this with my schedules." Almost everyone who has been engaged in meditation has had this kind of experience of low confidence. Even though it's normal to feel that way, it's not helpful, remembering that the purpose is not to downplay yourself or give yourself low self-worth but to focus on the present moment's happenings what it is. We all have the capacity to be serene, transparent, and mindful, so disengage your beliefs from judgments of good and bad meditations.

Sleepiness is another thing that happens to others as they try to meditate. This can happen when our mind is overpacked or because the body gets tired, and the need for rest is thereby exhausted. Nevertheless, there are competent methods to meditate on being awake. Straighten yourself in the place, open your eyes, try the walking meditation, and probably engage in listening to sounds rather than breathing as your anchor of concentration. You will be able to develop a sensation style to focus on; for example, first and foremost, get the breath in and out of your nostrils, then feel the diaphragm dropping and rising, and finally, cool air breeze right over your lips.

Most of the time, because we're used to being busy, meditation may seem banal and uninteresting at first, despite that, don't be too hard on yourself, just re-analyze your attention; take some out-breath, then in-breath and longer out-breath.

At first, longer duration of meditations might seem painful, such as dull cramps or backaches or sharp fleeting pangs in your leg.

Whatever it might be, give it a notice at first, and accept it. Know the truth, like any other, that it's a feeling and will inevitably go away with time. If it persists, then try to move your attention to another part of your body. If the pain continues badly, then you can see just your posture otherwise as supposed.

Every time you start a meditation practice, the main and crucial question you have to ask yourself is to be sure if you want to be guided or unguided. Preference for guided and unguided meditation varies from individual to individual.

Whatever suits you is what you later term preference for others, but exploring what each option entails is interesting.

Day 6. HEAL YOUR BODY IMAGE THROUGH CHAKRA

Your chakras can go a long way in helping you heal your body image. Through your chakras, you can affirm various aspects of confidence, courage, desirability, and self-worth to yourself. In doing so, you both harmonize and balance your chakras and improve your own connection to yourself and your body image. As you use this meditation, you are going to achieve two important things. First and foremost, you are going to experience a greater sense of balance within each of your chakras that is going to allow you to feel more at peace with your body. This is going to allow you to love and respect your body at all stages of your journey, even the ones where you may not be particularly happy with your body or where you may want to change your body.

Next, you are going to experience a sense of balance in areas where you cannot change your body and where no amount of exercising or dietary practices will change anything for you. Sometimes, there are parts of our bodies that we cannot change, and we simply have to learn how to love and accept them, even if we are not particularly fond of them. This does not necessarily mean that you have to like this part of your body, but it does mean that it is a good idea for you to stop hating this part of your body so that you can find peace and acceptance in it instead.

For this meditation, you will need about 15-20 minutes, and you can complete it either while lying down or while sitting with your legs crossed and your spine straight. If you choose to sit up, keep your hands on your knees, palms up, and keep your body engaged and activated. This way, you are balancing your chakras simply from holding this healthy and aligned posture.

The Meditation

Begin this meditation by taking a nice deep breath in, slowly filling up your lungs with fresh, nourishing oxygen, and then exhaling it slowly. Breathe as slowly as you can, feeling each breath getting slower and slower as you gently fill your lungs up with oxygen and then release that oxygen from your lungs once again. Allow yourself to naturally lengthen and slow down each breath so that you can feel deeply relaxed. As each breath grows longer and slower, you will feel yourself naturally sinking into a deeper and more relaxed state. With each breath, feel your relaxation and peace doubling as you allow yourself to completely embrace yourself with calm, gentle energy.

If you find your mind wandering as you work towards this relaxed state, allow yourself to gently draw your awareness back to your breath. Use the consistent and gentle flow of energy moving in and out of your lungs as a rhythm to keep your awareness focused and intentional. Take care to keep yourself as still, mindful, and engaged as possible while also allowing your conscious mind and body to relax completely.

When you are ready, send your awareness down to your root chakra. See it glowing bright red and flowing in a clockwise motion. As you keep your awareness in your root chakra, see yourself becoming aware of all of the body parts associated with your root chakra, including your: legs, feet, glutes, and bones. Allow yourself to lovingly send energy to each of these parts of your body as you mindfully accept them and express gratitude for them and all that they do for you. Send love to your legs and feet for holding you up and assisting you with walking or moving through life in a meaningful manner. Send love to your glutes for giving you a comfortable seat, and to your bones for holding your body together and upright. If you have any flaws within any of these areas of your body, send love to these flaws and accept them as they are. Accept yourself as you are.

Now, send your awareness up into your sacral chakra. See your sacral chakra glowing bright orange and gently flowing in a clockwise motion. As your awareness grows more attached to this part of your body, consider the parts of your body that your sacral chakra governs. Think about your sexual organs and your perception of your own attractiveness. Think about your adrenal glands, kidneys, and even your bladder. Send love and gratitude to each of the body parts that your sacral chakra governs. Accept these parts of your body as they are, and thank them for all of the work they do in helping you maintain a high quality of life.

Think about the parts that you can see and interact with, such as your sexual attraction. Send thanks to your body for being attractive, and gratitude for your ability to increase your attraction. Affirm your attractiveness and express gratitude for your increasing attraction. See yourself as having the attractive body that you desire, and see yourself as being desired by others for your attractive body, too.

Next, draw your awareness into your solar plexus chakra. Feel your solar plexus chakra glowing bright yellow and rotating in a gentle clockwise motion as you draw your awareness into this part of your body. Become aware of the parts of your body that your solar plexus chakra governs, such as your stomach, your digestive organs, and your diaphragm. Send gratitude to your solar plexus chakra for all that it offers you in life, and send love and acceptance to the parts of your body that it governs. Ask for forgiveness for always fixating on the extra weight that it carries and invite it to release that weight naturally and rapidly as you commit to loving and accepting yourself as you are. Visualize the weight naturally dropping off and your stomach taking on the shape that you have always desired.

Draw your awareness up now into your heart chakra, feeling it glowing bright green and rotating gently in a clockwise motion. Draw your awareness into your heart chakra and all parts of your body that are governed by your heart chakra, including your chest, your lungs, and your circulatory system. See yourself as having a desirable and attractive chest, strong muscles, and a healthy circulatory system. Feel your stamina increasing with each breath, and see yourself as having the level of fitness that you desire. Send love, gratitude, and acceptance to your heart chakra for all that it does for you, and to all of those parts of your body and how they support you in experiencing your best possible life.

Now, draw your awareness up into your throat chakra. See your throat chakra glowing bright blue and gently rotating in a clockwise motion. As you do, allow yourself to become aware of the parts of your body that your throat governs, including your neck, your ears, and your respiratory system. Send gratitude and love to the unseen parts of life that your throat chakra governs. Accept your throat chakra as it is, and visualize it naturally slimming as your throat and neck become shapelier and even more attractive. Appreciate your throat and neck for how they look now and for how they have served you all of your life.

Again, draw your awareness up and into your third eye chakra. See your third eye chakra glowing bright indigo and gently spinning in a clockwise motion. Allow yourself to become aware of the parts of your body that your third eye chakra govern, including your mind and your face. Feel yourself sending love and gratitude to your mind and accepting yourself for the beautiful and unique individual that you are. Allow yourself to accept and love your face and all of your facial features and the way they help you look unique and attractive. Send gratitude to your face for your ability to slim your body down and see the beauty in your reflection every time you look in the mirror. Appreciate yourself for who you are and for who you are becoming every single day.

Lastly, draw your awareness up into your crown chakra. See your crown chakra glowing bright violet and gently rotating clockwise. Become aware of your entire self and all that makes you, you, and send love, gratitude, and acceptance to yourself. Become willing to fall in love with yourself as you are, and feel how deeply connected you feel with yourself and all of life that surrounds you when you embrace this deep level of connection and love. Feel how peaceful and meaningful this is for you to fall into such a deep level of love and acceptance with yourself, including all that you can and cannot change, and all that you do and do not like about yourself. Understand that no matter what, you can choose to love yourself, even if you do not like everything about yourself.

Spend a few moments in this space, breathing and meditating into these feelings of love, acceptance, and gratitude that you are now feeling for yourself and your body. Then, when you are ready, awaken yourself by opening your eyes and gently shaking your limbs out so that you can bring energy and awareness back into the present moment. Allow yourself to approach the rest of the day and every day from here on out with great love, gratitude, and acceptance for yourself and trust that you can love yourself both now and later when you have achieved your ideal body image. From this place of love, acceptance, and gratitude, you will be far more likely to achieve your goals and feel truly happy and healthy in your new slimmer and stronger body.

Day 7. COMPLETE RELAXATION

Find a peaceable place to sit or lie down for complete relaxation, then breathe and pay attention. Notice as the air tides in through your nostrils and how your belly buzzes to the maximum and gently falls back to your spine as you breathe out. Allow gravity to hold you securely in place. Breathe as naturally as you can. Do not force your breathing and take notice if your breath is quick or slow and steady.

As you breathe in, accept gratitude and let warmth fill your lungs. Think of the things you are grateful for. Think of something that makes you feel happy and peaceful. Say to yourself, "I am thankful to be alive. I am secure and safe. I am confident and pure." Pay attention to your heart now. As you say these words to yourself, feel them deep within you. Give these statements positive energy and feed them with love. "I love myself; I can do anything I put my mind to. I trust that my brain, body, and soul are capable of providing me with what I desire most in life."

Breathe in now and fill your mind and soul with love and warmth. Imagine as you breathe in that there is a radiant light that fills your lungs before rapidly escaping your body. This light gives your patience, it gives you strength, and it provides you with the ambition and motivation to tackle the barriers that stand in your way. Breathe out naturally and notice as your body becomes heavier. With every breath that flows out, let go of negative thoughts; push those thoughts aside. You are good enough. You can do this. You are loved. You are special. Breathe out and release all of the tension that holds you back now. What other people believe and what you think are two different things. Say this now, "I believe in myself."

Count your breaths now. As you breathe in, breathe with your belly and count. One, two, three, four, and five. When you let go of this breath, make sure it is steady and slow. Breathe out, two, three, four, five. You are accepting this positive light to vibrate through your entire being. You are letting go of all the negativity that holds you back. Breathe in one, two, three, four. Breathe out one, two, three, four. And inhale for one, "I am happy," two, "I am strong," three, "I am kind," four, "I am brave," five, "I am driven to succeed." Breathe out now. You are counting your breath from one to five, slow and steady. Positivity embraces you now; you feel light and in complete control. Nothing can disturb you; nothing can bring you down; you are perfect the way you are. Repeat this step until you are ready to watch your thoughts flow in and out.

Bring focus to your inner thoughts now. What pops into your mind? If you have any negative thoughts, let them be there as long as they want to be without judging them. Watch them, and then let them go. With every in-breath, notice your thoughts pop in without judgment. These thoughts are neither positive nor negative. When you breathe out, just let go of all hostility and anger you might be holding. Let it escape into the universe and breathe in, one, two, three, four, five; you are accepting all honesty and trust within yourself that you can make it through anything. "I am resilient. I am beautiful. I am a leader."

If you notice any negative thoughts, just see them and replace them with positive, self-loving thoughts.

Breaking Barriers

Make sure that you are in a place where you are completely comfortable and will not be disturbed for at least thirty minutes. Have the room you are inset to a comforting temperature and make sure that the lights are low. Adjust your body so that your shoulders are relaxed, your arms are lying on either side of you, and your palms are facing the ceiling. You want to become as comfortable and relaxed as you can so that your focus is not on your body but on the meditation. Gently close your eyes and take a deep breath inward until you can no longer breathe in. Exhale slowly and steadily so that all of the air escapes your lungs. Repeat these two more times.

Notice how your mind and body are relaxing into this guided exercise now. Breathe naturally now and bring your attention to your breath. Notice as the air fills your lungs and escapes as quickly as it entered. Breathing is something we do every day that we often take for granted. It's one of the many gifts that life gives us. Just be mindful of this moment you are in right now. Don't worry if your mind wanders; that's natural. There is no wrong way to do this. Put trust in yourself that right now, you are not performing; you don't have to be perfect.

Bring your attention to your body and your weight now. Visualize in your mind what you look like and try not to judge yourself too harshly. You are who you are, no matter what you look like or how you feel about that. Erase the tension and negativity from your mind; just be present with yourself right now.

Say to yourself,

"I am beautiful. I am strong. I can do this. I will lose weight, and I will not let anyone or anything stand in my way. The only opinion I will accept is what I think and feel about myself. At this moment and in my future moments, I believe that I am beautiful just the way that I am."

Let your breath suck in all these thoughts and have your mind believe everything you tell yourself as if it was your last wish on Earth.

As you visualize your weight right now, I would like you to imagine that you are at the starting line of a race. There are people just like you are competing for success.

Say to yourself,

"I got this. I will not give up. I will succeed, and I will make it to the finish line. I will conquer my fears and overcome every obstacle that stands in my way."

In the background, you hear a coach shout, "Ready, get set..." Bring your awareness to your breath again. Inhale deeply and as you breathe in, get yourself fully committed and ready to take your first step toward losing weight. "Go!" Breathe out and visualize your feet, taking that first, second, and third step forward. Feel the pressure of your body press down on your legs and carry you forward. You realize this is hard, but you don't give up. You continue to jog ahead. Repeat this – "I know I can, I know I can, I know I can. I won't give up; I can do this."

You are now coming up to a bicycle, and as you get on it, you feel the bike hold your weight. You will not fall. Put your feet on the pedals and start cycling. As you cycle, you continue faster and faster. Your heart is racing from the much-needed exercise. You feel good. Your lungs begin to hurt, but you push yourself as you notice the wind flying through your hair. Notice the droplets of sweat cool your skin. You got this. You are coming to a curve in the course now. Turn your bike and follow the path to the finish line. As you look back, you can see people just like yourself competing to finish, and there are a few behind you and a few ahead of you. While exercising, take a steady breath in and push it out forcefully. You should hear a pushing sound coming from your pursed lips. Inhale and say, "I got this, I won't give up. I will succeed." You are coming to the finish line now, but the course isn't over yet. As you cross the finish line, you get off your bike in third place. Way to go!

Bring your attention now to your breath. You are breathing heavily, your heart is racing, your chest hurts, but it's a euphoric feeling. You feel free; you broke out of the cycle and crossed the finish line. As you take a look down your body, you notice your body has become thinner. There is a scale in front of you on the sidelines; you've lost ten pounds. The feeling you are experiencing at this very moment is breathtaking, so you want to try it again. Trust that your body knows you and what to do. Trust in yourself that you will get through this.

You get ready again and wait to hear the coach. Take a deep breath in for a count of five. When I count down, you can start your course. Five, four, three, two, one, and go! Let out your breath and feel your legs carry your ten-pounds-lighter body. This time it's a little more comfortable than the first round. Your breath quickens, and your heart speeds up. You can do this.

Say to yourself,

"I will complete this course. I am strong enough to conquer any barrier that stands in my way. This is hard, but nothing easy is worth doing. I got this."

In front of you now is a blow-up house with a wide opening. You crawl through this opening and are covered by colorful plastic balls. They are flying at you from all angles, and it becomes hard to see. Soon, you are swimming through these balls moving forward. You push these balls aside, and as you look up, you see another opening. "I got this,"

You say to yourself.

"I will make it through, and nothing can stop me now." As you reach the opening, you crawl through and are entirely on your stomach. You are in a narrow hole that you must army-crawl through to reach the end. Take in a deep breath now. Nothing scares you. Nothing can get to you. Imagine this hole the way everyone else bullied you or picked on you. You might have felt small, or enclosed, singled out, or trapped.

You have complete control. You can do this. You are coming closer to the light at the end now. Nothing can stop you. As you reach the end of the tunnel, you jump out and start doing jumping jacks and yell to the universe, "I did it!" You beat your fears, and you conquered the darkness, but your journey isn't over yet. On the right side of you are a glass of freshwater and a table with a scale right next to it. You down the water and step on the scale. You notice your weight dropped another ten pounds. As the euphoric energy escapes you, you feel happy and delighted.

As you look ahead of you, you see one more course twenty feet away and the finish line at the end. Take a step forward now. Walk or jog at your own pace. You got this. You have faced more difficult challenges before, so you are going to get through this one. Twenty steps later and you reach a potato sack, and five tires on the ground laid out in a straight line. You jump into the potato sack, and while holding it up, you jump into the first tire hole. Take a deep breath in, and now the second tire hole. Breathe out, jump into the third tire, now the fourth, and take your time. Breathe in and jump into the final tire.

As you jump out to finish, exhale slowly. You can feel your heart aching from the exercise. Pat yourself on the back; you're almost there. On the left side of the track, you notice weight balls that attach to your ankles and two five-pound dumbbells. You connect the ankle weights, pick up the dumbbells in each hand, and look forward. The finish line is ten steps away. Take a deep breath in. "I'm almost there, and I won't give up." Breathe out and take your first step. The weight around your ankles was the same amount of weight you carried at the beginning of the race. You notice how much of a difference this is and never want to feel like this again. Take another step forward and feel the sweat drip down the back of your neck. Feel the exhaustion.

Now visualize your ideal weight. Let that be your motivation to continue. With every step, you become more and more tired. Your body becomes more and more exhausted, but you don't give up. You keep moving forward; the finish line just steps away now. Take a deep breath in, and there is no way you are giving up now. You are so close to your ideal weight. You have almost accomplished your goal. You hear the people on either side of you cheer you on. Yes! You crossed the finish line and felt that it was all worth it as you step onto that scale beside you. And right before your very eyes are the numbers you have wanted to see for so long.

You did it! Congratulations! You are now at your ideal weight. Visualize what this looks like and take in the excitement. Visualize what feeling you would experience after completing your goal. Stay relaxed at this moment for as long as you would like.

When you are ready, come back to the present moment. Bring your awareness to your breath. Move each finger and wiggle your toes. Feel good as you remember your visualization. You completed your goal, and you didn't give up. That's what you will choose to do in your waking life every day. Everyone has obstacles, but you have the willpower and now the skills to beat everyone that gets in your way. You may open your eyes now.

CHAPTER 11:

Mistakes to Avoid

Mistake # 1: Deleting Fun Foods

I never take cheese," " I stopped chocolate completely," "Unthinkable to have sweets at home." These little declarations of war, we have heard them all, even pronounced. However, a determination is definitely not the key to lasting weight loss. Mind control over food is the basic error, arguably the heaviest and also the most common. By deciding not to eat the square of chocolate that you adore, you switch to cognitive restriction. In other words, it's the start of a relentless match against your body. And this control is fragile. A smell, tiredness, a blow of depression is enough to overcome it, sooner or later. Above all, instead of learning to recognize hunger, satiety, gustatory pleasure, you are moving away from natural sensations. We can even end up filling our hunger with a dish of green beans so as not to succumb to prohibited food. And, at the time of "cracking" (hearty dinner, snack, etc.), we enter a vicious circle:

- 1 / "I shouldn't, I'm going to get fat."

- 2 / "I will not eat more of the week."

- 3 / "I eat too much before being deprived of it."

Not sure, moreover, that this pattern is not repeated for several days in a row. What is more, the experience of two American researchers shows that we will eventually gain weight. According to their results, after a snack (a milkshake), the people tested spontaneously adjust, without calculation, the portions of their next meal. What the "restricted eaters" are incapable of.

The solution:

No longer believe in "foods that make you fat." For this, the nutritionist recommends an interesting exercise. A person who always ends lunches and dinners with yogurt or fruit, perceived as "authorized" foods, can replace them with two squares of chocolate, the famous "prohibited" food. By keeping this rhythm for six days (weighing before and after), she will have lost weight or, in any case, will not have gained it! Because, in terms of calories, the two squares of chocolate (dark or milk) are below the intake of fruit or yogurt. Result: chocolate will no longer be a "devilish" food.

The person will even find the desire to eat fruits and dairy products because they are good and not because they "make you lose weight.

Mistake # 2: Obey the Rule of Three Meals a Day

We have been told enough to believe it: You have to eat three meals a day. And, better still, a king's breakfast, a prince's lunch, and a poor man's dinner. The golden rule is actually much simpler and natural: you have to eat when you are hungry. We just haven't shown a relationship between the number of meals a day and weight gain.

Then, a morning calorie is the same as that of midday or evening. Studies have not shown that the body would assimilate cheese, butter, fish, fries, yogurt, fruit, protein, etc. differently. They consume the whole day's food ration all at once, even in the evening or at night. However, after a month on this diet, unless they are too rich, they do not gain weight.

The solution:

It is up to everyone to see whether they need to eat in the morning or not, a lot or a little. However, not forcing yourself to breakfast does not mean allowing yourself to throw yourself into anything at 11 am in the cafeteria or bakery. If the stomach is starving, it is better to wait until lunch while crunching an apple or taking a banana. What your brain will deduct itself from the next meal. Be careful, however, to make the difference with snacking! We eat because we are hungry. We snack because we want to eat. But small snacks are often minimized.

Mistake # 3: "Believe" in Light

Consumption of these products has only increased. Have people become less fat? No. "We now know that light and sweeteners will not solve the problem of overweight, obesity, and diabetes.

Diet products only "flatter the brain": you know you are eating a lower calorie product. But you lose in pleasure what you gain in satisfaction. A dietary cookie, "to taste, it's no longer a treat. And the 10 to 15% fewer calories compared to a normal cookie will not make a major difference, "he continues. Not to mention that, when it comes to salty snacks, "the lightened diet has the effect of distorting our taste, notes the nutritionist. Bread crumbs with fish flesh and a little oil."

The solution:

The war against sugar is no longer necessary. To his patients, Dr. Cohen advises instead to keep it, choose real sweets, and, for drinks, coffee or tea, add Stevia, a natural sweetener, for the most addicted palates with a sweet taste.

Mistake # 4: Eating Too Much Industrial Product

You apply to the letter the proportions that nutritionists recommend. But industrial or "processed" products are a real obstacle to weight loss. Breakfast cornflakes, for example, have nothing to do with grain from farmers' fields.

Children's brands have even recently been compared to junk food because of their high sugar content; a bowl may contain more than a donut, according to an independent American organization. Whatever the brand, cereal petals have a high glycemic index anyway, promoting an insulin spike and poor hunger control.

All forms of sugar that pass quickly in the blood consumed at breakfast are responsible for some of the vertiginous appetite before lunchtime. In this case, to opt in the morning for a meal based on "rye bread with a salty touch (ham, cheese, fish)."

The solution:

Whenever possible, prefer raw foods that you prepare yourself. "Instead of a tray of ready-to-eat grated carrots, you can buy the bag of already grated carrots at the supermarket, and even the vinaigrette sold next to it. It's all about dosing yourself. Nutritionists rely on the energy values of food alone, not those of prepared meals. Also, when a doctor advises a yogurt at the end of the meal, it is a natural one, not with fruit, coulis, caramel, or other. "This type of yogurt is the equivalent of three basic yogurts, 150 calories against 50," says the research director of Weight Watchers.

Mistake # 5: Running Away From the Bread

Bread makes you fat? No more than the rest. Regardless of the nature of the calories, it is their excess in the quantity that causes weight gain.

Moreover, in 1900, the average consumption of bread was 900 grams per day (against 110.5 g in 2010) without the era being marked by the emergence of overweight. Depriving yourself of it does not promote weight loss. It occupies a certain volume in the food ration. And eliminating it means it's going to be replaced by other foods, probably even more energetic.

The solution:

Keep it to accompany the meal or to taste, with a knob of butter (better than a cookie!). Whole or made from rye flour, it is even one of the foods to be consumed "without counting" from the Weight Watchers ProPoints2 program.

Mistake # 6: Not Being Followed or Encouraged

This is undoubtedly one of the elements of the success of the Weight Watchers method: regular meetings to take stock, strengthen your determination, discuss your difficulties, share recipes, solutions, tips, then go back to " real life "and hold on. The slimming program websites were not mistaken. All of them have a monitoring or coaching system based on e-mails to send back or explanatory videos.

This supervision of patients will soon be by text and will become daily. We will receive, at mealtime, a reminder of the type: "Remember to balance your plate in three thirds: vegetables, starches, proteins.

The solution:

The traditional consultations with a general practitioner, a nutritionist, or a dietitian in flesh and blood also have their card to play. During the meeting, they will have our full attention, and then we will be less easily lied to.

Mistake #7: Setting an Arbitrary Weight

You cannot - unfortunately - do what you want with your weight. Worse, there is not even a measuring instrument to determine which one it would be legitimate for everyone to claim. The only thing we know: the body will do everything to stay there! As with hormone production or body temperature, it is an internal regulatory system.

Also, in order to reach or maintain, not eating when hungry amounts to "fighting against inexhaustible and obstinate mechanisms. In other words, we will end up losing, inevitably.

The weight of form is that which one reaches by listening to oneself. Because the very function of appetite is to "help maintain a balanced weight," says the nutritionist.

The body is very precise. It calculates to the nearest calorie according to our needs and our expenses. Just as he knows precisely, once the taste is detected in the mouth, the quantity of mince pie, endive salad, or salmon toast that we need tame your hunger. It works.

We recognize it by its very specific manifestations: hollow in the stomach, gargoyle belly, nervousness, difficulty concentrating, spinning head. But the simple desire to eat, if it is upset, can cause anxiety, which signs are very close - wrongly - to those of hunger.

The solution:

Skip breakfast and postpone breakfast a little more each day to familiarize yourself with the range of sensations that range from the desire to snack until hunger. It is also she who must be in command during the meal. "We do not tighten up because we love, but because we are hungry.

Precautions

Losing weight quickly is never harmless for the body. Indeed, weight loss is always a test for all of the body's systems. For this reason, before considering a change in your eating habits, it is recommended to consult a health professional who may advise you to perform a blood test to verify that everything is fine. Also, to develop habits over the long term, it is generally recommended not to change everything all at once. Rather, take stock and focus on three areas for improvement at once. Gradually, you will then take on new lifestyle habits in the long term and very naturally. Finally, to lose weight quickly and well, it is essential to make a personal assessment and to precisely define your slimming goals. For that, do not hesitate to write down in a notebook the objective which you wish to reach and what motivates you to want to reach this objective. Also, you can write down the habits you want to lose and the ones you would like to have taken at the end of your food rebalancing. Planning and defining a course of action helps you lose weight faster and in an organized manner. This way, you will know exactly where you are going and why you are doing it.

Risks of Uncontrolled Weight Loss

Losing weight quickly should not be an end in itself. Ideally, your goal should be to lose weight permanently and healthily. That is to say, without risk to your health. It is recommended not to lose more than 1 to 1.5 kg per week for this to be sustainable.

- Anemia

- Chronic fatigue

- Melting of muscle tissue

- General weakness

- Hair loss

- Irritability

- Weariness

- Subsequent weight gain

- Chilliness

- Etc

CHAPTER 12:

The Change That Comes From Within

You're doing a wonderful job so far. You've already made a difference by making the decision to learn to master your emotions, understanding what they are, how they affect your lifestyle, and what you can do to make a change for the better.

The next strategy is going to focus on how you can sidestep your emotional triggers by changing your emotions and using them to help you grow instead.

How to Change Your Emotions

Change is something that rarely ever comes easy. When you're trying to change what is part of your personality, the very thing that makes you human, and something that has been part of your life for so long, it's going to be even more of a challenge.

That's okay, because the best things in life are the things which are worth fighting and struggling for, and in this case, learning how to master your emotions is something you're going to fight for because it promises you a much better life. With a happier life, not just for you, but for the people you love. Emotional triggers will always be there because you don't exist in this world alone. You constantly have to interact with people and even find yourself in situations that are less than ideal. It is bound to happen every now and then.

These factors are sometimes beyond your control, but there is something that you can control. You can control how you decide to respond. You can make a conscious effort to change your emotions, although it will take a lot of willpower to resist the urge to rise to the occasion and succumb to the temptation to react to what's provoking you.

It's going to be hard because you're going to have to go against your first instinctive response, to mindfully force yourself to react in a different way.

Changing your emotions may not be easy, but it is possible if you:

• Choose to Do Something That Makes You Happy

Those who struggle with their emotions are often unhappier than most, which makes it very hard to hold onto any kind of happiness.

When you're in a constant state of unhappiness, learning how to control anything becomes a challenge, let alone learning how to control something as powerful as your emotions.

Learning to master your emotions is not just about getting it under control; it is about reconnecting with yourself, too, and finding your happiness once more.

The best way to do that is to do something that makes you happy.

When you find yourself in an emotional situation, and you're struggling to get a hold of yourself, walk away and choose instead to do something that makes you happy. Each time you actively try to engage in an activity that brings you joy, you'll find your negative emotions ebbing away quicker with each effort you make. Harness the all-consuming power of happiness, because it's a good kind of emotion which will benefit you and everyone else around you.

A happier state of mind also makes it much easier for you to think with clarity, and in doing so, gives you a much better handle at controlling your emotions.

• Choose to Focus on The Solutions

Focus on the solution, not the problem.

The force of the emotions that we feel can still manage to get the better of us, even when we're trying hard to reel them in.

It is especially difficult because you're now trying to change the pattern of behavior that you have been used to for so long. The more you focus on the problem, the harder it is going to be to control your emotions, which is why you need to do the opposite.

Instead of focusing on the problems, turn your attention to the solution instead.

When emotions are running high, it is easy for someone else's anger, frustration, or any other emotion they may be experiencing to rub off on you (emotions are contagious, remember?), and this will disrupt your own attempts at trying to master your emotions.

It helps to focus on the situation at hand to help you find a solution to the problem.

The challenge here would be trying not to lose sight of the real issue that you should be focusing on.

When faced with an emotional situation or person, remind yourself that there must be a reason for it, and you need to find out what that reason is before you can attempt to find a solution for it.

Instead of thinking, "I'm so angry" or "I am furious," think about "What can I do to resolve this" instead.

There's always a reason and a trigger for every emotional outburst, and getting to the root cause of it is how to try to resolve the problem.

• Choose Not to Follow the Crowd

When everyone else is feeling emotionally charged up, it's not going to help matters in any way if you join the crowd and add fuel to the fire.

Instead, try an alternative solution where you are the one who continues to remain calm instead. Allow yourself to be the one who keeps a cool head on their shoulders and take on the role of problem-solver instead.

It's easy to let the emotions of others affect you, but the beauty of this situation is that you always have a choice, and you need to remember that.

If you choose not to follow the crowd, you're choosing to change your emotions. You now have the opportunity to provide that kind of solution for someone else.

• **Choose a Time Out When You Need It**

We all need a little space every now and then, especially when dealing with a highly emotional situation.

If you're the emotional one, don't hesitate to ask for a time out or a break if you need to remove yourself from the situation and take a few minutes to calm yourself down.

This is how you change your emotions by choosing not to feed into it even more and taking a step back, so you have a chance to breathe for a minute and try to calm your thoughts.

Emotions cloud your judgment and stop you from thinking straight, and you will be no good to anyone if you can't even think straight because you're too focused on how you're feeling to care about anything else.

The best thing you could do to provide a helpful solution will be to get some space if you feel like you need it. Recommend that they get some space, too, so everyone can come back and revisit the issue when they're not as worked up emotionally and willing to listen to reason.

There are times and a place for effective communication, and being emotional is neither the right time nor place. Take a time out if you need one.

• **Choose Open and Welcoming Body Language Responses**

Another challenging exercise in self-control and self-regulation is going to be making a conscious decision to remain calm, open, and welcoming with your body language, despite the strong emotional situation you may find yourself in.

Adopt body language mannerisms that are inviting, and you'll have a much better shot at getting your emotions under control quickly.

Body language is just as powerful as the words that you speak, and sometimes you could even end up making the situation worse without ever having said a word.

When someone is emotional in front of you, for example, and you roll your eyes and shake your head, you could end up aggravating the situation and making things worse, even if you never uttered a word the whole time.

As challenging as it may be, body language is just as important as trying to resolve social problems that are caused by emotions.

What you need to do to change those emotions is to adopt open and welcoming body language gestures, which include making good eye contact, not crossing your arms in front of your chest, not frowning, clenching, or muscles or display any visible indication that you may be feeling emotional yourself.

• Choose to Talk to Someone

We'll talk more about the negative effects of trying to suppress your emotions, but for now, one method of learning to keep your emotions under control is to talk to someone about it when it starts to feel like it might be too much.

Instead of keeping all those emotions bottled up inside you with no healthy means of release, choose instead to talk to a friend or family member with whom you're comfortable with.

Venting, as it is often referred to, can make you feel much better, almost like a weight has been lifted off your shoulders.

When that weight is gone, your head feels much clearer, and changing your emotions then becomes easier.

Friends or family members who know you well enough might be able to provide some form of insight too and even give you their feedback, which could prove to be useful advice.

• Using Your Emotions to Grow

Your emotions can do one of two things.

Either it will help you grow or become a better version of yourself, or it can hold you back and destroy your reputation.

The former opens doors to new and greater opportunities, while the latter will leave you with a reputation that you're someone others should stay away from when you're unstable and emotional.

To achieve the former, you need to begin cultivating a positive environment for yourself, one that is going to make it easier to nurture these positive emotions and help you grow.

Here's the twist - it's not all about you. That's right; growing your emotions is not going to be an exercise that is entirely focused on you.

This time, you're going to be focused on making others around you feel good, which in turn helps you feel good.

Humans are social creatures by nature, and doesn't it always feel much better when you know you've done something that makes a positive difference in someone else's life other than yourself?

That's how you use your emotions to grow as a person. This is what you need to do:

• Be Appreciative

There is nothing that demotivates you and other people around you quicker than a lack of appreciation.

Showing a little gratitude and appreciation every now and then can go a long way towards turning your emotions around when you're feeling terrible after a long day. Just remembering that there's a lot in your life to be grateful for despite all that is enough to put a smile on your face.

Simple phrases like "thank you" or "nice job," maybe even a "we couldn't have done it without you," can make a real difference in your morals and that of others you spend your time with.

• You Need to Be Engaging

No matter whom you interact with, be engaging, and go the extra mile to make a connection with them. A genuine human connection is what we all long for deep down inside, and there's no one who is ever going to tell you that they enjoy being lonely. No matter who you're engaging with, build a connection that is meaningful. With family, friends, and colleagues, out to them on a regular basis, congratulate them on little victories accomplished and remember special moments like their birthdays and anniversaries.

These efforts will go a long way towards keeping the people who matter happy, and in turn, you will feel a lot happier too.

CHAPTER 13:

The Power of Affirmations

Today is another day. Today is a day for you to start making a euphoric, satisfying life. Today is the day to begin to discharge every one of your impediments. Today is the day for you to get familiar with the privileged insights of life. You can transform yourself into improving things. You, as of now, include the devices inside you to do as such. These devices are your considerations and your convictions.

What Are Positive Affirmations?

For those of you who aren't acquainted with the advantages of positive affirmations, I'd prefer to clarify a little about them. A statement is genuinely anything you state or think. A great deal of what we typically report and believe is very harmful and doesn't make great encounters for us. We need to retrain our reasoning and to talk into positive examples if we need to change us completely. An affirmation opens the entryway. It's a starting point on the way to change. When I talk about doing affirmations, I mean deliberately picking words that will either help take out something from your life or help make something new in your life. Each idea you think and each word you express is an affirmation. The entirety of our self-talk, our interior exchange, is a flood of oaths. You're utilizing statements each second, whether you know it or not. You're insisting and making your background with each word and thought.

Your convictions are just routine reasoning examples that you learned as a youngster. The vast numbers of them work very well for you. Different beliefs might be restricting your capacity to make the very things you state you need. What you need and what you trust your merit might be unusual. You have to focus on your contemplations with the goal that you can start to dispose of the ones making encounters you don't need in your life.

It would help if you understood that each grievance is an affirmation of something you figure you don't need in your life. Each time you blow up, you're asserting that you need more annoyance in your life. Each time you feel like a casualty, you're confirming that you need to keep on feeling like a casualty. If you believe that you think that life isn't giving you what you need in your reality, at that point, it's sure that you will never have the treats that experience provides for others-that is, until you change how you think and talk.

You're not a terrible individual for intuition, how you do. You've quite recently never figured out how to think and talk. Individuals all through the world are quite recently starting to discover that our contemplations make our encounters. Your folks most likely didn't have the foggiest idea about this, so they couldn't in any way, shape, or form instructs it to you. They showed you what to look like at life in the manner that their folks told them. So, no one isn't right. In any case, it's the ideal opportunity for us all to wake up and start to deliberately make our lives in a manner that satisfies and bolsters us. You can do it. I can do it. We, as a whole, can do it-we need to figure out how. So how about we get to it.

I'll talk about affirmations as a rule, and afterwards, I'll get too specific everyday issues and tell you the best way to roll out positive improvements in your wellbeing, your funds, your affection life, etc. Once you figure out how to utilize affirmations, at that point, you can apply the standards in all circumstances. A few people say that "affirmations don't work" (which is an affirmation in itself) when what they mean is that they don't have a clue how to utilize them accurately. Some of the time, individuals will say their affirmations once per day and gripe the remainder of the time. It will require some investment for affirmations to work if they're done that way. The grumbling affirmations will consistently win, because there is a higher amount of them, and they're generally said with extraordinary inclination.

In any case, saying affirmations is just a piece of the procedure. What you wrap up of the day and night is significantly progressively significant. The key to having your statements work rapidly and reliably is to set up air for them to develop in. Affirmations resemble seeds planted in soil: poor soil, poor development. Fertile soil, bottomless event. The more you decide to think contemplations that cause you to feel great, the faster the affirmations work.

So, think upbeat musings, it's that straightforward. What's more, it is feasible. How you decide to believe, at present, is an only that-a decision. You may not understand it since you've thought along these lines for such a long time, yet it truly is a decision. Presently, today, this second, you can decide to change your reasoning. Your life won't pivot for the time being. Yet, in case you're reliable and settle on the decision regularly to think considerations that cause you to feel great, you'll unquestionably roll out positive improvements in each part of your life.

Positive Affirmations and How to Use Them

Positive affirmations are positive articulations that depict an ideal circumstance, propensity, or objective that you need to accomplish. Rehashing regularly these positive explanations, influences the psyche brain profoundly, and triggers it without hesitation, to bring what you are reworking into the real world.

The demonstration of rehashing the affirmations, intellectually or so anyone might hear, inspires the individual reworking them, builds the desire and inspiration, and pulls in open doors for development and achievement. This demonstration likewise programs the psyche to act as per the rehashed words, setting off the inner mind-brain to take a shot at one's sake, to offer the positive expressions materialize.

Affirmations are extremely valuable for building new propensities, rolling out positive improvements throughout one's life, and for accomplishing objectives.

Affirmations help in weight misfortune, getting progressively engaged, concentrating better, changing propensities, and accomplishing dreams.

They can be helpful in sports, in business, improving one's wellbeing, weight training, and in numerous different zones.

These positive articulations influence in a proper manner, the body, the brain, and one's sentiments

Rehashing affirmations is very reasonable. Despite this, a lot of people do not know about this truth. Individuals, for the most part, restate negative statements, not positive ones. This is called negative self-talk.

On the off chance that you have been disclosing to yourself how miserable you can't contemplate, need more cash, or how troublesome life is, you have been rehashing negative affirmations.

Along these lines, you make more challenges and more issues, since you are concentrating on the problems, and in this way, expanding them, rather than concentrating on the arrangements.

A great many people rehash in their psyches pessimistic words and proclamations concerning the contrary circumstances and occasions in their lives, and therefore, make progressively bothersome circumstances.

Words work in two different ways, to assemble or obliterate. It is how we use them that decides if they will bring tremendous or destructive outcomes.

Affirmations in Modern Times

It is said that the French analyst and drug specialist Emile Coue is the individual who carried this subject to the open's consideration in the mid-twentieth century.

Emile Coue saw that when he told his patients how viable an elixir was, the outcomes were superior to if he didn't utter a word. He understood that musings that consume our psyches become a reality and that rehashing concepts and considerations is a sort of autosuggestion.

Emile Coue is associated with his acclaimed proclamation, "Consistently, all around, I am showing signs of improvement and better."

Later in the twentieth century, this was Louise Hay, who concentrated on this point and called autosuggestions – affirmations.

Conclusion

If you think that what I prescribe is just a diet, you've got it wrong. Experts have long said that to keep weight off, and people need to make long term changes to their diet and activity levels. Remember that slow but steady wins the race. According to the CDC, those who lose weight at a pace of one to two pounds per week tend to keep weight off more successfully. Further, they emphasize how important it is to take steps to ensure you maintain your weight loss.

Hypnosis is different from normal "diets" because it doesn't promote temporary change. Hypnotherapy helps you resist going back to your old ways, but that doesn't mean that you don't also need to keep up your efforts. Hypnosis instills a tendency towards long term change, but if you don't fight to keep that change up, you're going to go back to how you were. Accordingly, take the messages you learn through hypnosis and reinforce them as much as you can after you've finished hypnotherapy. You can continue to use scripts on your own if you want to ensure that you maintain progress.

Too many people return to their original weights after they lose weight. Only about ten to twenty percent of people keep weight off and don't return to their original weight or higher after losing weight. This weight is often regained within five years, sometimes in as little time as just weeks, depending on how much you've lost. Thus, if you don't remain conscious of your habits, you may start to incorporate the ones that you'd ditched.

Carry all the changes you've made through even after you've stopped hypnotherapy. You probably won't want to continue hypnotherapy forever, but you need to keep up with all the dietary, physical, and mental changes that you've made on this journey because they are vital to your overall well-being and happiness. Don't let this journey end by returning to who you were. Continue on your path of growth.

Don't Forget What You've Fought for

Never forget the effort you put in once you got to your goal weight. You need to remember the time and energy you invested so that you feel motivated not to go back. You don't want to have to start all over and do that work again after you worked so hard to make progress. Thus, never forget that struggle, and when you want to return to old habits, remember how long it took you to lose weight and also remember the money you paid to get better (because no one wants to pay more money than they need to!). You don't need to go back, and you have the skills to keep moving forward.

Keep a picture of your old self handy. You can pull this picture out when you need a visual reminder of how far you've come. Remember that old person and know that you don't want to be him anymore. You've become a person that makes you happier, and there's no need to sabotage the better you. Respect your personal growth by loving the person you were without wanting to be that person anymore. You were fine just as you were in the past, but your changed self feels better, and that's the difference.

Remember how bad you felt before you made a change. You wanted to change for a reason! You weren't comfortable in your skin before you made the change, so you need to never forget that you changed for a reason. You wanted to grow as a person, and you accomplished this goal by dreaming of a better self and working to make that person a reality.

Think of how much better you feel now that you've made a change. Doesn't it feel exhilarating to take an issue and watch as it gradually improves? Of course, it does, so take that victorious feeling and carry it with you whenever temptation may strike. When you want to eat a whole bag of chips, think of how much better you'd feel if you didn't do that. Think of how good it will feel about choosing a snack that will fuel your body with nutrients and care. Use that feeling to maintain your good habits.

Promise yourself that you're never going to go backward. Repeat this message to yourself every day if you need to because if you tell yourself that it won't happen, your brain is likely to listen. You have to keep going forward, or you'll end up running in dissatisfying circles. It can be so easy to get stuck in the past and let everything that allured you into a false sense of security, but by relying so much on the past, you will lose sight of the present, and you will forfeit much of the happiness you could have by not seeing all the beautiful things that are right there in front of you.

Know that the future is yours for the taking. You decide what you want your future to be, and you build it. There are some variables in life that you have no power over, and those things can be terrifying and make you not want to think about the future. You get hurt, people die, you change jobs, etc. Lots of things will change in the future in ways you can't predict, but you have the power to take those changes positively or negatively. Any change can be used to better yourself in some way. You just have to determine how you will use that change to your advantage.

Stay Active

Humans need activity. It's important to keep doing things and accomplishing physical feats even if you've already met your goal weight. Once you've lost weight, you may be able to ease up on the activity, but it will hurt your physical and emotional health to quit being active altogether. Boredom is one of the biggest reasons people overeat, so keep yourself busy to avoid the pitfalls of having nothing to do but eat as you watch TV.

Continue your physical activity. If you've found physical activities that you love, don't quit them once you've reached your goal weight. Continue to let them better your life and drive you to be a happier and healthier person. Stay in tune with your body's needs and find power in all the wonderful things your body can do.

Challenge the activity you already do and try to keep pushing yourself. I bet that you can be doing more than you are. Don't let your workout regime become stagnant. Keep pushing your skills and building your body up. You should never be content with how you are right now. You can always do more and improve your physical condition.

Maintain hobbies that bring your fulfillment. Studies have shown that hobbies are good for your health and to reduce stress. These hobbies don't have to be physical, but keeping hobbies will give you purpose, and the projects help keep you motivated. You need to have outlets for your creative energy, which can be found through hobbies. Your hobbies should be recreational and have nothing to do with your work or other responsibilities. Hobbies such as constructing models, writing, or drawing are all just a few ideal options for people to consider. Some of the most common hobbies are games, collecting things, outdoor activity, or building things. The possibilities are endless!

Be mentally active. Finding pursuits that challenge your brain can be a strong way to keep yourself occupied. Maybe you like to complete puzzles. Maybe you like to write stories. Maybe you like to solve riddles. Maybe you like to read books. Whatever it is that keeps your mind active, do it. Your brain is a muscle, and you can train it just as you can other parts of your body, so don't neglect your brain. It will get bored if you don't keep it on its toes!

Spend time with people who make you feel good about yourself. Maintain quality friendships once you have lost weight. Don't find people who only accept you because you have lost weight or who will make you feel bad about yourself. Choose to spend your time with people who will keep you engaged in your relationships and feeling confident about those friendships. Supportive people are just as important when you maintain your weight as when you lose weight.

Being active is one of the best ways to maintain your weight, and it doesn't matter what methods you choose to keep you busy, but try to maintain several things that keep you staying strong and reaching for opportunities that make you happy and secure in your position in life. Being active will help you keep bad habits out.

Continue Making Goals

Goals aren't something that should ever stop. Throughout your life, you need to be making goals to continue to encourage you to live your life to the fullest. A person without goals is aimless. Michelangelo once said, "The great danger for most of us lies in not setting our aim too high and falling short, but in setting our aim too low and achieving our mark." This means that so many people have low expectations for themselves, so even when they reach their goals, they don't benefit from their goals because they haven't reached far enough and dreamed big enough to be satisfied.

So, don't stop making goals once you've lost all the weight that you wanted to lose. You don't have to keep wanting to lose weight, but if you want to keep your life on track, you need to continue to have objectives that you fight to accomplish. Don't be afraid to have goals because you'll feel a lot worse if you don't have them.

Hypnosis Is Always There

Hypnosis isn't going away. It's been practiced for hundreds of years and continues to grow as a practice. With how many celebrities turn to hypnosis to improve their lives, it will only become more developed as a therapeutic method. Further, with increasing apps and scripts on self-hypnosis available, further research will likely arise on the benefits of all types of hypnotherapy, showing how promising the future of this powerful force is. Humans have only just tapped into the power of hypnosis, so it's not going anywhere anytime soon, and you don't have to stop using it once you've lost weight.

If you're willing and able, you can continue to use hypnotherapy sessions or self-hypnosis to help focus your mind on maintaining your weight. Continued sessions, especially when you've first lost the weight, can help you stay on track as you get used to the permanency of the changes that you've made. Additionally, hypnotherapy gives you a dedicated time to relax and feel at peace, which everyone could use.

Furthermore, hypnotherapy can help you break other bad habits in your life if you'd like to continue your growth. Know that it's okay to need more treatment in other areas of your life. Maybe you're a longtime smoker, and you'd like to try treatment for that as well. Go for it! Some habits can be changed in just one session, and habits like smoking are one of those things that can require just a session or two to instill change. Thus, giving hypnosis a try for other mental health issues or bad habits that you have can be a life-changing way to keep you happy and healthy.

You can always return to hypnotherapy if you start to fall back on bad habits. It will always be there to give you the guidance and support you need whenever you want it. There's nothing wrong with having to continue treatment or start it again after a relapse. Change takes time, and some people are very resistant to it, but hypnotherapy is an ideal tool for not only those trying to lose weight but also for those trying to maintain their weight.

Take the Time to Embrace Success

One of the problems many negatively minded people experience is that they never take the time to appreciate success when it comes their way. Sometimes they are too afraid of jinxing that success to actually recognize it. Most of the time, however, they are unable to embrace success because their mindset is simply too negative for such a positive action. Mentally strong people, by contrast, always take the time to embrace the successes that come their way. This serves to build their sense of confidence as well as their feeling of satisfaction with how things are going.

Next time you experience a success of any kind, make sure you take a moment to recognize it. You can make an external statement, such as going out for drinks, treating yourself to a nice lunch, or some similar expression of gratitude. Alternatively, you can simply take a quiet moment to reflect on the success and all the effort that went into making it happen. There is no right or wrong way to embrace success, you just need to find a way that works for you. The trick to embracing success is in not letting it go to your head. Rather than praising your efforts or actions, appreciate the fact that things went well. Also, be sure to appreciate those whose help contributed to your success.

RAPID WEIGHT-LOSS HYPNOSIS FOR WOMEN

The Ultimate Collection Of Powerful Self-Hypnosis And Meditations For Weight Loss At Any Age. Transform Your Body Naturally And Feel Amazing In Just 30 Days

CAROLINE LEAN

Table of Contents

Introduction

Y ou don't automatically knock out all types of food with an effective weight loss program; you just become more aware of the food choices you make. This diet plan knows that sometimes you're going to want that piece of cake or that cookie, and telling you that you're not supposed to have it just makes the situation worse. The concept behind an Effective weight loss plan is to encourage you to have some of these snacks and goodies, as long as you incorporate them well into your diet.

When you go on a successful weight loss plan, a points system will be issued to you. It is to help you decide based on your current weight and how much you want to use in the process. These are the number of points you can use during the day, which can help you make better food choices. Every food you select will have a certain point value, and the intention is to remain within the points every day.

Now, as described, you're allowed to eat some of those sweets, but if you're at the end of the day and have only five points left, you could go for an apple instead of going for that piece of cake worth 15 and taking you over your target point. You get to determine whether to use the points, and there are plenty of manuals to help you see how many points each of your food choices are. When you want that piece of cake in the day (maybe you know you're going to a birthday party), you'll be able to budget in advance to select nutritious and balanced snacks that will keep you under your point limit without calories missing.

You'll need to be mindful of these issues. Some people get too excited about the weight loss and will try too much to limit their calories. That will seem like a smart idea; they believe that they can lose weight quickly if they only use half of their calories every day. But the issue here is that you could cut calories, but you also cut balanced foods that the body requires. You need to be careful about that.

There could be days where you're not as hungry, or you're too busy to eat as much as you would, and the percentages of your points maybe a little less. During these days, you should not force yourself to feed. But every day, you should try to get close to your total points so that you can provide your body with enough nutrition and calories to keep running.

When it comes to the foods you are allowed to consume on this diet plan, these points will be very important. Instead of focusing on the calories you consume, you'll be focusing on the points. Those points are based on the macronutrients and micronutrients within the food you expect to consume during the daytime.

If the food contains a lot of good macro and micronutrients such as protein, good carbohydrates, and healthy vitamins, you will find that they have a smaller number of points, and you will be able to consume more of them all day long. On the other hand, if the products are mainly calories, sugars, and saturated fats, they would rank higher in terms of the points you can use. The theory behind that is that you are motivated to consume some of the good foods when enjoying some of the bad foods, while some of those bad foods are allowed while you're on the diet plan on occasion.

These points are going to make the right choices when it's time to choose the foods you'd like to enjoy. You're going to be able to enjoy some of the sweets at times when you want to, but eventually, you're going to want to go out and eat the healthy foods as they fill you up more, you can eat more of them without having to use all of your points, and they're going to taste so good in the process!

CHAPTER 1:

Different Reasons for Being Overweight

Hypnosis clears the metabolic circuitry for weight loss prevention

If you are obese, you may be tired of reminding each person that reducing weight consumes less food and absorbs fewer calories. Each diet you may have tried, old and fresh. Often our bodies seem to have found a way of transforming a lettuce plate right into pound extra pound fat!

Sooner or later, many people who want to lose weight find their efforts complicated by aerobic systems that hold weight on the body regardless of just how one changes its eating habits.

If you are obese, or your close friend or customer, and consider losing some weight, please take the following set of questions:

- Can you sense that no matter how much you starve yourself, the weight just isn't reducing as rapidly as it should be?

- Do you discover that you eat less food than your slim good friends, and still don't reduce weight?

- Will you find that your food yearnings are also going up as the extra pounds begin to fall off? As if you starved to death rather than on a diet program?

- Do you end up inactive and tired when it comes to diet programs?

- Can you, at an unprecedented pace, get back all the weight that you lost from a diet?

If you answered "yes" to these questions, you probably have a subconscious metabolic program to maintain body weight rather than burn it off for strength as you should.

The good news is now below! There are many ways to handle this hypnosis program, so you don't have to fight your body to lose weight, other than your food cravings!

Initially, the causes of this programming will be investigated as much as possible.

Food metabolism is a complete mechanism by which the body absorbs and uses nutrients from food.

One of them is the function of the thyroid gland, the "master button," which, through hypnotic images, controls the speed of the metabolic process, we can show the development of thyroxine, the main metabolic hormone produced by the thyroid gland.

More thyroxine melts fat, leading to weight loss and more energy for you. There may be medical explanations for a thyroid condition, so we recommend a complete physical exam and a workable assessment of thyroid function before hypnosis training.

Essential pancreatic hormones are an additional key factor in the body's metabolic processes: insulin and glucagon. These primary metabolic and hormonal agents lead us to store or eliminate fat from our body. The food you consume can affect the activities of some hormonal agents. In the primary, most carbohydrates, including sugars, tend to induce insulin secretion, increasing the metabolism and storage of sugar.

Glucagons, produced after a low-carbohydrate meal, help with multiprotein and fats in the body. This is part of the reason that low-carb diets are preferred.

How does hypnotherapy help transform your food choices? Since all eating rituals are embedded in the subconscious mind, choosing to eat in various ways is usually enough to create long-term customizations in our eating habits. The image of hypnotherapy addresses and regulates these subliminal processes in a permanent and almost effortless way.

For a fact, coping with mental eating patterns is of vital importance. Researchers have discovered routine exercise, as low as half an hour a day. Hypnotic ideas can be used to improve one's motivation to practice as well as to enhance power and stamina. But often, it takes much more than straight hypnotic ideas to get more included again with the workout.

One of the clever processes that we use is to take you back to what you literally enjoyed doing as a child. You can pick one or two of those activities which you will surely appreciate once again! We use the power of Hypnosis to revive the playful enjoyment you experienced as a kid. We can go back to those terrible experiences that triggered us to turn off to exercise happiness and liberate the past self from these injuries.

As an example, a knowledge of being denied, humiliated, or hurt on the playground in a team sport can lead to one shutting down the need to play outside. Our rescue target allows the child to obtain comfort from the grown-up self and a promise of health and protection, along with an invitation to play outside with a grown-up in a new environment.

One of metabolic programming's mutual tools is hereditary. Some human ancestral lines (South Pacific Islander and Eskimos offer only two extreme examples) keep fat on their bodies faster because these features delivered well to their forefathers, especially in times of famine. It may be difficult for competent practitioners to change those genetic codes within our DNA. Through Hypnosis, however, we can convince the metabolic rate to bypass certain DNA programs and help us release fat. My clients have often said to me, "My entire household is obese!" This is the time to use details of hypnotic recommendations aimed at bypassing DNA shows.

Another common subject for those dealing with weight loss is that the subconscious mind can be scared to shed. Since if one's weight problems go away than one, weight might have to encounter other, more scarce problems. Another woman in Hypnosis told me that if she lost the weight she gained, she would have to "do something about my life, and I don't understand what to do!" At the Institute, we will check for these issues and have a treatment plan. One useful strategy that can be used from below is a path into the future self to figure out how to successfully fulfill one's life.

Another common motive that I have discovered among women clients with metabolic shows to store fat is the need of the body to shield itself from unwanted sexual developments by using fat. Most of my obese clients are victims of sexual harassment by young men.

Several others have gained weight within an unfulfilled marriage to silence their unmet sex-related demands. Many use weight as an excuse for not meeting men, and therefore run the risk of being rejected or deceptive. When you are unfamiliar with these subconscious systems, you can be buried deep in the subconscious mind and may be affecting your metabolism. Your hypnotherapist will help you locate the problems and restore them. I was personally effective in saving clients from early sexual assault trauma, which typically resulted in dramatic weight loss without any visible dietary improvement.

Let us look at an instance whereby a woman is willing to lose a few pounds to achieve the desired weight. She keeps trying different diets and manages to put off some of them, but soon she may be frustrated when it happens that the weight keeps recurring, and she does not know how she can successfully manage the weight and achieve permanent results. There is a great possibility that such a woman can rely on guided meditation for weight loss. Instead of facing the frustrations she had faced earlier while trying different programs to lose weight, this time around, she would be happier because of maintaining her weight for the long term. Such is the power of guided meditation, and this many people nowadays have resolved to use different programs that are based on meditation to achieve various goals, including losing weight. When this woman decided to experiment with several minutes of guided meditation for weight loss, it took a few weeks when she discovered that she could not do this during weekends, as it would disorganize her. She decided to be disciplined during the other days of the week following some of the meditation techniques. The program was successful for her, but after a few weeks, things started being tough for her at the workplace, and she felt the stress was mounting. It was so severe that she started experiencing periods of hunger frequently and even ate a lot due to emotional stress. When this happened, she chose to add several minutes to her program, and diligently followed them throughout the five days of the week.

She aimed to change her life for the better by losing weight and attaining the body she felt was comfortable for her. That is why the mantra phrase she chose was, "I aim to change my life." This is a phrase that is repeated several while maintaining focus on the phrase without any disruption. She continued to use the program, and things were now starting to get straight. The whole program was a wonderful experience for her, and since she had chosen to do it for six weeks, she was happy with what she got and even decided to continue. Even after doing the program for six weeks, she continued and did not stop, and after the other six weeks, things weeks, things were different for her. She realized that she had lost all the weight she wanted, and it gave her the confidence she did not have earlier while handling difficult things in life. Since she saw that the program was helping her a lot, she decided to use it while focusing on other goals she wanted to achieve in life. She wanted to maintain her happiness and be enthusiastic. She had to feel the way she had earlier felt before she hit a difficult road full of stress in her job. She followed various techniques and continued to follow her programs well and with discipline until she achieved success. Eventually, she succeeded in achieving her goals and now feels her life is much better. She uses the same techniques to achieve various goals that she might have.

Let us consider the case of John gained a lot of weight from when he was a kid. He was overweight before he decided to use to meditation program. Why did he develop weight problems when he was a child? Psychological issues influenced him, and it contributed to her eating a lot leading to unwanted weight gain. Worse for him, he did not succeed in stopping his habits when he became an adult. He joined many groups and organizations advocating for diet change, but he could not find help because it was only temporary, yet he wanted permanent results. He even went and stayed in diet canters, whereby he succeeded in reducing weight, but soon, he found himself gaining even more and more weight gain. The change was only for a few months, and soon the problem escalated. When it could not work at all, what he did was to hate himself, and he was never comfortable when he struggled to pass people, especially when they were in crowded areas. The weight became a major problem such that he lacked confidence, and every time he felt this, he would result in eating more and more food, and the problem would continue to haunt him.

CHAPTER 2:

Weight Loss Without Diet

ow often did you try a diet? We don't remember how many ways we struggled to lose weight. As an "ordinary" girl, during the 47 years of our life, we have tried to lose weight for a long time. Sadly, we do not belong to the metabolism of people who allow them to eat anything without gaining weight. While we enjoy food and drink, my body turns any extra calories into fat. But-and here is the good news-we have handled my weight effectively over the years. We are 1 75 meters tall and weigh about 60 kilograms (its 5 feet 9 inches, 132 pounds for the United States). If we can, you can, too. You can. My secret: Forget about all diets and please your soul and body.

My qualification: You might tell me about my credentials for the subject "weight loss without diet": we're not a food expert. We served as a professional journalist for newspapers and radio in Germany for a decade, but we are now specialized in information collection and processing.

We have also been struggling with weight problems for many years. When we grew up, we passed a two-year "Anorexia nervosa" phase, although we were not correctly diagnosed and treated as such at this stage. Fortunately, it didn't last long enough. When we were divorced at the age of 29, my binge eating disorder reappeared. This period we received a lot of supportive psychotherapy.

So, from a layman, we dare say that diets make you fat.

Although, if you are super-rich and can afford your chef or diet caterer, this rule may not apply to you. However, for the average person who follows a diet, it is too restrictive to succeed for a long time. Who needs to weigh every bit before eating? What wants to eat what a diet tells you exactly? A diet does not leave space for urges and appetites, so a diet makes us continuously feel dissatisfied and restrained.

I firmly believe that a slim body can only be a satisfied, well-nourished body. Our bodies convey in cravings their desires. When a strawberry thought makes my mouth water, we suppose that my body needs a strawberry, and only a strawberry can give me the satisfaction that makes me feel good and better.

The body gets used to a low-calorie intake if you adopt a diet. Once you start eating normal again, your body packages happily, and all your effort is lost. This is particularly true for any fasting or crash diet: once we fasted for three weeks absolutely and lost our weight. Nonetheless, my slim body lasted just one week.

When we began again to eat, my body jumped at all the calories it was denied-a very frustrating experience, not to mention the exhausting mental fight for three weeks to refrain from eating.

According to my experience, you have to understand why your body looks like it before you lose any extra pounds.

There are many explanations for overweight, but we dare say: the bulk of overweight we bear is ingrained in our subconscious. Explanations for overweight: We prefer to pile on pounds if we take life too hard. Will you put on your shoulders too much responsibility? Do you like to do more than you could? Or are you suffering from depression without it being realized?

We have to dig within ourselves if we want to shift our weight. Perhaps you have just too much enjoyed the culinary pleasures of life and thus put in additional pounds. On the other side, why do you need food or drink to relax?

It may sound transparent and pseudo-psychological now, but we were there, and we know what we are talking about. If you have been seriously struggling with your weight for many years, you must seek the help of a good psychotherapist or get psychological assistance in all ways. A friend's sympathetic ear cannot be underestimated.

Only when you find out what makes you fat you will lose weight.

I think one of the main factors for accumulating pounds is the multitude of chemicals that are incorporated into fresh food. First and foremost, there are the different glucose and malt syrups that go straight into your blood from your mouth into your hips.

Then all the preservatives make the digestive system have cable. Only consider the essence of a preservative: its purpose is to prevent bacteria from spoiling food. Sadly, our digestive system also works with bacteria. We cannot believe that food swamped with preservatives can easily be digested or provide our bodies with enough nutrients.

If you like overeating, you eat a lot of unhealthy fats. Have you ever checked what type of oil a restaurant kitchen uses? We dare to say that anyone who wants to stay healthy ought not to eat fast food or restaurants every day.

Another source of overweight can be an undetected digestive system infection with the yeast. Yeast infections are now common, and you can easily catch them in any public place. They're really difficult to get rid of. Candida albicans tend to penetrate the digestive tract and absorb food from our food. This can lead to regular food cravings and binge eating.

How to stay slim or lose weight: after this, let me show you how we keep my weight free of diet, and we are fond of eating and drinking. For all people who claim that there are foods that make you lean, we would like to say this (it's hard to gain weight eating just leafy and green beans, of course, but who wants to live like that?): The only food that doesn't get into your mouth does not make you fat.

If you want to lose weight, minimize the amount that you eat-but don't deny anything to yourself. Bring your appetites and cravings, whether it's chocolate or French fries. Don't overeat this sinful pleasure. Stop following a little slice of cakes or some French fries. The stomachs are habituated creatures: once you are used to smaller portions, you are comfortable with less. Permanent loss of weight is always a slow process, so you should be ready to eat less for a long time.

1. **Move**. If people ask me how we can stay slim over the years, we answer: we don't overeat, and at least three days a week, we go to the gym. There is no option for exercise at all. Our bodies have to function well. Use increases the heart rate, which gives our cells more oxygen and nutrients. The workout increases our metabolism and hormone production. You feel good and comfortable after a good workout. What kind of exercise you do doesn't matter; it's essential to move your body and pump your heart. We never thought of me as a sportsman, but we like to exercise in the gym because we feel so good afterward. Fortunately, exercise is very addictive: after the workout, you start to enjoy the great feeling.

2. **The magic of love**: the simplest way to lose weight is to fall out of love. Usually, if we fall in love, we lose a few kilograms without notice. This way of losing weight cannot be programmed, unfortunately, though you can fall in love with yourself. When was the last time you got mimicked? How did you say to yourself how good you were the last time? Have you ever looked at your bare breasts and told yourself how gorgeous you are? Remember: Gender is one of the best slimming and slimming practices. If you are lucky enough to live with a girlfriend, do all you can to spice up your sex life. Many publications are available. Just check what works for you. There's no cause to worry if you're alone. Sexual activity with your self can always be a healthy and slimming workout, anywhere. You know best what turns you on. Be your very best friend and lover.

3. **Avoid sugar and pure carbohydrates: without the natural fiber, the blood flows directly from your belly to the sugar, white flour, rice, and other cereals**. They increase your blood sugar levels so that you boost until the sugar is consumed, and you get drop-in energy. Then you need some more sugar to raise you. DA diet rich in sugar and empty carbohydrates keeps you eating all day without ever being satisfied and full. The occasional ice cream, cookie, or cake, of course, belongs to the pleasures to be enjoyed–but not regarded as a natural part of a healthy diet.

4. **Avoid high foods**: it is, of course, good to have a meal of five or six times at parties or just when you feel like it. Without indulgences, what would life be? However, it is better to keep your meals small and eat

them more often daily. Stretch the calorie intake and don't eat too late throughout the day.

5. **Stop hunger pangs**: don't wait until you're thirsty; keep on eating. When your stomach grumbles and you need something to eat, you tend to eat too fast. It takes about 20 minutes for our brain to realize that we filled our stomachs, and it helps to eat slowly and to chew carefully.

6. **Satisfy your cravings**: try to satisfy this urge when something is making your mouth water. Your body tells you what it has to do. Cravings are one of the manifestations of our bodies. As stated earlier: If you want to eat strawberries (or a chocolate bar or hot dogs) in any way, follow your will.

7. **Minerals and Vitamins**: Make sure that you have enough vitamins and minerals on your doctor's advice by taking supplements.

8. **Then the obvious thing**: don't drink too much alcohol, eat plenty of fruit and vegetables, and rest enough. If you cannot sleep properly, you may have anxiety and a hormonal imbalance, feel tired or depressed. Go to the doctor and get assistance. Consult online and ask your doctor about your symptoms.

CHAPTER 3:

How to Lose Weight Fast Without Working Out

In today's market, there are so many different choices that it is natural to be skeptical, but what if I could show you a method that works? Are you in discovering the secret to losing weight quickly that the Hollywood elites have been hiding for years? Are you part of those being frustrated with their inability to lose weight, regardless of the program? I will share a secret with you that is not commonplace knowledge, and few people are aware of it. Here are ways to lose weight without workout:

Modifying Your Diet for Weight Loss

Most people can maintain their current weight or even lose weight, simply by learning to change their eating habits. However, opposed to traditional fad or crash diets, it can benefit your body in terms of health for the sleep of your life. If you are a person who consumes food because of emotional or spiritual problems, then you need to have these issues addressed. You will be able to make very little progress with your weight loss if there is an underlying issue. Many people also eat when they are experiencing times of stress. You must learn to modify these habits as well. Various diets and weight loss programs promise delivery of quick weight loss. However, most crash diets are unhealthy.

They strip the body of water weight and muscle tissue. These are two key ingredients that the body needs when it comes to burning body fat. With a crash diet, you may see an initially large loss of weight on the outset. Your body will eventually send itself into starvation mode when it realizes it is not getting the appropriate amount of nutrients and food. With your metabolism in starvation mode, it becomes increasingly difficult to lose weight. This is the point where most people abandon their diets altogether. To lose weight permanently, you must be prepared to modify your food intake.

Do you know why the vast majority of dieting methods are highly ineffective?

Unfortunately, these programs attempt to do too much, essentially pulling and pushing your body, eradicating any chance of success; what happens when you attempt to push and pull something simultaneously? Simply, nothing at all, opposing forces in different directions cancel out their energies. This is an illustration of what effect the majority of dieting programs have on your body, and why they always fail. To help your body shed the extra weight, there are two key maxims you will need to do:

- Reduce your daily calorie intake.

- Burn off your body's fat reserves.

However, these two concepts are actually at odds with one another. If you choose to reduce your daily caloric intake, your body begins to burn less fat. Unfortunately, this is how our body copes. This is a survival mechanism that kicks on to help guard against dangerous circumstances, such as famine.

Maintaining Your Weight Loss

You have ever had the experience of being so-called successful at losing weight following being a member of a slimming club for a few months, only to regain all the weight that she lost when you stop attending regularly.

It seems as if it is almost like a plot to keep you paying to keep on going to the slimming club; otherwise, you find that you can't maintain your weight loss.

So, to maintain the success you feel you've added, you need to do more than just regularly go to a slimming club or follow a diet in a newspaper.

It's about changing your mindset about your weight and realizing that diets on their work. Yes, if you follow what is written, or what you're told and you will lose some weight. However, the weight is in many, and in most cases, regained very quickly once you decide you're going back to a "normal" diet. If diets don't work, then what can you do to be the way that you would like to be, and be healthy too.

- **Eat regularly**: You may have tried to lose weight by skipping meals entirely. This doesn't work because your blood sugar level drops, and you begin to crave lots of sugar and other simple carbohydrates. As a result, he will probably find yourself eating too much high calorie, high fat, unhealthy food and, as a result, find it anyway kudos goes back on very quickly.

- **Eat healthily**: If you think about is actually what you're eating and try to make your diet as healthy as possible, without being fanatical, then you will have a much better chance at being able to control your weight by controlling your mindset. Eating healthily means having a balanced diet, eating plenty of fresh fruit and vegetables, low-fat protein, healthy fats such as olive oil and avocado, and plenty of complex carbohydrates. It also means cutting right down on food containing sugar and white foods such as white flour, white rice, and white pasta and eating instead more whole-meal foods.

- **Relax frequently**: If you tend to eat more when you feel stressed, take a few moments when you feel the stress building to close your eyes and take some slow breaths in as you breathe in relaxation and breathe out any tension.

- **Listen to your body**: Learn to listen to what your body tells you it needs at any time of the day and allow yourself to have whatever it seems to need, even though at the same time being aware of the healthy guidelines mentioned above.

Get Enough Sleep for Weight Loss

When we think of the most important things that our bodies need, sleep is right up there with food, water, and oxygen; the amount of sleep you get daily can have a dramatic effect on your health and weight. But do we know how must sleep we need?

As a general guide, most adults should be aiming to get around 7 - 8 hours a day. Our bodies are all different, and some people may find they function at their peak on 6 hours of sleep a day while others may need around 9. Sleep deprivation, however, is a big problem, and if you are only managing around 4-5 hours a night, then your body is being deprived of sleep.

Let's firstly look at the benefits of getting a good night sleep:

- **Sleep Naturally Repairs Your Body**: Extra protein molecules are produced while you are sleeping, which helps to fight infection, and your immune system repairs cells.

- **Sleep Reduces Stress Levels**: A good quality sleep can help lower blood pressure and levels of stress hormones in your body.

- **Greater Concentration**: A good night's sleep will allow you to concentrate better the following day and will also aid memory function.

- **More Relaxed**: A good sleep will mean you wake up more refreshed and relaxed.

If you are not getting enough sleep on a regular basis, then all of the above benefits will be reversed. So, this may mean waking up emotion groggy, emotion more stressed, and unable to concentrate. You will also be more prone to illness and higher blood pressure. You may think that being deprived of sleep and emotion tired may result in a loss of appetite and weight loss, but the truth is that a lack of sleep may lead to weight gain.

Sleep helps to keep in check the hormones in your body that control your appetite, so if you are not getting enough sleep, then your appetite will increase, and you will feel even hungrier. Sleep deprivation will cause your body to have reduced energy levels, and your body will crave high-fat content foods that may give you a temporary boost. These foods tend to be high in calories and salt or sugar; they will not fill you up because they lack nutrition and will leave you sluggish and hungry again very soon.

Nothing will set you better for the day than a good refreshing sleep followed by a well-balanced breakfast. To aid your sleep, try to limit your consumption of alcohol and spicy foods. Try and unwind naturally before bed with a nice long soak or some relaxation exercises. Try to avoid using alcohol as your main way of unwinding and relieving stress.

If you are looking to lose weight, as well as eating a sensible and balanced diet and taking regular exercise, you need to be getting a good night's sleep every night.

CHAPTER 4:

Women's Complicated Relationship with Food, Emotions, and Stress.

W omen are not taught or encouraged to meet their own needs. Instead, they put the needs of their families, friends, and even their work before their health.

You Eat What Is Necessary

At times we eat not because we are hungry but because food is available. The same way you make random decisions to purchase items you don't need in a supermarket in the same way we purchase food at times. For instance, you might recently have acquired a job, and it's your first time to acquire some financial freedom. You find that there is that expensive restaurant you have wanted to go to, but you couldn't afford it since you had money at that particular time. Now that you can afford it to visit it frequently and purchase food that you do not need but you are buying just because you have the money and food is available. Most of the bad decisions that lead us to eat food that we do not have to eat can be avoided if we focus our thoughts on getting that which is necessary. This process will require an individual to acquire some personal discipline. Before you purchase any food, you ask yourself if it is really necessary. See if the food that you are taking will add any value to your health. After asking yourself such a question, you get to know the right thing to do based on your response to the questions. It is an easy process that will save you from consuming some carbs that make you add unnecessary weight.

It Helps You Avoid Emotional Eating

You might fall into the category of those people that eat anytime they feel stressed out, or any time they have some negative thoughts. You find that anytime you are angered or someone makes you feel sad about yourself, all you want to do is eat. In the process of wanting to eat more, you start adding some weight. You could be consuming some cards, refined carbohydrates, and fast foods.

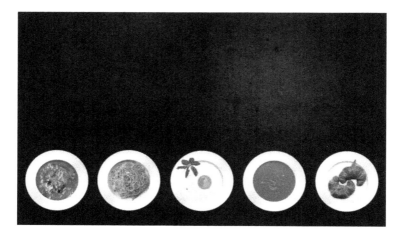

The body acquires more food than it needs. For instance, the glucose levels increase, and it is unable to convert all the sugars into energy. As a result, the individual adds extra weight since the sugars are converted into fats. Meditation allows you to challenge negative feelings and stressful thoughts. You get to understand the cause of the challenges that you are facing. In a calm state of mind, you can come up with a possible solution for the issue that you are struggling with.

If it is beyond your control, you can learn how to accept the situation as it is and let it not affect your feelings negatively. When you learn to do this, you can avoid emotional eating, and in the process, lose weight.

Helps Us In Making The Right Decisions Regarding Food

We live in a time where people are becoming creative with food. People are trying out new recipes to see what can work and what cannot. We are having increased production of processed foods as people venture into the food business. They want to make money and provide foods that people will love and will make them keep coming for more. They learn their target audience and give them what they want. Most people will eat something just because it is sweet, and they like how it tastes in their mouths. You might be hungry, and you are looking for something to eat. You have the decision to choose a healthy meal or eating an unhealthy meal. Y

ou know the benefits of taking a nutritious meal, and at the same time, you understand the disadvantages of taking an unhealthy meal. Meditation allows you to make a better and more informed decision regarding your life choices. Some of these life choices are in the decisions we choose to make for the meals that we want to take. Most times, we overlook the power of such decisions and the impact they could have. Meditation allows you to consume that which is necessary at that moment. In this case, you chose to make a vegan meal over some processed food. In the end, you are healthy, and it helps you lose extra weight since you only take foods that are well utilized by your body.

Improves Your Mode Of Eating

How do you chew your food? Did you know it can influence your weight? Some of the things we do look simple, and you would not expect them to have any effect; surprisingly, how you chew your food matter. When you chew your food fast and swallow it immediately, the food particles are not well broken down. The body might find it hard to utilize the contents of the food, and much of what you consumed becomes waste. After the food leaves your mouth, it goes through other processes.

The body may not be able to break it further, and hence it becomes extra bulk in your body. When this happens, the body converts it into fats, and you end up gaining weight. You might have consumed a little amount of food, but due to your poor mode of eating, you add some extra weight.

Meditation allows you to concentrate while chewing food. Once the food particles are completely broken down, it becomes easier for your body to process them. In the process, each nutrient content present in the food consumed is well utilized by the body.

Afterward, there will be no extra food that needs to be converted into fats. It prevents you from adding excess weight, and in the process, you get to lose weight.

You Realize The Effects Of Certain Foods On Your Body

Once we consume food, our bodies respond to what we have consumed. It could be a negative or positive response. Different foods generate different feelings. We may not believe what some of these feelings are unless we focus our minds on realizing them. The power of meditation is that it allows you to focus, concentrate, and point out certain things that need your attention. This is an easy thing to accomplish; you only need to evaluate how your body reacts to the foods that you consume. After consuming some foods, you will notice that some make you feel energized while some make you feel tired. Anytime you overeat, there is some sudden feeling of tiredness. You feel like your body is full, and all you want to do is take a nap or rest. This is a sign that whatever you ate was unnecessary, and hence the body will not use it. As a result, most of what you ate will be waste that your body needs to eliminate. In that process, you add some extra weight as the excess food becomes excess fat in your body. On the other hand, if you eat and immediately feel energized, it means that your body was receptive to the food that you consumed. It can convert much of it into energy, and each component present in the food is well utilized. This is beneficial for the wellbeing of your body and can help you in loss of weight and prevent you from adding unnecessary weight.

It Helps You Realize Your Cravings

A variety of things can cause various food cravings that we have. You might be busy viewing posts in your various social media accounts, and all of a sudden, you come across a picture of a good-looking hamburger that seems to taste as good as it looks. Immediately, you develop a need to eat some. Before you saw the picture, such a thought had not crossed your mind, but now that you have seen it, you suddenly want to have some. As a result, you automatically develop a craving for a hamburger. You might find yourself walking to get fast food to get some, or you might want to order some online. The craving makes you make suddenly rushed decisions to eat, which can contribute to adding some extra weight. Some cravings are generated from wanting to consume the foods that we like eating. You might be an individual that loves taking tacos. All you think of any time you want something to eat is how you will get those tacos that you love so much. Being aware of some of these cravings can help you in avoiding them. Meditation helps you to realize the cravings that you have. After conducting an evaluation, you can find out if some of these cravings are beneficial to your body. If you realize that they are doing more harm than good, you get to avoid them.

You Get To Realize When You Need Food And When You Are Full

At times we confuse cravings with hunger. There is a difference between wanting to eat chocolate when you are hungry and wanting to get some food when you are hungry. The chocolate bar contains some sugars that make you full once you consume them. You might be having a busy day at the office, and you grab a lunch bar during lunchtime, and it's probably all that you will eat at that particular time. In that moment of choosing what to eat, you can still decide to eat a healthy meal that will still satisfy the need at that moment. Meditation allows you to distinguish between when you have a craving, and when you are really hungry. This allows you only to eat when necessary. You avoid eating foods that are not helpful to your body, and as a result, you are highly unlikely to gain weight. On the other hand, mediation allows you to know when you are full. Earlier, we stated that we, at times, eat just because food is available and not that we are hungry. With the help of mediation, you can easily know if you are eating food just because it is available or if you for sure need to eat. Such minor decisions are major when it comes to weight loss as they ensure you only eat what your body requires.

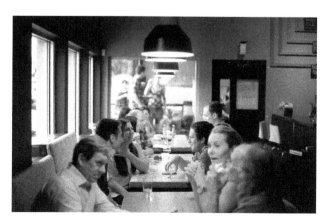

You Formulate The Good Eating Habits

There are certain ways in which we consume our food. Some of these ways are not beneficial and cause us to create more harm to our bodies. Most of the time, we ignore the time factor as far as eating is concerned. We barely look at the decisions we make regarding food, and all that we do is make some rush decisions. Having an eating routine is very important. Nutritionists are constantly advising us on the right ways to consume our food. For instance, it is wrong to drink water immediately after a meal. You first have to allow the food to settle; then, you take your water after some 30 minutes.

On the other hand, they advise that fruits should be consumed before meals for them to benefit your body rightfully. When you consume them together with the meals, they may not have the huge impact they would have if; you had consumed them before the meal. Some of these healthy facts are simple and easy to follow; we just choose not to.

CHAPTER 5:

The Holistic Approach – Making Decisions About Diets

Relationship with Food and Weight Loss

Our stomach is a muscle. Although it is a fist-size, it extends relying upon the measure of food eaten. Anyway, fist-size is genuinely what we have to eat to fulfill our hunger. This size applies to bit food - this is the thing that goes into the stomach. Eating fist-size healthy suppers when you are hungry is a way to get thinner.

Anyway, it isn't always simple since specific individuals create "unique" associations with food. Some of them are:

1. **Eating to numb negative emotions**. Food can never tackle your problems, and it can't make you feel in any capacity. You are in charge of the way you feel. Understand this and quit eating for emotional reasons. It will be likewise useful to have different side interests, for example, sewing, stitching, crossword fathoming, and so, rather than emotional eating, you could transform into your preferred pastime. Attestations, perceptions just as stress reduction techniques, can likewise help stop this unfortunate habit.

2. **Being on starvation diets and after that, binge eating**. This can create an endless loop: blame related to binge eating at that point desensitized with more food, and all weight-related endeavors are destroyed. Eating well parcels as opposed to starving and dealing with emotional eating can help with this.

3. **Eating regularly or eating substantially more than should be expected to fulfill the hunger**. These are habits unfavorable to the weight loss process and should be unlearned. Don't eat while accomplishing something different (sitting in front of the TV, for

instance). Eat deliberately, gradually, getting a charge out of each piece. Along these lines, you will eat only enough to fulfill your hunger.

It is critical to give yourself some time to supplant the old habits that don't work well for you: changing habits requires time and tirelessness. Try not to feel blameworthy if, eventually, you pursue your undesirable eating habits - return to your weight-loss diet.

Is Stress Eating Sabotaging Your Midlife Weight-loss EFFORTS?

Have you at any point utilized food to make yourself feel better - stress eating to deal with negative emotions, instead of to fill your stomach? Dessert following an awful day, treats after a contention or heavy crunching when you are overpowered, to divert and comfort yourself.

Utilizing food now and then to comfort, to reward, or to celebrate isn't an awful thing. Be that as it may, when food and eating are your essential adapting to stress system when your first drive is to open the cooler whenever you're forlorn, vexed, angry, overpowered, depleted, or exhausted or some other emotional indications of stress, you stall out in an undesirable cycle where the genuine fundamental feeling or problem is never addressed.

We as a whole endeavor to feel right somehow. Feeling stressed means feeling terrible, no questions about that. Stress eating is a way to smother or mitigate negative stress emotions, for example, uneasiness, outrage, dread, fatigue, pity, and depression. Both significant life occasions and the issues of everyday life can trigger stress that leads to stress longings and possible weight increase and by and significant medical problems.

Eating may feel good at the time. However, the problem that activated stress is still there. Furthermore, you regularly feel more regrettable a short time later: liable or remorseful than you did before as a result of the excessive calories you devoured. You beat yourself up for failure and not having more self-discipline.

With the fact that the arrangement isn't determination or even the most current diet - when you are a lady beyond 40 years old, you may have seen that diets and physical exercises don't resolve middle-age weight problem, there substantially more to consider - awkward hormonal nature, a decline of bulk and more slow digestion and... Stress.

It's a snowball effect: additional calories you devoured as an aftereffect of stress eating - eating for others that physical hunger reasons, unavoidably prompts 'lethal weight' - stress fat. The stress fat gathering around the stomach area isn't just stylishly terrible yet more awful again - it prompts metabolic disorder, degenerative maturing infections, and untimely maturing, which are solid stressors necessarily.

Aggravating the problem, you quit learning sound ways to deal with your stress, you have an increasingly hard time controlling your weight, and you feel progressively weak, vulnerable, and miserable over both food and your stress.

Whatever emotions drive you to overeat, the final product is frequently the equivalent. The stress-activated emotions return, and now you need to deal with extra stress - additional weight.

Is it safe to say that you are prepared for change? Great! Mindfulness is the initial step to change.

Is it safe to say that you are a stress eater?

- You eat more when you're feeling stressed or eat to lessen stress.

- You eat when you're not physically hungry or when you're full.

- You feel the inclination to eat when you have significant activities to complete, and you are running delayed.

- You eat to feel better (to quiet and calm yourself when you're tragic, distraught, exhausted, on edge, and so on).

- You use food for stress relief, rather than exercise or different stress reduction techniques, since it's simpler.

- You reward yourself with food.

- You consistently eat until you've stuffed yourself.

- You don't set aside effort for stress relief since you have an excessive amount to do.

- You overeat quickly and need starches.

Do you perceive yourself? We genuinely don't have the foggiest idea why a few people battle with an incredible sweet tooth, and others don't during stressful times. Be that as it may, there are a LOT of ways to address stress and manage it superior to food.

Is it accurate to say that you are hungry for more responses to address your stress and stress eating? There are a LOT of ways to address it and manage it better.

Techniques Hypnotherapy Use For Weight Loss

Every case is not the same as everyone got their reasons as to why they want to reduce in mass; there are some recommendations that you might come across:

- You must envision your body the way you want, or to the level of fitness and health you want to attain.

- Just try to think of how you will feel with your new appearance and health.

- Think about how to be there effortlessly.

- Have a look at how you are improving daily.

- Think about how energized and confident you will feel.

- When you get to know that with more exercise, It's the more you will be exercising, and it will be much easier.

The methods have been put up to encourage and inspire you and assist you in taking charge of your choices. When you have negative thoughts about some foods being unhealthy, then hypnotherapy for food addiction can be of help to cut out such negative thoughts. With the help of weight reduction hypnosis, then you can enjoy the taste of healthy meals and stop craving for fatty and sugary foods. Hypnosis for the mass loss will assist you in adopting a healthier life pattern and happier mentality by tackling the deep feelings that bring about the creation of your feeding habits.

Your Probable Mass Loss Blocks

Many people are trying and failing to lose weight for several whys and wherefores. Reasons which can also be referred to as "secondary gains" are most of the time insensible, thus being difficult for you to overwhelm them. When you have focused on reducing or cutting your mass, then you must look at the belief that has kept your mass for that period. Most of us have beliefs where we think about ourselves, value, and what we want as humans. Insensible characters will take away your emotional opinions towards yourself.

A clinical hypnotherapist, Amreeta, explored the hurdles humans can experience when trying to cut mass. Most of you will gain comfort when you don't make any change, thus feeling secure just being the way you are. You may want to reduce mass, but the insensible things are baring you from making them happen. Hypnotherapy for mass reduction helps to solve such reasons, thus making patients have a break from hurdles that prevent you from reducing mass over the years.

Comfort Eating

When you are still an infant, you will associate eating with the help of your mother. A lot of professionals have been able to prove that the association never gets over; thus, when life gets stressful, you can look back at the previous days of full dependence. From this point, emotional eating can be hectic. At times you can get yourself going for a chocolate bar after a tiresome day or having a takeaway when you are all alone and sad; this can make you a relaxed eater. When you are a comfort eater, then there will be some difficulties in cutting your weight as you will have been compatible with food, and without it, you can't be able to handle your sensations.

Hypnotherapy will assist you in addressing this, make you learn how to handle negative sensations in a way that won't bring about comfortability in your feeding. The greatest change you can have is being less bothered about feeding. You can still have fun, but teach your body to eat only when you are hungry and not when the brain feels like and wants to appease feelings. Hypnotherapy has assisted so many people in stunning their passionate eating.

CHAPTER 6:

Working in Harmony
(Mind, Emotion, and Body)

Perfect Mind, Perfect Weight

Perfect thoughts and ideal weight." The term may seem like a fantasy to you. Which is the ideal mind or ideal weight? They're the realistic conditions you'll be able to utilize as you pursue fat reduction. "Realistic?" You inquire. "How can anything be 'ideal,' let alone my burden and my ideas about my burden?" Well, recall what we said about the strength of believing and belief. Is it serving your curiosity to desire or hope to anything less than perfection on your own? Indulge us for some time as we clarify why you're able to think your mind and burden because "perfect."

Perfect fat is your weight that's ideal for you. It's the weight that's attainable and consistent with everything you need and precisely what you're ready to give yourself and accept yourself.

More to the point, your ideal weight provides you with the healthy entire body, the human body which goes effortlessly, and also the one where you are feeling great about yourself and joyful.

And what're ideal thoughts? You presently have a mind. It's flawless. But there can be a few ideas in that ideal thought of yours who are providing you with undesirable outcomes. There can be something that you keep in your mind, possibly habits or routines, which provide you with undesirable outcomes. However, you may use your ideal head to match your ideas to offer you precisely what you desire. It's possible to use your head to accomplish the bodyweight that you desire.

In the Twinkling of an Eye

Your current body is the consequence of your ideas and beliefs. You've behaved out these ideas and beliefs by your lifestyle, which generated your current weight. You haven't made any errors, regardless of what you may be thinking of yourself; instead, you've just experienced undesirable outcomes.

These undesirable effects are an immediate effect of misaligned ideas and beliefs about yourself, which are very patterns of behavior or lifestyle. The Rapid Weight-Loss Diet is all about utilizing your perfect thoughts

To align your ideas to provide you with the results you desire. You honestly can use your head to accomplish the bodyweight you desire. Let's take a look at a few of the learning which has occurred in your life, which has let you know where you're now together with your body weight.

Do you wake up one afternoon, and you had been using the additional pounds?

Or could it be a slow accumulation with time?

Or perhaps you've understood nothing else as early youth. Whatever the situation, there are lots of factors that made your body:

- Food options
- Eating customs
- That the self-critic in you
- Economic history
- Psychological history
- Impact of household
- Impact of buddies
- Cultural heritage

These and several other variables were discovered in your life and eventually became the beliefs, which subsequently became routines of activity that generated your body.

In other words, consider what you did understand about your youth, about eating and food.

- What kinds of grocery stores did your household buy?
- What foods did your kids cook, and were they typically ready?
- Can you eat only at home or often grab food?

Have you been served fresh, healthy, high-calorie foods, or can you eat mainly processed and extremely processed foods, fried foods, and "junk" foods?

- Was their aware focus on nutrition, or has been there any irresponsible disregard for that which your household ate?
- What did you find out about eating mindfully?
- Were you educated that healthful food options led to healthy bodies?
- Did anybody teach you how you can understand what's healthy food and what's not?
- Are your meals selections based on which tasted or seemed high or priceless?
- Can your loved ones or college instruct you about healthy lifestyles and audio nourishment, or has it been the "nutrition education" through TV advertisements and food makers' advertising?

What exactly did you learn as a kid? What're your beliefs about eating food, along with your entire body? Analyze your own socioeconomic or socio-cultural roots and see if they had an effect on the way and what you've learned to consume. Over thirty-five Years Back, sociological research pointed out weight issues in the working and lower class according to their intake patterns of what's been known as "poverty-level foods," like hot dogs, canned meats, and processed luncheon meats.

Cultural groups also have been analyzed to understand their nutritional patterns and meals, like eating with lard or ingesting a diet of fried and high-fat foods, which can lead to higher body fat loss. These influences can readily be accepted because they're "regular" into the category, of course. Then let's take a look in the teen years. During adolescence, are there some changes in your weight loss? Just as a boy, have you been invited to pile more food on your plate? "Look at him, consume! Certainly, he will develop to a large guy!" (There's a telling metaphor) Or are you currently admonished to eat? When you're a budding young woman, did a Smart girl take you under her wing and then discuss with you that the marvel of menses and the wonderment of body modifications, such as the organic growth in body fat with all the evolution of breasts and broader hips?

Were you conscious during puberty, which, unless the body improved body fat by 22 percent, it wouldn't correctly grow and create menses? Or was that "hushed up" within an awkward improvement? It was likely during adolescence which you heard there's a stigma involving obese individuals. Ponder the encounters and influences which are forming your body. In high school, the athletes at college sports have always been a healthful weight and are the cheerleaders and homecoming queens.

What ancient beliefs regarding your popularity and self-image could have formed from your social interactions in high school? What did you understand about physical activity, and what customs did you produce? Have you been introduced to physical activity as part of a healthy lifestyle, through family or sports outings of walks or hikes? Or was that the blaring TV a regular fixture, enticing everybody to the sofa? Next is a matter which most people have never been aware of throughout their development.

As you're growing up, has been that the attention of self-care based on trendy clothes, makeup, and hairstyles, or about healthful food, routine physical activity, along with spiritual and intellectual nourishment? What about today? Spend a couple more minutes writing down the aspects that appear to be accurate for you in the past couple of decades. What influences and experiences formed the ideas, which turned into the beliefs that turned into your body?

After high school, you moved away from the house. Suddenly you're no more captive to your family lifestyle. Can you be aware of your options, or can you start eating with blow off? If you input into a close connection, just what compromises or arrangements about foods and physical activity did you input into too? Most associations develop from similar pursuits, including food preferences and eating styles. In the end, the relationship comprises eating routines and tastes, which are a consequence of compromise.

Have your connections encouraged smart food choices and healthy eating? Maybe you've experienced pregnancy. Can you learn the way to get a wholesome pregnancy and then nourish a healthy infant within you? Or did you put in pounds? After giving birth, how did your lifestyle assist you in recovering your typical fat or suppressing it? If you were more active in the league or sports games, did your livelihood or family duties take priority and eliminate these physical fitness tasks from your regular? Can you correct exercise and diet so, or even did the fat begin to collect? Did an accident, injury, or disease happen that disrupted a standard physical action that has been supportive of healthy fat?

Because you can see, the way you got to where you're now was no crash. You heard from the folks about you--or you also consumed out of the surroundings --the best way to create food decisions, the way to eat, and the way to look after yourself emotionally and physically. Whether the thoughts you heard were tremendous and healthy or not so high and not as healthy, they became your own beliefs and eventually became you and the own human body because it is now. Bear in mind, and you didn't do something wrong; however, you need to experience the outcomes of eating and living, which have been consistent with your ideas and beliefs.

Through time, what's been your answer to individuals and their opinions about your weight loss, bad or good? Can you go out and purchase a fantastic pair of sneakers, or do you consume to facilitate psychological distress? Maybe you even heard the latter response in your youth.

Did your mom ever provide you with a plateful of food to comfort you when you're miserable? These are learned answers, and they may be unlearned and replaced with new answers and routines to make your ideal weight. Just ask, "Just how long does this happen?" We inform you, "In the twinkling of the eye," For the minute that you understand that you need it sufficient to get anything to possess it, it's completed. You've just altered the management of highly efficient energy in you, which will be directed at figuring out how to attain the outcome which you need: your ideal weight.

Your Perfect Mind Relearning

It's simple to comprehend how you got or "heard" to contemplate over your ideal weight. And it'll be simple to create new decisions, to relearn new routines, and also to make new and much more healthful habits. How can we learn? We understand by mimicking another individual, analyzing books with different tools, and practicing the activities that create the outcomes we all seek. The best and lasting learning entails repetition and practice. The best way to practice is essential. Pretend for a minute that you're a violinist. You're searching for a grand symphony operation in New York.

The critical thing is that you're giving your focus on practicing correctly.

Heal Your Relationship with Food

As you can see, the desire to reduce sugar is not easy. It becomes not only our habit, but we also become physically dependent on it. It disturbs our health and even our overall functioning as individuals in society.

A Simple and Magical Solution Does Not Exist

Yes, some foods are healthy and which can replace sugar, but it takes discipline and a change of lifestyle.

In the morning, after a night when you don't eat, your blood sugar level is the lowest, and we should eat a meal that provides a constant increase of sugar to avoid hunger attacks. This meal should contain a combination of protein and complex carbohydrates (bread, pasta) because they are digested slowly.

This is about enough for me to start the day. Fruit also causes relatively rapid rises in blood sugar. Therefore, it might be better to eat it in the afternoon after lunch, but with a gap as it is quickly digested and absorbed best on an empty stomach. This will help in the afternoon when our energy is lowered, and will not have such a yo-yo effect on blood sugar as chocolate or ice cream.

CHAPTER 7:

Emotional vs. Physical Hunger

Emotional hunger and physical hunger are two very different things. Many individuals may claim that they're just trying to fill their empty stomach whenever they take a ton of food out of the fridge. However, they may only be trying to fill their empty heart or, at least, to make their mind of something. It's easy for many not to see the differences, especially when they're depressed, stressed out, and troubled. It will help you determine which is which. If you're still stuck in a cycle of emotional hunger, frustration, and negativity, you're encouraged to note the things explained below.

Mindless Eating Usually Follows After Emotional Hunger

Mindless eating is characterized by a lack of awareness of what's going into your body or the amount of food you're stuffing yourself with. After several hours, you may have already consumed a whole bag of chips or an entire pint of ice cream without paying much attention and without thoroughly enjoying the meal. You're emotional, not necessarily hungry.

Emotional Hunger is Sudden

Emotional hunger does not follow a specific schedule. It will hit you instantly, filling you with a sense of urgency that's simultaneously overwhelming and very tempting. Since emotions are also quite challenging to manage and predict, emotional hunger can surprise you in many instances. On the other hand, physical desire is gradual. Unless you haven't eaten in a very long time, you wouldn't want to eat as soon as possible. The hunger builds up because since your last meal this morning, you haven't had anything to eat. There's still an hour away before the lunch break, and your stomach's already rumbling a bit.

Being Full Won't Satisfy Emotional Hunger

Physical hunger can be satisfied when you've had your fill. After a healthy amount of food, you can continue being productive or doing various activities. On the other hand, emotional hunger continues to demand more and more. You're led to eating more because the bad or negative feelings haven't been addressed yet.

You're so focused on drowning your sorrows and disappointments with different types of "Comfort Food" that you forget about your body needs. You're already full if you'll consider your physical needs, but your heart and mind aren't made yet. For so many reasons, they won't be done until you gain much weight; until you see what you've become because of emotional hunger. Once you're full, but your body's still searching for more food, consider the possibility of being emotionally hungry. Some people fall into a dangerous cycle of binge eating because they don't want to admit that they're emotionally troubled. They turn to food because they think they're just hungrier than usual. This isn't the case most of the time, though.

Specific Comfort Foods are sought during Emotional Hunger

Physical hunger can be satisfied with virtually any type of food. Those who are simply hungry can get by with a vegetable salad with steamed tuna. Healthy eating is also considered—most likely, even preferred more than unhealthy choices. You just want to respond to hunger and healthily get to such a goal. Emotional hunger craves for specific and usually unhealthy snacks.

Guilt, Regret, or Shame Usually Follow After Emotional Hunger

People know what's wrong and right for them. When they make healthy food choices, they are filled with satisfaction and genuine joy because they know they're taking good care of themselves. They eat only when they are hungry, and they don't let their emotions dictate their food choices.

Sadly, for those who are emotionally hungry, guilt, regret, and shame can become frequent companions. After you finish that giant bag of chips or that extra-large coke, you're filled with so much sadness because you know it's not right. You're guilty because once again, you've allowed yourself to get caught up in the moment. You're also ashamed because you weren't strong enough to make the right decision.

The Causes of Emotional Eating

Childhood Habits

Look back at your experiences with food as a child. How did your parents associate food or eating to various circumstances in your life? If you were rewarded with food whenever you did something right or unusual, you must have unconsciously considered food to be a reward for good behavior.

Another way of looking at it is if your parents gave you sweets or a tasty meal whenever you were feeling down. In the early years, his perspective on the role of food in his life is primarily influenced by his parents or guardians. Essentially, the overall view of the family towards food also creates a foundation for the young one's view of food when he grows older. Emotionally-based childhood eating behaviors, which on develop into habits, usually extend to adulthood. It's also actually possible for someone to eat based on nostalgic feelings. Eating because you remember how your dad grilled a couple of patties when you were younger feels good.

Influence of Social Activities

One right way of relieving stress is to meet with your close friends or loved ones. Their presence and their tolerance for your food choices gives a great feeling. You feel at home with them, and because they may also be eating due to emotional hunger, you may end up doing the same.

There's a high tendency that overeating may occur because you're in the company of overeaters. You just decide to do what they're doing because all of you are going through tough challenges. You may want to empathize with them.

Another reason why overeating or binge eating may occur during social gatherings is nervousness. Things can get even worse if you're encouraged by your loved ones to eat a lot. They don't mind your current body mass because they love you too much to see you not eat and just sit at a corner.

Emotion-Stuffing

Food turns into medicine, which isn't as effective as it's viewed to be. People just want to bury their negative emotions under a massive pile of food. When they break up with someone, they turn to food. When they lose one of their loved ones, they think of the best way to stuff themselves up. When things don't go according to plan, a local binge eater shows his immense faith in the local supermarket and his great adoration for his refrigerator.

A Feeling of Emptiness or Extreme Boredom

Some people eat a ton of food just because they're bored. When they have nothing to do, they most likely don't even try to look for some activity to keep themselves busy. Boredom is sometimes a sign of laziness.

Since an individual doesn't want to do what he's supposed to do, he ends up feeling empty. Instead of using this time to be productive or to help himself, he turns to food. This behavior can also turn into a habit if not detected, admitted, and addressed promptly.

Stress

Have you ever noticed that stress can also make you hungry? It's not just in your head. Having chronic stress in this past-faced and the chaotic world often leads to increased cortisol levels, the stress hormone. Cortisol will trigger cravings for salty, sweet, and high-fat foods. These types of food will give you a burst of energy and pleasure, which is why they're so tempting to consume. The more stressed out you are, the more likely it is for you to turn to unhealthy food.

Unfortunately, so many things can act as stressors, so it's also a challenge for several people to handle themselves. At the workplace, school, and even at home, certain things stress people out. Avoiding stress would be another issue altogether, but making wise decisions on managing yourself during tense situations can make a difference.

Using Awareness or Mindfulness to Beat Emotional Eating

You either eat with your emotions or with your mind. You can't work with both. This is why mindful eating is considered to be the exact opposite of emotional eating. Awareness is a powerful tool in defeating binge eating. Once you become less nervous and more rational about problem-solving or self-management, you'll be able to overcome this seemingly unbeatable foe.

You simply have to start with the identification of the triggers of emotional hunger. After that, you should look for better alternatives. As you work on these, you're also encouraged to savor the eating experience. Lastly, remember to live in the present.

Identify Triggers of Emotional Hunger

Many things can trigger emotional eating. Whatever triggers your emotional outbursts or fills you with negativity are the same factors that influence your diet. It may be challenging to accomplish this step, but you can seek assistance from your loved ones.

You can do it, though. You just have to believe in your ability not to be biased when assessing yourself. Be more observant of your day-to-day activities and regard your problems through positive lenses.

Push pessimism away because this will hinder you from seeing the picture. Instead of thinking that you'll just end up counting your problems, see it as an effective method of analyzing your enemies to take them down.

Great soldiers or warriors are aware of what they're feeling during various circumstances. They know what they should do because they look at every detail.

Find Alternatives to Address Negative Emotions

Emotional eating isn't the only path toward relief. It's not even a unique path to begin with. Instead of eating to your heart's content whenever you're feeling down, look for other ways to lift yourself. The most excellent solutions to emotional hunger are of love.

This essentially means that if you do things that you're passionate about, you can feel more fulfilled and satisfied. The list of things that can make you happy indeed isn't only filled with different types of food. You will find other things to do in your free time and during those tough moments.

The alternatives need not be expensive. They don't even have to cost you a dime. Simply meditating a few times a week, talking to a good friend, or walking at the park every day can make the blues away.

Savor the Eating Experience

Some say that obesity isn't a massive concern in France because they know how to enjoy their food. They're able to avoid a wider waistline by having a full grin whenever they're eating. Generally, the French enjoy eating as much as they have fun cooking a variety of healthy and hearty meals.

You may not be a professional cook or chef, but you can choose to savor the eating experience whenever you're at home or eating out. You can have fun eating, exploring the different flavors and textures of the meal before you.

Binge eaters "enjoy" food in a different way. They use it to conceal severe emotional struggles. Instead of eating healthy and doing away with their hunger, they use food to break out of their gloomy state. Unfortunately, they're not free. If you seek freedom, one effective way of achieving it is to savor every bite and not rush to the refrigerator during a crisis. Enjoy your salad, steak, or whatever it is in front of you. Don't eat more than you're supposed to because your sadness and disappointments won't vacate your heart because your stomach's filled with so much food.

CHAPTER 8:

How Hypnosis Works

Hypnosis has been purported to work very effectively in several different habit-breaking protocols and has undoubtedly been promoted as a right car for dieters.

If you are open-minded and are ready to believe that the power of the hypnotic idea is real and is going to provide you with a helping hand in your weight loss journey, you are much most likely to see it work. If you think that hypnosis works, and consequently go through hypnosis as a mechanism to assist you to lose weight, you are far most likely to lose weight than a doubter would be.

There are entire bodies of work appearing around this "biology of belief" concept that your inner inclination is the essential element to the success rate you will see when attempting treatments of any kind.

As part and parcel of a good dietary routine, and in a supporting function, if you believe that a proper hypnotist can implant in your "inner ear," a suggestive incentive to follow through on your diet, by all methods, do it! If you believe that just investing a couple of hours under the watch-eye of the extremely best mental magician is going to melt off the 20 pounds you've gotten for a long time, well, you are going to be bitterly dissatisfied. You do need to select an excellent diet plan also! With that said, if you are a supporter, like I am, in the absolute power of the mind, go for it. And make sure to share your success like the rest of us do, often! It keeps everybody determined, slimming down, and sensation fantastic.

Bridging the Gap to Success

Hypnosis and weight-loss are a successful pair. Whereas lots of people try to tackle slimming down on their own, merely through self-discipline and motivation, and end up stopping working, weight loss hypnosis can supply the missing out on link that will eventually lead to success. By having the ability to soothe us down mentally along with by taking on the physical procedure that may be impeding our efforts, hypnotherapists and hypnosis downloads make the entire journey much more accessible, more satisfying, and, eventually, more gratifying.

One needs never to think that it is their fault if they are not able to get down to their preferred weight. Hypnosis and weight loss are a distinct pairing that can tackle our subconscious to assist significantly in losing weight. When you believe about what is involved in the process of losing weight, using hypnosis for weight loss makes a lot of sense. In essence, we are breaking routines, behaviors, beliefs, and desires that we have held firmly for several years. Just thinking of dieting is enough to make anyone feel denied and, therefore, contributes to the level of difficulty that is being experienced. For that reason, it is essential to discover a way to make the experience simpler and to find out a way to unwind throughout the whole course of dropping weight.

Research studies show that hypnosis, when used correctly, can have a considerable effect when used for weight-loss. A 9-week study of 2 weight management groups - one of which was executing hypnosis as a tool showed that the group that used hypnosis continued to reveal results more than two years later on. Adding hypnosis to any present weight reduction procedures you're currently doing, such as workout and healthy consuming, increases your chance of dropping weight by 97%.

Weight-loss is challenging; however, weight gain is natural. Experts will inform you that a diet plan and exercise are the only way to shed the undesirable pounds; yet, not everyone has the time to sign up with a fitness center, and the tension of life can lead to poor food choices. Hypnosis and weight loss can assist you in developing a more favorable self-image. You will still be you, only better and healthier. Using hypnosis can help you feel more unwanted and not just about food, however, also in your day to day life. When you can conquer stress, you will no longer turn to food for comfort, therefore adopting a much healthier general mindset. Hypnosis can also help with favorable thinking. You should never underestimate what a positive outlook can attain.

How does it Work?

Since they lead a sedentary way of life, the factor that individuals are obese is not. It's merely because they have a desire to consume more than "regular" people. When our bodies feel full, then we are supposed to stop wasting.

For obese individuals, when they feel full and are no longer starving, they continue to eat. For lots of obese people, this is one of the couples of satisfactions that they can get.

Since it resets an individual's relationship with food, Hypnosis is useful. Food is supposed to taste good. That's what kept us alive for thousands of years - a craving to head out and get food to please the appetite with. When you are no longer starving, then you need to stop eating.

How Successful Is Hypnosis?

The majority of clients require a few sessions of hypnosis for it to have an impact. Many individuals report that they can start to reduce weight quickly.

Unfortunately, in the long term, a lot of patients will return to their old habits. Although they were "taught" how to treat their food, ultimately, they did not decide on their own to deal with food as it should be processed, and they slip back into old methods of overeating.

How Hypnosis for weight reduction works

The answer is that your motivation to modify your habits to decrease or lose excess weight and keep it off must be genuine. No number of Clinical Hypnosis sittings is going to be of any assistance to you if you are not ready yet to do what it takes to lose the weight.

You will discover that, unlike cigarette smoking, we all need food to stay alive, and for almost everybody, eating tasty, fun food is pleasing. Sadly, what makes many people's mouth-watering is not necessarily excellent for you. We frequently consume for pleasure, as a kind of satisfaction, centering ourselves on the gustatory feeling as we overgorge ourselves with no regard to those signals from our tummy.

However, the truth is, as soon as you eat way too much on processed food, you generally don't feel well, even

We could use this reality of life as a part of the hypnosis treatment for weight loss. Well, every food is a mix of chemicals that act on our physical structure. We require to recognize that truth and find out to select foods that work on our body in health-positive and sound method to feel great.

Hypnosis has to do with an idea(s), and part of it is the post-hypnotic idea that deals with you unconsciously when you have an impulse to eat what you acknowledge that you ought to not. The particular plans used are customized and developed on the very first examination in the commencement of treatment.

When you had the food, the core of post-hypnotic tips is to get you to reroute your attention to how you will feel later on. If the diet produces a lousy feeling once you eat it (and your body currently acknowledges this), your subconscious mind broadcast to your mindful account a message that effectively specifies: "I do not wish to consume this because I do not wish to feel later on."

This mechanical action to decline things or matters that make us feel bad is imprinted into the subconscious, and with the help of hypnosis, we learn to deal with or handle such impulses and yearnings. You will also find out brand-new behavioral routines that become automated with the practice of Self Hypnosis.

The usage of post-hypnotic tips helps to direct both departments of the mind, conscious and subconscious, for individuals with weight reduction issues, to develop a greater motivation for exercises such as exercise and reduce the number of calories they consume daily to attain their aim for weight reduction.

Furthermore, analytical hypnosis might be used to reveal any prospective unconscious, undesirable emotional sensations that you might be squeezing down with food. In some circumstances, people use food as a means to dull underlying psychological harming. This needs to be dealt with and resolved.

The usage of Food is not planned to be an anesthetic

A couple of sessions of hypnosis with a qualified therapist can cause those favorable cognitive procedures. To discover self-hypnosis the proper way, the most efficient thing to do is to have some Person-to-person hypnosis sittings with a qualified, scientific hypnosis professional in his/her office. By using self-hypnosis, you can help yourself along so that you can preserve your weight reduction objectives, correct weight, and your brought back health.

Attempt It At Home

If you can't manage hypnotherapy, or simply aren't comfy working with a hypnotherapist, you can carry out hypnotherapy on your own.

If you're trying to reduce weight through better sleep, write something like, "I will have my teeth brushed and be in bed by 10 p.m. I will choose not to watch TV and go to sleep. I will rest comfortably." If you wish to eat more veggies, compose something like, "I will eat a vegetable with every meal."

"So numerous people are used to multimedia nowadays, music can assist get you in the zone," she includes. Open a voice recorder on your phone and read your affirmations aloud.

When you have your audio recording all set to go, listen to it every day in the early morning and at night when you're preparing yourself for bed. The recording should simply be background noise. You do not need to be actively listening, considering that your mind will play along unconsciously.

After a week or more, the statements you've been listening to will begin to change the chatter in your head and ideally assist you in making healthier decisions with less of a conscious battle.

CHAPTER 9:

How Meditation Works

Meditation is the art of quieting the mind. It's the art of awakening our consciousness. Meditation helps us shift from a consciousness bound by a small ego to a deeper sense of self. We will achieve peace of mind, relaxation, and a positive attitude about ourselves and the world if we meditate properly. When we have a healthy mind and increased self-esteem, the rest of our being will benefit too. We will find better health when we can be comfortable no matter what life throws at us.

"If your meditation is very high and intense, then you must have a quiet conversation with love."-Sri Chinmoy Meditation refers to a state of body relaxation and mental concentration. Many who practice meditation are reporting that they note a change in focus, concentration, attention, and a more optimistic outlook.

Meditation practice is most commonly used as a part of meditation and other metaphysical disciplines. One of the benefits is that you don't need any special equipment or location to do meditation.

The basic concepts of meditation are similar. There are several ways in which it can be performed. The most important, and sometimes the hardest, a part is to relax your mind and avoid following any distracting wandering thoughts. It is the negative thoughts which are polluting the mind. You will find harmony and relaxation in a hectic day by learning to keep them out. Training to keep your mind quiet helps you to concentrate on deeper, more positive thoughts that motivate you to enjoy life more.

When you stomp down life's fatiguing alleys, life always resembles a rat race. Workplace tension, frustration at home, and intense soul fatigue add up to build a peculiar state. Sometimes the busy workers thought they'd handled their lives better if the day had 36 or more hours in it.

Yet, several risks arise from persistent stress and anxiety. Indeed, almost all modern illnesses are somehow connected to a stressful lifestyle. Meditating is the best way to counter fatigue and tiredness. Now meditation will only produce great replenishing results if you do it in the right way. Too many people know meditation's common benefits, but very few know how to meditate. If this is the first time that you intend to engage in any meditation exercises, it is recommended that you meet with a qualified trainer or someone who is experienced in such techniques. Here are a few basics of meditation for beginners to support.

How to Prepare

You need to make some arrangements before meditating. At first, try to secure in the early morning at some time. The explanation for this is that a person is usually in his best mood and health in the morning. You should perform this exercise with an empty stomach. And if you prefer meditation evening, make sure you didn't take any food at least three hours before the session. You are taking a cool shower before meditating is always healthy. This will help you to concentrate better.

The Right Ambience

You need a great ambiance for proper meditation, which is serene and calm. Choose a place to get yourself some solitude. A mild, calming fragrance would be of great help in this. Space light should be dim, and the session should not be disturbed by noise.

Right Posture

Posture is also an essential factor influencing the action. With a sitting position or lying position, you can do it all. Yet the beginners also fall asleep while they are lying on the floor or mattress doing this. Hence beginning with a sitting posture is advisable. The typical method of meditating is to sit cross-beamed on a mat or a flat mattress in a posture called Lotus. But if you have knee pain or other discomforts, consider sitting on a chair that holds the back and neck straight.

Breathing exercises and tips

Few special breathing techniques that are mandatory at the time of the sessions. Deep breathing is one of the most common meditation techniques, where both the process of inhalation and exhalation is long and slow. You should try to focus on thinking about one specific thing. Besides these, there are other strategies that you can get from any book or other tools on "How to Meditate."

Meditation is the best way to calm your mind and rejuvenate the damage to your soul as well. Practice it daily and track the results over a short period.

Below are a few tips to help you learn to practice the art of meditation.

- **Bring some comfortable clothing on first**. Close-fitting trousers and tight clothes are likely to be something of a nuisance. Find something to wear that lets you relax without having to worry about being pinched or pulled.

- **You can then play some good and calming instrumental music**. If you listen to music with lyrics when you are meditating, you are likely to start singing along in your ear, which will not help you concentrate. To help them concentrate, some people think it helps to have a candle or other item to look at. Many tend to close their eyes to help avoid anything that might disrupt their mental comfort.

- **Sit in a snug spot**. Putting a pillow under your bottom could help you sit up straight and balanced. When you think you can stay awake during your meditation period, you can always lie in bed or on the couch. What is crucial is that the place helps you to relax as you concentrate.

- **The position or location may also be helpful**. Select a place that is free from disturbance inside your home. A place where temperature and appearance are both relaxed and friendly. Some decorate a specific part of a room only for meditation purposes.

- **Switch your mobile phone off the Screen and the ringer**. You may want to set the timer on your phone, so you'll know when it's time to stop without having to check every minute to see how long it has been. If this is a new activity for you, simply schedule it for 5 minutes and start developing your meditation skills. As you develop your ability to concentrate and quiet your mind, you can extend your meditation practice.

Now that you are ready, what are you going to do?

- **There are two rising meditation methods**. One focuses on the air, during mindfulness instruction, that is also a technique taught. You just focus on the air as you inhale through your nose and softly exhale through your mouth. Reflect on the wind feels when it gets into the body. See it as it moves through your lungs, giving life to your mind, and then see it as it leaves your body.

Any time an outside thought comes into your mind, accept it but don't act on it, just return your attention to your breath for the time that you set it. The other common approach is to imagine a healing beam of light that hits your eyes, bringing to your mind and body a wave of relaxation and peace. Let it search gently across your body, starting at your head and slowly going all the way to the tips of your toes. When you feel any stress or discomfort, just imagine the soothing beam the dissolves discomfort and stress in your body.

- **There is no downside to meditation practice**. No physical exertion or special equipment is required. If you have any mobility problems, just sit in a chair, providing you with the support you need to feel secure and relaxed.

Meditation has been shown to relieve tension and to be helpful in many ways, such as changing a person's outlook on life. It is easy to do, and yet difficult because, at the same time, you are learning to relax and control your thoughts. Take 5 minutes a day and do a week or two of meditation practice. You can do it for free, and the benefits you get will significantly improve your life!

CHAPTER 10:

How the Mind Works

We are, on the whole, going far and wide with a significant debilitation on our hands. Also, what his impairment is, is that we are not utilizing the full power of the mind to further our potential benefit. What you must know is that at present, as you are perusing this article, all you are doing is maybe utilizing about 15% of the power of your mind. Even at ideal yield, you are just utilizing about 40% of the mind to the best of your bit of leeway.

You have to realize that science and medication have been around for quite a while, they, despite everything, have no clue what is going inside the mind. Without a doubt, they can distinguish which projection goes where, yet they don't have a clue what is happening inside. For the majority of the brain, they are making what is referred to in the network as taught estimates, and this is something that you ought to be distinctly mindful of. You ought to likewise be distinctly mindful of the way that there is something many refer to as the self-awareness industry, and this has been around for quite a while.

They also have been attempting to open the privileged insights of the mind, since they solidly have confidence in the way that the mind is the most important thing in the world of the human framework. With the power of the mind readily available, you would have the option to have full command over your body, your feelings, and you can likewise clean yourself of any interruptions and wrongs inside your body. Presently how this is done is to open the power of the mind and use innovation to improve certain segments of it. There are sure ventures on the planet that have been investigating this. For one, there is the subconscious business, which is investigating super recurrence incitement to influence the subconscious, the most powerful part of the human mind.

At that point, there is the brainwave entrainment industry, which is utilizing figured out sounds to influence a recurrence following impact in the brain, and what they are doing is to expand the brain utilizing its electromagnetic waves that the neurons inside the cortex are creating every day. We can likewise look to increasingly progress restorative and logical techniques for the Dream Machine, autogenic, bio criticism, and the utilization of attractive acceptance.

These are on the whole techniques that are being utilized to open the power of the mind and give the human species a bit of leeway in the futile way of life that is the present reality. In this way, you ought to be intrigued because there is great progress being made into opening the insider facts of the mind. A portion of this innovation is as of now accessible online for your utilization, and you can give them a shot at no hazard to you. These are attempted and demonstrated ways that you can expand and tune the mind to do what you need it to do.

Kinds of Mind Control

Mind control has been around for a long time now. Individuals have had both interest and fear of what might occur if somebody were ready to control their minds and cause them to get things done without wanting to. Paranoid ideas proliferate about government authorities and others of power utilizing their abilities to control what little gatherings of individuals are doing.

Indeed, even some legal disputes have been raised utilizing the reason of brainwashing as a clarification for why they carried out the wrongdoing they are blamed for.Despite the sensation of mind control that has been depicted in the media and the motion pictures, there is little that is thought about the various kinds of mind control and how every one of them works. This section will investigate a smidgen about the most well-kinds of mind control as a prologue to clarifying increasingly about this fascinating theme.

While there are various sorts of mind control that can be utilized to control the planned casualty, there are five that are most normally thought of. These incorporate brainwashing, hypnosis, manipulation, persuasion, and deception. These will all be examined underneath.

Brainwashing

Brainwashing is the main kind of mind control to talk about. Brainwashing is essentially the procedure where somebody will be plotted to abandon convictions that they had in the past to take new standards and qualities. There are ways this should be possible, even though not every one of them will be viewed as awful. For instance, if you are from an African nation and, at that point, move to America, you will frequently be compelled to change your qualities and beliefs to fit in with the new culture and environmental factors that you are in. Then again, those in death camps or when another tyrant government is assuming control over, they will frequently experience the way toward brainwashing to persuade residents to track with calmly.

Numerous individuals have misconceptions of what brainwashing is. A few people have progressively suspicious thoughts regarding the work on including mind control gadgets that are supported by the legislature and that are believed to be handily turned on like a remote control. On the opposite side of things, some cynics don't accept that brainwashing is conceivable at all and that any individual who claims it has happened is lying. Generally, the act of brainwashing will land someplace in these two thoughts.

During the act of brainwashing, the subject will be persuaded to change their convictions about something through a mix of various strategies. There isn't only one methodology that can be utilized during this procedure, so it very well may be hard to place the training into a flawless little box. Generally, the subject will be isolated from everything that they know. From that point, they will be separated into an emotional expression that makes them defenseless before the new ideas are presented. As the subject retains this new data, they will be rewarded for communicating thoughts and considerations which oblige these new thoughts. The compensating is the thing that will be utilized to fortify the brainwashing that is happening.

Brainwashing isn't new to the society. Individuals have been utilizing these methods for quite a while. For instance, in an authentic setting, the individuals who were detainees of wars were regularly separated before being convinced to change sides. Probably the best instances of these would bring about the detainee turning into an exceptionally intense believer to the new side. These practices were new in the first place and would frequently be upheld, relying upon who was in control. After some time, the term brainwashing was created, and some more methods were acquainted, all together with making the training increasingly all-inclusive. The more up to date methods would depend on the field of brain science since huge numbers of those thoughts were utilized to exhibit how individuals may alter their perspectives through persuasion.

Numerous means accompany the brainwashing procedure. It isn't something that is going to simply transpire when you stroll the road and converse with somebody that you have recently met. Most importantly, one of the primary necessities that accompanies brainwashing being fruitful is that the subject must be kept in confinement. If the subject can be around others and impacts, they will figure out how to think as an individual, and the brainwashing won't be compelling by any means.

When the subject is in segregation, they will experience a procedure that is intended to separate themself. They are informed that all the things they know are bogus and are caused to feel like all that they do isn't right. Following quite a while of experiencing the entirety of this, the subject will feel like they are awful, and the blame will overpower them. When they have arrived at this point, the operator will begin to lead them towards the new conviction framework and personality that is wanted. The subject will be persuaded that the new decisions are, for the most part, they're thus, it is bound to stick.

The entire procedure of brainwashing can take numerous months to even years. It isn't something that will occur in only a discussion, and generally, it won't have the option to occur outside of jail camps and a couple of secluded cases. It will broadly expound on what happens during the three primary phases of brainwashing and how the entire procedure happens.

Generally, the individuals who experience brainwashing have done so when somebody is simply attempting to convince them of another perspective. For instance, if you are in contention with a companion and they persuade you that their thoughts bode well, you have experienced brainwashing. Without a doubt, it probably won't be abhorrent, and you had the option to consider everything intelligently, except you were as yet persuaded to change the convictions that you held previously. It is extremely uncommon that somebody experiences genuine brainwashing where they will have their entire worth framework supplanted. It will ordinarily happen during the way toward coming around to another perspective, whether or not the strategies utilized were persuasive or not.

Hypnosis

The following kind of mind control that is notable is hypnosis. There are a variety of meanings of what hypnosis is. As indicated by the American Psychological Association, hypnosis is a helpful communication where the trance specialist will give proposals that the member will react to. Numerous individuals have gotten comfortable with the methods of hypnosis on account of famous exhibitions where members are advised to do crazy or irregular assignments. Another type of hypnosis that is picking up in fame is benevolent that utilizes this training for its helpful and health advantages, particularly with regards to the decrease of tension and torment.

On certain occasions, hypnosis has had the option to diminish dementia indications in a couple of patients. As should be obvious, there are a variety of reasons that hypnosis can be utilized. Where it begins to become mind control is the point at which the trance specialist can suggest recommendations that can be destructive or change the way that the member demonstrations in their environmental factors.

For a great many people, when they catch wind of hypnosis, they consider an individual in front of an audience who is swinging a watch to and fro to place the member in a daze. If you have been to a phase appear for diversion, you may have a few pictures in your mind of the absurd demonstrations that the members performed. As a general rule, the individuals who are experiencing what is viewed as genuine hypnosis are experiencing a procedure that is different from this picture. This implies the subliminal specialist attempts to get the member into a modified perspective, so they are increasingly open to recommendations that are given.

CHAPTER 11:

The Hypnotic Method Of 21 Days with Daily Statements

The 21-day entrancing technique with day by day certifications

Would you like to free your life of uneasiness, show your fantasy list, and praise the energy surrounding you? In case you're not kidding about utilizing the Law of Attraction, one of the best approaches to supercharge your inspiration and center your essentialness is to follow a 21-day challenge plan! You can use this methodology with any objective, regardless of whether little or extraordinary. Its motivation is to give you honed center and upgrade your capacity to show anything you desire.

Keep perusing to find your free printable sheet and manual for the 21-day challenge just as point by point clarifications of the specific activities and strategies to utilize every day.

Day 1: Clear Your Mind

Go through this day discreetly, doing fundamental breathing activities, and purposely relinquishing any burdens that may have been keeping you down of late. You need a fresh start to draw in energizing new things. Here is a straightforward breathing activity to kick you off today.

- Take a deep breath in through the nose. Fill your lungs and feel your stomach grow. Hold this for 4 seconds.

- Discharge the breath through your mouth, similar to you is letting out a significant moan.

- You're completely done! Rehash as regularly as you have to.

Day 2: Make Space in the Life

Look at your living spaces and clean up things that help you to remember negative considerations or bind you also firmly to the past (for instance, protests that help you to recall past connections). Encircle yourself with things you partner with good faith, development, and enthusiasm. These aides may likewise help you while doing a 'spring clean' of your home.

- Instructions to Declutter Your Home: 9 Questions To Ask Yourself When Tidying

- Instructions to Improve Your Bedroom For MAX Energy Level

- 150+ Things To Throw Away Today

Day 3: Explore Your Goal

Consider what you trust you need. Presently ask yourself these inquiries...

- For what reason do you need it?

- Do you need it?

- When thinking about your objective, envision it showing in various ways until you get a feeling of the particular purpose you're genuinely taking a stab at.

Day 4: Put Your Goal into the Words

Investigation with methods of stating what you need to show.

Change the words around until you simply realize you've found the correct ones. Record them and put them up someplace you can see.

One helpful method is to put them by or on your restroom reflect!

Day 5: Make a Step-by-Step Plan

Note down each progression you'll have to take to meet your definitive objective.

This assists with guaranteeing you're progressing in the direction of something achievable and makes each stage concrete and genuine in your brain.

Day 6: Create a Dream Board

This engaging activity just expects you to pick magazine patterns, photos, and words that best speak to the thing you need to pull in and join them such that you find moving. Be as imaginative as you like!

For instance, if you are attempting to show your perfect partner, you may cover your fantasy board in pictures of sound connections, you know. You could likewise include statements of what you are searching for in an accomplice. You can utilize physical arrangement for this, for example, using photos and patterns as portrayed above or utilize online assets. Numerous individuals like to utilize locales like Pinterest as a type of fantasy board. Get more motivation for your fantasy board today with your free dream board toolbox!

Day 7: Pick a Manifestation Song

Discover a tune that catches all the sentiments you partner with your fantasy. For instance, you may pick a triumphant song of praise in case you're moving in the direction of a vocation or wellness objective, and a fantastic melody in case you're searching for adoration. Play it, move to it, sing it, and associate with it.

Day 8: Basic Visualization

Put aside, in any event, ten minutes in a tranquil spot where you won't be upset and focus on building a maximally striking picture of the thing you need. Here are the absolute most helpful hints for improving your perception procedures:

Envision not just the sight and sentiment of the thing you need to show yet, besides the various faculties. Picture the scents, sounds, and sensations as well.

The utilization of reflection or hypnotherapy can likewise help dig further into your representation by shutting out interruptions and expanding your core interest. You can likewise utilize craftsmanship, composing, and music for perception! Draw, paint, or write your vision. Centerfold girl your work in a generally noticeable region, so you are helped to remember it regularly. Submerge yourself in this procedure, permitting yourself to feel it as if it's going on. It before long will be!

Day 9: Design Your Affirmations

Utilize the expression (or expressions) from day four to assemble attestations that fortify your conviction that you can draw in what you need. Let's assume them into the mirror, grin, and let them resound. You'll likely get the best outcomes on the off chance that you state them consistently. For instance, attempt a portion of the accompanying positive every day certifications:

- "I acknowledge my capacity."

- "All aspects of my life are copious and filling."

- "Each experience I have is ideal for my development."

- "I merit adoring. There is love surrounding me."

- Make sure to get a definitive assertion to manage in your one of a kind LOA toolbox!

Day 10: Write About Your Dream

Let your psyche meander unfiltered and record as much as possible about your fantasy. For instance,

- What it resembles.

- Why you need it.

- How it'll be to live it.

- Try not to blue pencil yourself by any stretch of the imagination, regardless of whether you get negative musings or emotions sneaking in.

Day 11: Uncover Negative Thinking Patterns

Check whether you can spot regions where constraining convictions and suspicions may hold you down and gaze them in the face. It is astounding what the number of our contemplations is subliminally negative! Take a stab at asking yourself the accompanying inquiries...

- Which are your uncertainties and tensions?

- How 'reasonable' are your presumptions?

What messages did you get when you were youthful that may lead you to figure you can't show your wants? At the point when you figure out how to respond to these inquiries, you can begin to reveal why you have explicit reasoning examples you do and how to recognize and battle whenever you get yourself on edge.

Day 12: Challenge Negative Thinking Patterns

For each constraining conviction you found in the past exercise, record a clarification of why you hold it. At that point, compose another, positive reasoning that you need to use to supplant the negative old one. You can utilize these to structure new attestations or simply look at the definite rundown once every day.

Day 13: Take Stock of the Value you have

Days 11 and 12 can be hard, so go through day 13 on self-care and consider things that support your confidence. On the off chance that it helps, take a stab at checking ten things you love and incentive about yourself. You have the right to have all that you need!

Day 14: Connect With an Object

Discover something that speaks to your objective, for example, a stone, a bit of gem, or an adornment. Practice a perception while holding the article; at that point, ensure that the thing remains with you for the rest of the 21 days. It will ground you and help you to remember your latent capacity. Additionally, consider examining the various advantages of gem recuperating. A scope of different gems and stones can help center the Law Of Attraction work and lift your appearance power.

Day 15: Multi-Perspective Visualization

Add another layer to your perceptions by envisioning your fantasy from an outsider point of view. Notice new subtleties, develop a much increasingly amazing and energizing picture of what you'll accomplish.

Day 16: Start a Gratitude Journal

Record 3-5 things that cause you to feel appreciative every day or every week, contingent upon your way of life.

The reason for this errand is to fill you with vigorous positive imperativeness that causes you to vibrate at a high recurrence and improves your capacity to draw in progressively positive things to you.

On the off chance that this is hard, make sure to consider what you underestimate every day.

Things may not stand apart as something to be thankful for, yet envision your existence without specific things.

Day 17: Revisit Your Plan

Come back to the arrangement you made on day five and consider where you are. Does anything have to change? Alter as vital and be satisfied with the means you've taken.

Day 18: Look for Signs

The Universe regularly conveys signs to direct you towards the things you need; however, to see those signs, you have to get to your instinct. Today, keep your eyes stripped for rehashing expressions, incidents, or shock solicitations. These sorts of things may help you on your way. (P.S. Make sure to likewise pay a one of a kind psyche to these seven great karma signs and otherworldly change manifestations!)

Day 19: Give Love

Commit the day to consideration, empathy, and liberality, causing companions and outsiders the same to feel great. This, similar to your appreciation diary, encourages you to vibrate on a recurrence of wealth as opposed to one of need, placing you in the perfect space to show what you need. Here are only several thoughts of interesting points doing today just as instructional exercises to assist you with accomplishing the immediate objective:

- 20 Actions Of Kindness That You Can Do For Loved One's Today

- Step by step instructions to Be Kind To Yourself

- 10 Exercises You Should Try For Increased Happiness

- Step by step instructions to Help Someone With Depression And Anxiety

Day 20: Live "As though"

Plan like you will have an accomplice, investigate excursions like you'll have the cash to pay for them, or buy garments like you'll fit into them how you need. This limits the vibrational hole among you and the thing you need.

Day 21: Release What You desire

At last, you have to figure out how to consider them to be in life all things considered and acknowledge that the Universe will send what you need precisely when you need it. Put stock in your capacity to show, yet discharge your longing and have a sense of security in the information you can and will have the life of your dream.

CHAPTER 12:

The Program
(30 days Meditation and Hypnosis)

Visualizing your path through meditation

While meditation can be undertaken just about anywhere at just about any given time, there are certain guidelines that you need to follow if you want your meditation to be as effective as possible. However, keep in mind that meditation is meant to be flexible.

The idea is not to create a rigid system that you will find difficult to follow. Meditation is meant to be easy and adaptable to adjust it to meet your specific needs.

Attuning to Physical Sensations

The physical world around you impacts your mind. This is a fact that we are all aware of.

What we don't necessarily notice is that just as the physical world impacts our mind, our mind, in turn, also impacts our physical form. In the world of meditation, this form of comprehensive understanding is referred to as body sensing.

Think of the last time you were happy. In addition to feeling mentally excited, how did you feel on a physical level? Were you in pain? Did you find it difficult to move? Or did you feel uneasy for some reason?

Odds are you didn't feel any of this — why? When you are happy and relaxed, you don't feel physically unwell. You tend to feel lighter and more physically relaxed. At the same time, the exact opposite happens when you are dealing with some sort of emotional upset. You might feel nauseous or uneasy when you're freaking out before a major exam, for example. Or maybe you tend to feel lethargic when you are depressed or dealing with huge amounts of mental stress. Your body is a reflection of your mind. If you feel happy, your body is also happier, and you are more at peace. Whereas, when you are distressed, your physical form tends to manifest in a way that reflects that negativity.

When you decided on your essentials, you made a list of what was non-negotiable for you. That list contains the most important things in your life, your bottom line. You also made the conscious decision to let go of emotional baggage and mind clutter that no longer serves you. In doing that, you eliminated stress. We can now work on removing it from other areas.

Stress comes from the mental and emotional strain caused by unfavorable or challenging circumstances. Sometimes a little stress can be good for us. It can push us to try harder or improve upon ourselves. When we are attempting to live a more mindful life, stress is not in the equation. Eliminating as much stress as we can is detrimental to our health and well-being and must be done to live mindfully. Now is the time to make yourself and your stress level a priority to keep this journey less complicated. Nothing can be done thoroughly and efficiently under stress, and making others aware of your intentions is one way of bringing down your stress level.

Sometimes, your friends and family are a source of stress for you simply by being in your life, because their stress can become your own. You have to decide that you will not let their troubles become a source of agitation for you. It is possible to be comforting and understanding without taking on other people's problems. If you are eliminating stress, the first worries to go need to be those of others.

You are not able to change their circumstances by feeling the emotional strain. It has never worked, and it never will. So let the stress of others go. When you are approached with another person's stressful situation, take the time to acknowledge what they are sharing with you, and let them know that their feelings are important. If a way to eliminate their stress comes to mind, share it with them, if you like.

Let them know that you hope the best for the matter, and treat them with kindness. If you find that their troubles come back to your thoughts, recognize that this is simply you feeling empathy, and let them know that they are on your mind. Maybe you can even ask how things are, and if they have resolved the matter.

Keep yourself from actually feeling the stress, because it could help them more in the long run, anyway. Your mind, free from stress, works more efficiently, and with all of the decluttering you have been doing, perhaps you will come up with a viable solution to their problem. Eliminating stress has a ripple effect, just like a lot of the other things you have learned thus far.

Now we are back to self. One of the most prevalent causes of stress in human beings is finances. Some would say money is the root of all evil. I say it is the bane of peace, but only if you allow it to be. Take most of the stress surrounding finances out of the equation by making everything you can automatic. We live in an amazingly effortless time where automated systems and paperless billing are commonplace. Wherever you are financially right now is what you are working with, so just make as many of these financial responsibilities as little as part of your everyday life as possible. Work with your financial institution and others to set up all that you can to be automatically deposited, paid, withdrawn, and recorded. Designate one day a week to check into things to be sure they are in good working order but don't keep this plan in your daily thoughts. Write the weekly financial check down on your schedule like you have learned so that you truly remove this part of the stress of finances from your thoughts until it's time to address them. Getting your finances in order and putting the responsibilities associated with them in a safe place to be revisited takes the thinking out of it for the most part, and gets rid of that portion of stress.

Another source of stress is the everyday, mundane tasks that do not deserve the amount of significance they get. Back to the idea of auto-pilot, what other routine things can be put in that mode? Ask yourself how you can eliminate stress for each part of your day simply by taking the guesswork and over-thinking away. How does your day begin? What can you put on auto-pilot?

As you prepare yourself to practice meditation, one of the things you are going to want to ensure is that you are working on your ability to understand what your body is saying to you. The easiest way to do this is by practicing body sensing. Body sensing not only allows you to control your central nervous system and allow your mind to achieve a deeper form of mental and physical relaxation, but it is also known to boost your body's natural resilience. This work will help develop your ability to experience a more solid and constant sense of wholeness and well-being, in a manner unattached to your external obstacles.

Emotional Focus

As you prepare to embark on your meditative journey, another factor that you are going to need to look into is Emotional self-focus. One of the core objectives of meditation is to promote self-care. Meditation itself is known to have extremely therapeutic properties. Emotion-focused therapy is a short-term psychotherapy approach that is commonly included in most meditative guides. The logic applied here is simple - emotion-focused meditations are meant to identify and cull the innate emotions the participant has. This form of the elimination of a specific emotion may be problematic to a person's growth and development, since eliminating a specific emotion in its entirety can cause people to developmental blocks.

Research has shown that emotion-focused therapy helped participants identify with themself, which in turn allowed them to better manage their emotional experiences. Mental health issues such as depression, complex trauma, etc. have shown improvement when associated with emotion-focused meditations, which is why it has been used specifically to help individuals with the internalized stigma of sexual orientation, for example.

As you practice using the provided meditative guides, you must focus on trying to attain a specific goal during the meditative process. This ensures that you are focusing on self-care and self-awareness. As you grow up, you will find that it is much easier to focus on the needs of other people rather than those of your own. However, even though this is commonplace, simply put, it is not right. Remembering your own needs and feelings is just as important as tending to those of others. Furthermore, it is equally important that you ensure that your self-sacrificing mindset doesn't lead to you suppressing your own emotional needs and depriving yourself of the help that you require.

Meditation can only help you once you have begun to consciously focus on your wants and needs. Keep in mind that the goal you set for yourself is an important part of your meditation. By using your meditative goals and manifesting empathy, you can attune yourself to the needs of others. But this ability can only truly manifest when you have come to terms with your own needs and have accepted yourself for who you are. Once you start to take care of yourself better, you'll be better equipped to take care of others as well.

You deserve to be happy and are a good person. These are the thoughts that you need to live by.

Identifying and Dealing with Bodily Pain

Another important factor in preparing for a meditative lifestyle is clarity in terms of what you are working towards. Let's say, for instance, you are working toward dealing with physical pain. You are going to need to know specifically what kind of pain you are trying to deal with. Understanding the basis and depth of your pain will help you choose which meditative guides are going to be most effective for you.

When it comes to dealing with bodily pain, you must make it a point to understand which pain management technique would be best suited for your ailment. Body-scanning allows an individual to mentally "x-ray" their body, identify their points of pain and then address or heal them as they go.

Another important form of pain management meditation is the mindful-movement technique. This technique teaches individuals to use mindful-movements, such as standing in a specific posture and then proceeding to go through a list of physical actions, including rotating your hands and shoulders, stretching your arms, and breathing in and out at specific intervals. This type of focused breathing is another common pain management technique that can assist individuals with relaxation issues and chronic pain.

CHAPTER 13:

Day 1 Guided Meditation –
A Visualization of a New You

Before you can begin using mind exercises and meditations to do things such as help you burn fat, you need to make sure that you set yourself up properly for your meditation sessions. Each meditation will consist of you entering a deep state of relaxation, following guided hypnosis, and then awakening yourself out of this state of relaxation. If done properly, you will find yourself experiencing the stages of changed mindset and changed behavior that follows the session.

These exercises will involve a visualization practice; however, if you find that visualization is generally difficult for you, you can simply listen. The key here is to ensure that you keep as open of a mind as possible so that you can stay receptive to the information coming through these guided meditations.

- **Relaxation sequence** – imagine yourself relaxing each part of your body in turn until you are in a fully relaxed, comfortable state

- **Visualization** - Imagine waking up in the morning of your future, getting out of bed, how does your body feel, imagine each part of your body feeling how you want it to be

Imagine yourself getting dressed, what kind of clothes are you wearing, do you look at yourself in the mirror, what do you see?

Imagine yourself going through your daily routine, eating healthily, getting up, how do you behave to other people, how do they treat you.

Imagine yourself reaching the end of your 'future' day.

Start by gently closing your eyes and drawing your attention to your breath. As you do, I want you to track the next five breaths, gently and intentionally lengthening them to help you relax as deeply as you can. With each breath, breathe in to the count of five and out to the count of seven. Starting with your next breath in, Count 1-10.

Start repeatedly counting from 1-5. Do this three times, while inhaling and exhaling.

Now that you are starting to feel relaxed, I want you to draw your awareness into your body. First, become aware of your feet. Feel your feet relaxing deeply, as you visualize any stress or worry melting away from your feet. Now become aware of your legs. Feel any stress or worry melting away from your legs as they begin to relax completely. Next, become aware of your glutes and pelvis, allowing any stress or worry to fade away as they completely relax simply. Now become aware of your entire torso, allowing any stress or worry to melt away from your torso as it relaxes completely. Next, become aware of your shoulders, arms, hands, and fingers. Allow the stress and worry to melt away from your shoulders, arms, hands, and fingers as they relax completely. Now, let the stress and worry melt away from your neck, head, and face. Feel your neck, head, and face relaxing as any stress or worry melts away completely.

As you deepen into this state of relaxation, I want you to take a moment to visualize the space in front of you. Imagine that in front of you, you are standing there looking back at yourself. See every inch of your body as it is right now standing before you, casually, as you simply observe yourself. While you do, see what parts of your body you want to reduce fat so that you can create a healthier, stronger body for yourself. Visualize the fat in these areas of your body, slowly fading away as you begin to carve out a healthier, leaner, and stronger body underneath. Notice how effortlessly this extra fat melts away as you continue to visualize yourself becoming a healthier and more vibrant version of yourself.

Now, I want you to visualize what this healthier, leaner version of yourself would be doing. Visualize yourself going through your typical daily routine, except the perspective of your healthier self. What would you be eating? When and how would you be exercising? What would you spend your time doing? How do you feel about yourself? How different do you feel when you interact with the people around you, such as your family and your co-workers? What does life feel like when you are a healthier, leaner version of you?

Spend several minutes visualizing how different your life is now that your fat has melted away. Feel how natural it is for you to enjoy these healthier foods, and how easy it is to moderate your cravings and indulgences when you choose to treat yourself.

Notice how easy it is for you to engage in exercise and how exercise feels enjoyable and like a wonderful hobby, rather than a chore that you must force yourself to commit to every day.

Feel yourself genuinely enjoying life far more, all because the unhealthy fats that weigh you down and disrupt your health have faded away. Notice how easy it was for you to get here, and how easy it is for you to continue to maintain your health and wellness as you continue to choose better and better choices for you and your body.

Feel how much you respect your body when you make these healthier choices, and how much you genuinely care about yourself. Notice how each meal and exercise feels like an act of self-care, rather than a chore you are forcing yourself to engage in. For your wellbeing.

When you are ready, take that visualization of yourself and send the image out far, watching it become nothing more than a spec in your field of awareness.

Then, send it out into the ether, trusting that your subconscious mind will hold on to this vision of yourself and work daily on bringing this version of you into your current reality.

Now, awaken back into your body where you sit right now. Feel yourself feeling more motivated, more energized, and more excited about engaging in the activities that will improve your health and help you burn your fat. As you prepare to go about your day, hold on to that visualization and those feelings that you had of yourself, and trust that you can have this wonderful experience in your life. You can do it!

Daily Weight Loss Motivation with Mini Habits

Once you have set your plans, written your affirmations, chosen your mantras, begun to practice all the meditation and mindfulness techniques you have learned, what is next? Like anything that you have invested in, it is important to perform maintenance. Being able to reach and stay at your goal weight is only part of the picture because what you are working on is a total lifestyle change. You want your habits and your decision-making to match the life you want to be living. Let us recap the methods you have learned and show you how to apply them to the future of your new self.

Making Habits Count

We spent a lot of time thinking about the importance of habits. It can be hard to see the behavioral patterns in our lives until we try to change them. By making a conscious decision to take something that is not conducive to weight loss and replacing it with a habit, you have already taken a step towards improvement. It is said that no one can change unless they want to change, and that is very true.

Habits are the key that can tie all of your other efforts together. You can make a habit of reading your affirmations and reciting your mantras. You can replace a television or video game habit with exercise and meditation. You can break the habit of eating convenience foods by mindfully making a shopping list. Everything we have talked about in this entire book can be tied back into making, breaking, or replacing a habit.

Positive Words for a Positive Outcome

Here is just one last reminder to think positive! We talked a lot about the power of positivity and how it can impact everything you do. Words do have a tremendous amount of power, which is why mantras can be so vital to reaching a weight loss goal.

When you learn to apply mantras to your goals, you are assigning power to positive words, and when you shun the negativity of others, you are taking power away from their words. Do not let your life be a power struggle. Use strong, upbeat words to describe yourself. Be sure that if a sentence contains both negative and positive statements, that you phrase your words to frame and emphasize the positive component.

It can be difficult to change your mindset, and it will take work. But do not get discouraged and do not allow negativity to rent any space in your brain. Every day is a new day to wake up and commit to positivity. Think carefully about your words and mind, how you speak to and about yourself.

By making a conscious effort to be positive, you will have a great day and another, until being positive becomes your new way of life.

Taking Time for Meditation and Mindfulness

You may be wondering how you will make time for all this positivity, habit formation, and affirmation reading. Now we are going to add meditation and mindfulness to the mix. We do only have so many hours in the day, but all these elements are so crucial to reaching your goals. So how can you do it? How do you find the time to stick to your plan?

The answer is, you make time. When you commit to change yourself, there will be sacrifices. You can try getting up a half-hour early or carving out time after work.

If you have a support system around you, ask someone to watch your kids while you go to the gym or take them off the school bus to have a few extra minutes to yourself in the afternoon. Where there is a will- and you have the will- there is always a way.

You can combine your affirmation and meditation time into your wake up and bedtime routines—practice mindfulness in the shower. Recite mantras during your grocery shop.

You can, and you will find the time. Yes, things like yoga and visualization can be a little time consuming, but the more you practice all your techniques, the more efficient you will become. Be creative about how you spend your time. If you need to make yourself a loose schedule of when you are going to practice your self-hypnosis methods, it will help you stay on track.

Tying It All Together

You have probably decided what methods you would like to use to aid you on your weight-loss journey. Any of the techniques outlined in this book will be useful tools for you as you move forward. But what happens once you reached your initial goal? You do not want to slip back into your bad habits or let go of the positivity you have injected into your life.

CHAPTER 14:

Day 2 Prepare Meditations

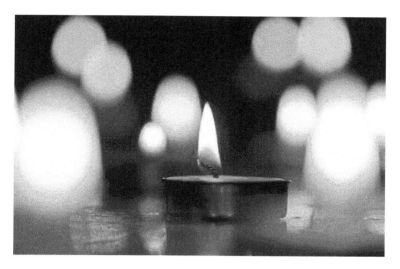

Program: From your 'future self' notes, write meditations that start with "I am…" "I enjoy…" "I feel…" and then "for this/these reasons I choose to only eat healthy food." Write as many as you like on sticky notes or paper, and stick them on to a board or somewhere visible.

Write them down on a piece of paper or have notes with them on them that you leave throughout your house. Remember to practice your breathing exercises that we have learned through the other mindset exercises and keep an open mind as always.

- Losing weight is more than just looking good to me. I understand that I need to live a healthy lifestyle to feel better all of the time.

- I know how to lose weight, and actually, I choose to do this naturally because it helps me be healthier.

- I know exactly what I need to do to get the things I deserve from this life.

- I am capable of reaching all of the goals that I set for myself, and I am the one who decides what I do next with my life.

- I recognize that it's important for me to be patient throughout this process.

- I can wait for the results because I know that I will get everything that I want in the end.

- I do not punish myself because I don't achieve a goal as fast as I had originally hoped.

- I nourish myself throughout this process.

- I constantly look for ways to encourage myself and build my self-esteem because I know that is what is going to help me feel the best in the end.

- I can control my impulses.

- I know how not to act on my greatest urges.

- I recognize the methods that will help me to enable myself to work harder in the end.

- I am happy because I know how to say no.

- I can turn away when I'm confronted with an impulse.

- I am stronger than the biggest cravings that I have.

- I am proud of my ability to have a high level of willpower.

- I trust myself around certain foods and recognize that what tempts me does not control me.

- I look at the things that I already have in my life instead of only paying attention to things that I don't have.

- This is the way that will help me better achieve everything that I desire.

- I do not allow distractions to keep me from getting the things that I want.

- I can stay focused on my goals so that I can create the life that I deserve. In the end, even when I am tempted by something or somebody else, I know how to push through this urge and instead focus on my goals.

- I will wait for everything. Love is coming to me because I know that, when it does, I will feel entirely fulfilled.

- I am enjoying the journey and the process that it takes to get the body that I want.

- I recognize that small milestones are worth celebrating.

- I do not wait for one big goal to be reached to be happy with myself.

- I look for all the methods needed to achieve greatness in this life.

- I understand that a temporary desire to eat something unhealthy is not worth giving up all of my goals.

- I know how to distract myself from my biggest cravings so that I can do something healthy instead.

- I recognize that doing something small is better than doing nothing at all. Even on the days that I don't want to go to the gym, I do something at home to work out so that I can at least accomplish something minor.

- Just getting started is the hardest part for me, but I know how to work through those feelings now.

- I am emotionally aware of what might be holding me back so that I don't allow myself to be tempted by distractions.

- I control my feelings and my urges so that I don't do anything that I regret.

- I am happy because I am knowledgeable about the things that make me who I am.

- I forgive myself when I do act on an impulse.

- I don't punish myself or deprive my body of the basic things that it needs just because I did something wrong.

- I sacrifice certain things that I want, but never to a point where I cause punishment or torture on myself.

- I am successful because I am dedicated.

- I have strong willpower because I am successful.

- I move through my life with gratitude and always look to appreciate the things that I have around me.

- I can pick myself up when I'm feeling weak.

- I am appreciative of even the hard parts of my life because they create the person that I am.

- I am an important and powerful person.

- I have control over my body, and nobody else does.

- I recognize my weaknesses, but in the same breath, I am very aware of my strengths.

- I balance my life with these things.

- I empower my strengths and thrive when I am in an environment that helps me grow.

- I recognize my weaknesses, and I always look for ways to turn them around to live more happily and healthily after.

- I cook meals for myself because it makes me feel healthier and stronger in the end.

- I am going to get the dream body that I want because I can recognize things that might be healthy or unhealthy for me.

- I move my body at least once a day.

- I always feel better after I agree to a workout rather than if I try to avoid one.

- I can give myself rest when I need it. I don't push myself when I'm too stressed out because I know that this isn't going to help me get the things that I want.

- I can always find motivation and passion within myself.

- I set my own goals, and I set newer and bigger ones after I achieved ones that I already completed.

- I do not procrastinate with my goals. I know exactly what I have to do every single day to reach these goals, and I always look for ways to go above and beyond as well.

- I am constantly improving the methods that I use to live a healthy lifestyle.

- I self-reflect productively so that I can find real solutions to any issues that I might face.

- I don't let what other people think to take over how I see myself.

- I am not afraid of judgment from other people because I know that not everything negative that somebody thinks about me is true.

- I make the right decision for my body.

- I understand that even if I make wrong decisions, sometimes they all play a vital role in making me the person that I am today. These struggles are something that I had to undergo to become the powerful individual that I am.

- I am constantly losing weight because of all this dedication and passion.

- I feel lighter, happier, and healthier.

- I am free.

- I am pure and clean.

- I am collected and calm.

- I am peaceful, and I am happy.

- I heal myself through my weight loss.

- I take everything bad that I did to my body in the past and turn it into something good, as I exercise and make healthy choices. I'm focused on pushing through my biggest setbacks to achieve the things that I deserve.

- I do not sit around and fantasize about what I want anymore. Instead, I know exactly how to get this.

- I believe in myself because I know that this is going to be the most important part of my journey.

- I trust my ability to lose weight, and I'm not afraid of what will happen if I don't.

- I know how to say these affirmations to myself when I feel better.

- Other people like being around me. Others recognize my hard work. Others know that I deserve to have good things in my life. When I listened to my body, I can thrive. I recognize the things that my body tells me to get the best results possible.

- I feel good, and I look even better.

- I look great, and I look incredible because of this. Not only does losing weight help my body to look better, but it also helps my soul, and that is something that can show through so easily to other people.

- I choose to do things that are good for my body.

- I value myself, and I have virtue in all that I do.

- I add value to other people's lives, as well. I motivate myself, and therefore, I know how to motivate other people.

- I am not afraid of anything. The worst thing that can happen to me is that I stop believing in myself.

- I will always be my best friend.

- I will always know how to encourage myself and include confidence in everything that I do.

- I love myself, and I am proud of the body that I have.

- I am perfect the way that I am, and I am beautiful.

- I am happy, I am healthy, and I am free.

- I am focused, I am centered, and I am peaceful.

- I am stress-free and thankful.

- I have gratitude and love.

- I am attractive, and I am perfect. There is nothing that I need to punish myself for.

- I accept everything that I am.

- I love myself.

- I am healthy.

- I am happy.

- I am free.

CHAPTER 15:

Meditation With Positive Affirmation

N ow I am about to take you on a journey of visual imagery and relaxation to a far-off place. Enjoying vibrant and compelling images, you will hear powerful and positive statements that will endorse many feel-good affirmations that will improve your perception of yourself and improve your overall wellbeing.

We tend to turn to food whenever we are stressed in life. When problems overwhelm us, most of us tend to stress-eat, and then we experience a cycle of guilt and regret. In time, this cycle can impact how we feel about ourselves.

During this guided meditation, you will remember how to feel good and understand your connection to food. During times of stress, you will learn to release tension and experience all that is natural and spontaneous.

The experience of this guided meditation will be enhanced if you find yourself a comfortable and ventilated spot.

Ensure that there is no disturbance from anything or anyone for thirty minutes.

Mental guided meditation and hypnosis are strong and powerful ways to help heal and protect one's psyche from external and internal harm. This, however, is not the only benefit that they have. Mental exercises aside, hypnosis, when done properly, can help convince the brain to accelerate and begin the process of physical healing, and as such, can be used to help heal the human body in its entirety.

This is, of course, not an alternative to conventional medicine or medicinal drugs as prescribed by professionals. Still, when used in conjunction, it can rapidly increase one's likelihood of survival from fatal diseases and, more importantly, can help individuals deal with day to day pain like old injuries or even terminal illnesses.

So, are you ready to walk into your hospital?

Hypnotic Guide to Self-Healing

Once again, like most of the other forms of healing that we will be dealing with here, hypnotic healing tends to lead the listener or practitioner into a deep guided trance, which can be dangerous if one is around or handling heavy machinery.

Make sure you find yourself a good, quiet place where you can comfortably sit down in a stiff back chair or on a stool, with your legs bent at the knee, and sit down.

As you seat yourself, hold your knees close together and straighten your back, as if you were in a schoolroom.

Breathe in deeply and release.

As you release, focus on the various points of pain in your body, and identify them in your mind's eye.

Relax.

Breathe.

Now, as you work on your breathing, slowly focus on entering a deeper state of consciousness.

Relax your body and breathe.

Once again, you are at the end of a tunnel.

Keep walking down the tunnel, and as you do, notice the faint glow of light at the end.

As you are walking down the tunnel, allow your body to follow your mind into a deeper state of consciousness, and relax every muscle in your body, starting from your feet up to your face.

Remove your tongue from the roof of your mouth and relax your face.

You are now at the end of the tunnel, and like before, a strong oak door is before you.

Open the door, and enter into the light.

As you enter through the door, the strong hospital lights blind you.

You can smell the strong acidic smell of sanitizer.

Keep walking through the crowded halls until you see a room on your left labeled X-Rays.

Enter the room, and go stand in front of the massive machine.

Now exit the room and walk over to the next room.

You will find a massive projector displaying an X-Ray of your entire body on the screen.

Look carefully at the image.

You will notice that certain parts of the X-Ray are glowing with a sharp red light.

These are your points of pain.

Identify them in your mind.

Breathe deeply, and focus on your breathing.

Inhale again, and as you do, travel with your breath down to the first point of pain. As you arrive, look around you, inside the hollowed veins and across the muscles and bone, you will find flashing red lights causing pain to shoot through your body.

Go closer and press your hand across the light, covering as much of it as you can.

You will find a soft blue light is covering your hands; use it to cover the red lights. Apply the light again and again over the red areas, like a gel concoction, and as you do, breathe deeply in and pull the pain, all the way down to the point of pain, harness the pain to your breath and powerfully expel it through your mouth.

Breathe deeply.

Exhale.

Practice this again and again.

Then, once you can feel the pain subside and see the light dim, move on to the next point.

You are healing your pain with the power of goodness and light as it courses through your veins.

Positivity must radiate from your being, and you must believe deeply in the power it holds.

You are strong and healthy.

You are vibrating with vigor and happiness.

You are not afraid.

You are not in pain.

You are whole.

You are complete.

Once again, breathe deeply, and focus your breathing.

Inhale again, and travel with your breath down to the next point of pain.

As you arrive, identify the red lights of pain and pinpoint their origin.

Once you see them, walk over and cover them with the blue gel-like concoction spreading from your hands.

Breathe deeply, harness the pain to your breath, and powerfully expel it through your mouth.

Breathe deeply.

Relax.

As you finish going through each point of pain, repeat the following –

I am strong and healthy.

I am vibrating with vigor and happiness.

I am not afraid.

I am not in pain.

I am whole.

I am complete.

The oak door is beckoning you; as you step beyond it, walk back out the tunnel, and I will count to three.

On the count of three, you will have exited the tunnel and will be clear-minded and fresh, as well as healthy and whole.

One.

Two.

Three.

You are healthy and whole, and your mind is clear and fresh.

You will feel better and better each day.

CHAPTER 16:

Day 3 Meditation to Burn Fat

Our bodies were designed to burn fat. It is the way that they provide the body with energy when we haven't given it enough through the foods we eat. We require more energy when we workout, so our bodies will burn more fat during these processes. Though it can sound so simple on paper, it will be rather challenging to always include these things in our lives. This meditation is going to help guide you through the journey of getting the body you want with a visualization exercise to help you see your goals laid out clearly. Listen to this first when you are in a relaxed position in case you become calm to the point of sleep. After you know how you react, you might include this when you are doing yoga or another form of light exercise to help keep you grounded and relaxed.

Fat Burn Meditation

Narrator: This is a visualization meditation. I am going to take you on a mindfulness journey through your body. To start, ensure that you are somewhere that you can be fully relaxed. You don't want to have any distractions around, and the only thing that you are going to focus on now is the air that is coming in and out of your body.

Narrator pauses for 3 seconds

Narrator: Let your mind go blank. As thoughts begin to creep in, gently push them out with each exhale—focus on nothing else other than the air that enters your body, and how it exists.

Narrator pauses for 3 seconds, breathing in and out

Narrator: When we count down from ten, you are going to imagine that you are in the middle of the woods. There is a light trail, and you are walking down it.

Breathe in for one, two, three…

And out for three, two, one…

You will be in the woods in ten, nine, eight, seven, six, five, four, three, two, and one.

Narrator pauses for 3 seconds

Narrator: You are walking through the woods, noticing everything that surrounds you. There are trees, birds, and even a little stream that you can hear the water running from.

You are feeling incredibly good at this moment, healthy and focused. You haven't eaten in a little bit, but you aren't very hungry just yet. You felt your stomach grumble, but it was just a small signal that you need to eat. Nothing is causing you pain or discomfort. You are focused on right now only, and nothing else.

You are walking up a hill now, a slight incline. You feel the burn start to occur in your legs. As you continue to walk, you begin to realize that your body is starting to burn fat.

You don't have to tell your body to do this. You don't have to take a pill to do this. Your body knows how to do it on its own.

You supply it with healthy food that doesn't add as many calories as you need for energy to your body, meaning that you are burning fat faster.

You put it through workouts to burn fat. The combination of both of these is helping you to lose weight.

Narrator pauses for 3 seconds

Narrator: You won't notice in the mirror immediately after burning the fat, but you are feeling it immediately in the way your body functions. Each time your stomach growls, you feel it. Every time you take a step, you feel it. As your body is continuing to get stronger and stronger and push you closer and closer to the goals that you want, you feel lighter and lighter.

Your body is burning more and more fat. You are becoming more and more relaxed, focusing only on your breathing and the good feeling circulating through your entire body.

Narrator pauses for 3 seconds

Narrator: You are only burning fat. You aren't doing anything to add fat, which means that your body's only option is to use what is already there as an energy source.

You consistently make choices to burn the fat from your body. You are always looking for ways to become lighter and lighter. You feel as your waist is getting slimmer and slimmer.

It feels good to drop the weight. It feels amazing to finally let go of all that has been holding you back.

The more weight that you are burning, the easier it is to lose even more. There is nothing that is going to keep you from getting the things that you want in this life. You are working with your body to get the things that you have been hoping for.

Narrator pauses for 3 seconds

Narrator: You continue to walk through the woods with the realization that you are a part of nature, just like all that surrounds you. Your body was made to keep you as healthy as possible. Now, it is time to train your brain so that it is optimized for health as well.

Your brain will try to do what it thinks is right for your health. It wants you to eat ice cream, so you feel better right now. It wants you to sit on the couch instead of the workout so that you can save your energy. Your body is only thinking of the "now."

You are training your brain to think about the future. You are accepting all that surrounds you, and that you are a part of this nature just like the rest. You are connected to the earth and feel the natural processes flow through your body. You are highly aware of all of the things that you need to do to keep your body as healthy as possible.

Narrator pauses for 3 seconds

Narrator: Your body feels better and better the further that you walk. Sometimes you feel a slight strain in your legs, but nothing that is painful. It is simply your body doing its best to burn as much fat as possible. It is your body working hard. It is a good pain, one that makes you feel healthier, stronger.

You have water with you that you take a drink of. This is the fuel that helps to keep your body going. You provide it with everything necessary to continually work hard.

Your body will always burn fat. It is designed to use what you already have stored within you. Each time you make a healthy choice, it makes you feel healthier.

Every time you do something good for your body, you are burning fat. You continue to burn fat, always feeling lighter and lighter.

Narrator pauses for 3 seconds

Narrator: You are more relaxed now. Your mind understands what it needs to do to be healthy. You are starting to feel lighter every day.

The forest around you is fading.

As we come to the end of the meditation, remember to focus on your breathing. You will either be able to drift off to sleep or move onto other meditations needed for a weight loss mindset.

As we reach ten, come out of the forest and back into reality, where you will be focused only on burning fat and losing weight.

Narrator counts to ten

CHAPTER 17:

Days 4, 10, and 17 Hypnosis

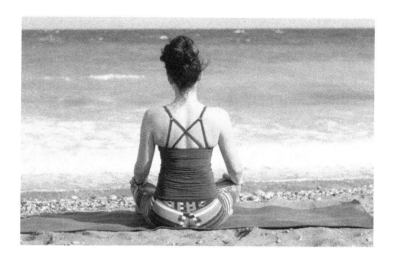

Self-Hypnosis Session

Now we will go over ten simple and concise steps to perform a successful and fruitful, and positively effective session of self-hypnosis. I will list the steps first and follow up with a step-by-step breakdown featuring a brief and easy to understand the description of what each step should entail for you in your journey.

- Step 1: Preparation of Self

- Step 2: Preparation of Time

- Step 3: Preparation of Space

- Step 4: Preparation of Goal and Motive

- Step 5: Relaxation of the Physical Body

- Step 6: Relaxation of the Soul and the Mind

- Step 7: Realization of Trance

- Step 8: Active Repetition of Mantra or Performance of Script

- Step 9: Preparation for Exiting the Trance State

- Step 10: Returning to Earth

As you read those steps, I'm sure they bring forth images in your mind. It may seem apparent already what you have to do, and ideas for how to guide yourself through this self-hypnosis you are preparing for are blossoming like wildfire in your mind. Let us go more in-depth to further prepare and become aware of all that you can do to make your self-hypnosis as easy and effective as your soul will wish to better yourself in the most transformative way possible.

Step 1: Preparation of Self

So, as you are aware, one of the first and foremost goals is to become as relaxed as possible before, during, and after entering the trance-state. Relaxation is the key that helps us enter the trance-state, and the trance-state further facilitates relaxation of the entire being both during the active self-hypnosis and afterward, for positive benefits of your being. To achieve the most successful self-hypnosis possible, we must first prepare ourselves, our minds, and our physical bodies, for what we desire to achieve, a state of heightened relaxation in which we can become hyper-aware of the inner machinations of the mind, to achieve a closer union with them, to bond with them, and to converse with them on the most intimate level possible. The popularity of this music exists because people desire for sounds that will lull them into a more peaceful state. Maybe you would like to try something like this. Some people prefer silence; some people prefer peaceful noise, a sort of hypnotizing drone that guides them into a more relaxed state of being. White noise, be it from a fan, a laundry machine, running water, or a white noise machine made specifically to fill the air with a light white noise, can also be effective for this purpose. Anything that has the desired effect on you will serve this purpose. Another thing you can do is to drink a nice herbal tea of your choosing; find a blend that is relaxing to you as an individual. Some common choices would be lavender-orange teas or chamomile teas. These will set a space internally for you to prepare yourself for entering your trance-state.

Step 2: Preparation of Time

It goes without saying that if an alarm clock goes on when you are in your trance-state, the effectiveness of your self-hypnosis session will be largely inhibited. It is necessary, if you wish for an effective and transformative session of self-hypnosis, that you make sure a certain amount of time is allotted where you will be safe, secure, at peace, and uninterrupted by your daily responsibilities. Many things can get in the way of this. Common inhibitors of time include children, chores, spouses, day-to-day noise, and work. If you have children, maybe you can have a relative or a reliable babysitter, watch them for a certain amount of time. Maybe you could ask your spouse to take the children out for an hour or two and explain to them your intentions of performing a transformative inner-journey that requires the utmost relaxation possible. Situations in which you have a large burden of responsibility, ironically, are the types of situations that can make necessary long and fruitful journeys into self-hypnosis. It takes planning and cares to make sure that, while all responsibilities are met, there is a designated and a specified time for you to go into your journey with the utmost confidence and care that you will be able to do what you need to do and come out the other end as enlightened as possible.

Step 3: Preparation of Space

It also should go without saying that a crowded, busy subway station at peak times of the day is no place for you to go about your most effective journeys into self-hypnosis or the trance-like state. The place is of the essence. Just as your body temple must be totally clean and prepped and ready for the ascension, so must your surrounding area be prepared for you to feel as comfortable as possible to allow for the most successful transition into a strong and malleable trance-like state, allowing for the most successful self-hypnosis possible? As always, it is different for different people, depending on beliefs, religion, and personal comforts. Feel free to experiment and find what makes you most comfortable. No one knows how to make you as comfortable as possible, like yourself. Trusting yourself is both one of the biggest keys and one of the biggest goals of self-hypnosis in general, so you must trust yourself here.

Step 4: Preparation of Goal and Motive

One of the critical factors of self-hypnosis is having a plan for what specific change or changes you wish to enact once having entered the trance state, and how you plan to achieve them. This is where the narratives you wish to express, the prayers, or the mantra or mantras you wish to repeat to yourself, come into play. What do you hope to achieve in your self-hypnosis session? It is always different for different people and at different times. But there is always at least one goal, and preparation for achieving that goal is a must when it comes to performing a successful and fruitful and transformative self-hypnosis session. Imagine you are about to have a very important conversation with a very important person in your life. You are crossing a river one stepping stone at a time, putting one foot in front of the other, and you will make it across if you stay steady, attentive, and aware of your surroundings. Be calm, be collected, and be prepared for what you are about to do.

Step 5: Relaxation of the Physical Body

Now we begin. There are many schools of thought on the best ways to relax the body. One very common through-line in all of these is the act of deep, conscious breathing. Breathe in, breathe out, be aware of your breaths, be in control of each one of them. The goal here is mainly to become aware of every single voluntary and involuntary action of the physical body and slow it down. Feel your heartbeat. Be aware of it. Envision, it slows down. Relax. Expand the space and the length of each breath. Focus on certain areas of the body and watch them become more and more still.

Step 6: Relaxation of the Soul and the Mind

So, to relax the mind, we can perform a series of steps very similar to those shown when relaxing the body but carried over to another plane. Just as in relaxing the physical body, our goal was to become aware of all voluntary and involuntary actions of the body, to slow them down to a point where they are more malleable and understandable, so too here, we must become aware of all the voluntary and involuntary actions of the mind, to slow them down to a point where they are more malleable and understandable. It is like slowly zooming in with a microscope, so things that were once small, almost invisible, become very large and monolithic. Our goal is to achieve a state of hyper-awareness.

Step 7: Realization of Trance

Now you are here, and you have willfully affected the realization of the trance-like state that is the initial aim of a good, effective session of proper self-hypnosis.

Don't be afraid to reach out and touch the light. Fully immerse yourself in this experience that you have prepared for. Know that you are achieving a very important and personal goal and be glad and grateful and ecstatic and proud of where you are. Feel the ball of light at your core, your solar plexus, emanating out like a shining star, like the sun, like the soil. It may be orgasmic. You may be taken aback by the power you have tapped into, the infinite potential. Focus on the awareness of the self and see who you are.

Step 8: Active Repetition of Mantra or Performance of Script

Now you have journeyed into space. Speak.

Speak the words you wish to speak to yourself. Each repetition of the mantra will completely change the landscape that you have found yourself in seismic waves. You will feel growing energy completely under your control swarm over your entire being and beyond. You are in charge here. What you say goes.

You are the ruler of this land, and you are going to take care of it well and make sure it is a prosperous paradise. Watch the negative thoughts, the images, the shadows, the memories you feared, the people you hate, the guilt, the pain, watch it fade into dust and evaporate before your very eyes, melted into oblivion by the sheer overwhelming power you have achieved.

Step 9: Preparation for Exiting the Trance State

Just as when you fully submersed, take a moment after you are done with your action to appreciate the beauty of what you are witnessing. Just be here now in this state. It is an eternal state. You will leave, and you will go back to the physical world, but this state will stay untouched, eternal, waiting for you to return. This is heaven. Know that you are about to return, and you are about to feel very different than you have ever felt before. Embrace these differences. It may be odd and imperfect at first, but it is a learning experience. The physical reality still awaits you as always—a different eternal experience. The rest of your life will be spent juxtaposing these two very different and very real planes and finding the perfect balance where you are in absolute control, yet in total surrender and synchronicity.

Step 10: Returning to Earth

Open your eyes. Where are you? Who are you? You may feel like this is something equally new as the realm you have just left. But there is a feeling of familiarity. You are awakened to the infinite possibilities of life. You see that your perspective can change in infinite ways, and with that change in perspective leads a portal to infinite different realties experienced through the multi-faceted crystal that is existence. You may be stunned. You will be changed.

CHAPTER 18:

Day 18, 20 Hypnosis Session for Weight Loss

S tart by taking a deep breath in.... then let it out slowly. Make sure that you are seated comfortably and that you are somewhere safe where you can relax for twenty minutes or so. During this session, you will ignore all daily noises like the telephone ringing, traffic sounds outside, or any other sounds except for sounds of alarm. If you hear an alarming sound, you will immediately come out of the trance state with no residual sleepiness.

Relax... take another breath in....and out. Let go of all of the stress that you are holding onto. Relax... breathe in... and out.

Start by relaxing the muscles in your feet and legs. Think of each muscle one by one and let them all just let go and relax. Feel a warmth spreading from your toes up to your calves... feel the warmth go to your thighs, and as it moves across your body, feel each muscle group that it reaches completely let go and relax.

Relax your stomach muscles... and moving up to your chest and shoulders. Feel the warmth move up your body and relax... breathe in...and out... now your neck muscles are feeling warm and relaxed. Feel all of the muscles in your face relax completely.

Imagine yourself at the top of an escalator. As you step onto the escalator, you realize that you are passing numbers on white signs on the way down. The first number is 10. As you pass each number, you will fall deeper and deeper into a relaxed state. Take another deep breath in...9...the escalator is moving you slowly forward and down...8...you are becoming more and more relaxed each time you pass a number...7...relax your body completely and let go of everything...6...you reach the halfway point of the slow-moving escalator...5...you are very relaxed now...completely relaxed...4...you feel as if you are floating down the escalator becoming more and more relaxed...3...you can see the bottom. When you reach it, you will become even more deeply relaxed than you are now...2...you reach the bottom of the escalator...1...breathe in...and out...very relaxed now...

With each of the suggestions that I give to you, you will become more deeply relaxed than before. Each of these suggestions will stay in your subconscious, and they will be used to influence your behavior when you awake...continue to relax as each suggestion is given...

You no longer have to eat too much food to feel the good feelings about yourself that the food provides... your feelings are good as they are...

When you feel an emotion, your response is to eat. However, you don't need to do that. When you feel anxiety, you should slow down and try to find the cause. You don't need to overeat to solve anxiety. Overeating will not solve the problem; it will only make it worse. If you feel depressed, that means that it is time to spring into action. When you feel frustrated, what you have been doing may not be working, and instead of eating, try something else. If you feel stressed, you will not become less stressed by eating. Instead, try to relax and take things one by one as they come. If you feel the emotion of loneliness, try to surround yourself with people instead of food.

Eating will not satisfy these emotions. When you feel these emotions, your response will be to do something other than eat. In the future, you will find it easier to understand these emotions, and you will not feel compelled to eat. Your feelings are there to guide you through life, and each one means something different. Your response to these will no longer be to eat. Instead, you will allow each emotion to happen and then take action.

In the future, you will be free from the cycle that you have fallen into in the past. Eating will not solve any problems, even temporarily, and will only make you feel worse. Eating should only be done when you are hungry, and you should eat until you are no longer hungry. When you find yourself tempted to make large portions, you will have the willpower to say no, and you will be very satisfied with the amount you have.

When you have other emotions, they are not hunger. Those are simply emotions, and eating will not make them go away. You will remember these things when you awake. As I count up from 1, you will start to feel more awake, but still, remember all the suggestions given…2…you are coming up…3…you are starting to feel less relaxed and more alert…4…when you awake at the end of the count, you will feel refreshed and ready to continue your daily activities…5…you are more awake now…6…7…8…9…you will wake up completely refreshed on the number 10…

Self-confidence is essential to progress well in your life. Not enough confidence prevents you from going to the maximum of what you can do and from developing fully. But too much self-confidence, pretension will shut your doors. Self-confidence is, therefore, good as long as you don't go to extremes: be honest with yourself and trust yourself. How to successfully achieve this goal? With only a little practice.

Nothing is sexier than a woman who radiates confidence!

CHAPTER 19:

Days 19, 25 Mindful Eating Meditation

A ll too often, we eat well beyond what is needed, and this may lead to unwanted weight gain down the line.

Mindful eating is important because it will help you appreciate food more. Rather than eating large portions just to feel full, you will work on savoring every bite.

This will be helpful for those people who want to fast but need to do something to increase their willpower when they are elongating the periods in between their mealtimes. It will also be very helpful for individuals who struggle with binge eating. Portion control alone can be enough for some people to see the physical results of their weight-loss plan. Do your best to incorporate mindful eating practices into your daily life so that you can control how much you are eating.

This meditation is going to be specific for eating an apple. You can practice mindful eating without meditation by sharing meals with others or sitting alone with nothing but a nice view out the window. This meditation will still guide you so that you understand the kinds of thoughts that will be helpful while staying mindful during your meals.

Mindful Eating Meditation

You are now sitting down, completely relaxed. Find a comfortable spot where you can keep your feet on the ground and put as little strain throughout your body as possible. You are focused on breathing in as deeply as you can.

Close your eyes as we take you through this meditation if you want to eat an apple as we go through this, which is great. Alternatively, it can simply be an exercise that you can use to envision yourself eating an apple.

Let's start with a breathing exercise. Take your hand and make a fist. Point out your thumb and your pink. Now, place your right pinky on your left nostril. Breathe in through your right nostril.

Now, take your thumb and place it on your right nostril. Release your pink and breathe out through your nostrils. This is a great breathing exercise that will help to keep you focused.

While you continue to do this, breathe in for one, two, three, four, and five. Breathe out for six, seven, eight, nine, and 10. Breathe in for one, two, three, four, and five. Breathe out for six, seven, eight, nine, and 10.

You can place your hand back down but ensure that you are keeping up with this breathing pattern to regulate the air inside your body. It will allow you to remain focused and centered now.

Close your eyes and let yourself to become more relaxed. Breathe in, and then out.

In front of you, there is an apple and a glass of water. The apple has been perfectly sliced already because you want to be able to eat the fruit with ease. You do not need to cut it every time, but it is nice to change up the form and texture of the apple before eating it.

Breathe in for one, two, three, four, and five. Breathe out for six, seven, eight, nine, and 10.

Now, you reach for the water and take a sip. You do not chug the water as it makes it hard for your body to process the liquid easily. You are sipping the water, taking in everything about it. You are made up of water, so you need to constantly replenish yourself with nature's nectar.

You are still focused on breathing and becoming more relaxed. Then, you reach for a slice of apple and slowly place it in your mouth. You let it sit there for a moment, and then you take a bite.

It crunches between your teeth, the texture satisfying your craving. Amazingly, this apple came from nature. It always surprises you how delicious and sweet something that comes straight from the earth can be.

You chew the apple slowly, breaking it down as much as you can. You know how important it is for your food to be broken down as much as possible so that you can digest it. This will help your body absorb as many vitamins and minerals as possible.

This bit is making you feel healthy. Each time you take another bite, it fills you more and more with the good things that your body needs. Each time you take a bite, you are deciding in favor of your health. Each time you swallow a piece of the apple, you are becoming more centered on feeling and looking even better.

You are taking a break from eating now. You do not need to eat this apple fast. You know that it is more important to take your time.

Look down at the apple now. It has an attractive skin on the outside. You wouldn't think by looking at it about what this sweet fruit might look like inside. Its skin was built to protect it. Its skin keeps everything good inside.

The inside is white, fresh, and very juicy. Think of all this apple could have been used for. Sauce, juice, and pie. Instead, it is going directly into your body. It is going to provide you with the delicious fruit that can give you nourishment.

You reach for your glass of water and take a long drink. It is still okay to take big drinks. However, you are focused now on going back to small sips. You take a drink and allow the water to move through your mouth. You use this water not just to fill your body, but to clean it. Water washes over you, and you can use it in your mouth to wash things out as well.

You swallow your water and feel it as it begins to travel through your body. You place the water down now and reach for another apple slice.

You take a bite, feeling the apple crunch between your teeth once again. You feel this apple slice travel from your mouth throughout the rest of your body. Your body is going to work to break down every part of the apple and use it for nourishment. Your body knows how to take the good things that you are feeding it and use that for something good.

Your body is smart. Your body is strong. Your body understands what needs to be done to become as healthy as possible.

You continue to drink water. You feel how it awakens you. You are like a plant that starts to sag once you don't have enough water. You are energized, hydrated, and filled with everything needed to live a happy and healthy life.

You are still focused on your breathing. We will now send the meditation, and you can move onto either finishing the apple or doing something relaxing.

You are centered on your health. You are keeping track of your breathing. You feel the air come into your body. You also feel it as it leaves. When we reach zero, you will be out of the meditation.

20, 19, 18, 17, 16, 15, 14, 13, 12, 11, 10, 9, 8, 7, 6, 5, 4, 3, 2, 1.

You should work and invest time and effort into reaching your desired body weight, not because of some thin body ideal circling around and not because of other people around you, but because weight gain in addition to helping you be more satisfied with your body image, also brings numerous health benefits which are crucial on top of all other weight loss effects on your life.

The truth is that you do not have to lose some excess amount of weight to experience weight loss health benefits as losing only several pounds can make a huge difference.

For instance, losing ten pounds for a person weighing two hundred pounds improves her overall health state, makes her feel better, more energized, and much more.

Losing only ten pounds can rapidly ease up on your joints, remove some pressure off your knees as well as remove pressure off your other lower body joints, which can wear out easily when you have to carry around those additional pounds.

Additional fat accumulated in the body can also cause various types of chronic inflammatory disorders as chemicals contained in the body, which tend to do tissue damage while damaging your joints as well.

Therefore, losing weight can prevent this from happening as well as reduce your risk for developing arthritis at some point later in life due to your weight.

Losing those extra pounds also can decrease your chances of developing some types of cancers. There is one study showing that a female who lost at least five percent of her body weight lowered her chances of developing breast cancer by twelve percent.

There is no clear proof that losing weight can protect you from other types of cancer, but even the slightest weight loss progress decreases the chances of developing breast cancer.

For instance, overweight females who lose extra pounds also tend to lower their hormone levels, which are linked to the development of cancer cells, including androgens, insulin, and estrogens.

If you are more likely to develop type 2 diabetes, weight loss is your way to go to delay or even prevent it from occurring.

Moreover, in addition to losing weight in these cases, moderate exercise for at least thirty minutes per day is also highly recommended.

On the other hand, if you have already been diagnosed with diabetes, losing those additional pounds can help you in many different ways, such as keeping your blood sugar levels in control, lowering your odds of the condition causing some other health issues, and lowering your need for taking all of those medications.

By losing additional pounds, you can also lower your levels of bad LDL cholesterol just by embracing healthy dieting options.

Unlike balancing those LDL cholesterol levels, balancing those levels of good HDL cholesterol is harder, but not impossible by losing body fat and by exercising regularly.

Just as you can balance your cholesterol levels, by losing those additional pounds, you can also bring down your triglyceride levels, which are responsible for transporting energy and fat storage throughout the body.

High triglyceride levels mean you are more likely to have a stroke or heart attack, so moving closer to those healthy triglyceride levels is crucial for maintaining an optimal health state.

Those who are overweight and struggle with high blood pressure can make a huge change by losing those additional pounds.

As you know, having excess body weight puts the body under more stress, so the blood starts pushing harder against the artery walls.

In these cases, the heart needs to work harder, as well. To avoid suffering complications related to high blood pressure, trimming only five percent of your total body mass can make a massive change.

Another dieting tip for lowering high blood pressure includes eating plenty of low-fat dairy products, plenty of foods and veggies, and cutting down on salty foods.

CHAPTER 20:

Re-Program Your Mind

1) Visualization

If you want to reshape the reality of your life, start by visualizing how you want your ideal life to be. Our subconscious mind's main language is emotions and images. Write a script of your ideal life and then play it like a movie in your imagination. The more detailed, vivid, and emotional you make it, the more your subconscious will think it is real because it cannot tell the difference. Remember, the subconscious is your captive audience. You can transfer your ideas from your conscious imagination to your subconscious to make success happen for you. Do your visualization for 10 to 15 minutes daily. For visualization, you can also use a vision board, which is covered in.

2) Affirmations

The trick to saying affirmations that work and can program your subconscious mind is confidence and perceived truth. Simply put, although our subconscious does not know the difference between real or fantasy, our affirmations should not raise internal objections because it is too farfetched. For example, if you are currently broke and unemployed, it might be a stretch for your subconscious to believe the affirmation "I'm going to be a billionaire by this December" as compared to "The ideal job is already mine. My finances are improving every day."

- Write affirmations that have corresponding feelings, focus on the positive, and have no opposing views.

- Face a mirror, take a deep breath, and speak your affirmation a few times in the morning, noon, and evening. When saying your affirmation, focus on the meaning and feeling of your words.

- Another method is to write your affirmation several times on a piece of paper daily.

- Repetition and feelings are the keys to reinforcing affirmations to your subconscious.

3) Listening to brainwaves audio program

Neuroscientists have discovered that different types of brain waves can influence our creativity, habits, behavior, thoughts, and moods.

There are five types of brain waves:

a) Beta brain waves are associated with our waking consciousness and are important for our state of alertness, logic, and critical reasoning.

b) Alpha brain waves are present in deep relaxation, meditation, or dreaming states. This is also the optimal brain wave when we need to program our subconscious mind for success, as it is when our imagination and visualization are at their peak.

c) Theta brain waves are present during light sleep, REM sleep, and meditation. These are also optimal waves for mind programming, vivid visualization, creativity, and insight.

d) Delta brain waves are the slowest brainwaves that happen during deep, dreamless sleep and transcendental meditation. During these brain waves, our body is healing and regenerating.

e) Gamma brain waves are the fastest brainwaves, which are associated with high-level processing and insight.

For subconscious programming, you can use either alpha or theta brain waves to help you while you are doing your visualization work. There are many apps and online audio programs that you can download, such as Brain Waves - Binaural Beats, Brainwave Tuner Lite, Banality, edenBeats for Android and iPhone users.

4) Hypnosis

Typically, in hypnosis, a qualified hypnotist will put you in a relaxed and suggestible state before programming positive and empowering messages into your subconscious mind.

Techniques for Health

We explained the emotions that harm our health and the mind-body connection where we feel an emotion, and it activates certain neural pathways in our brain. Whether you're looking to improve a specific area of your health or your total wellbeing, the first step is to be aware of negative emotions that might be hampering your health. This step is like removing the weeds from your garden before you can start planting good seeds. The good news is, once you have identified these negative emotions, you can work towards healthy subconscious programming.

- Be aware of your inner dialogue because every feeling, thought, and emotion carries energetic effects that can influence your body. For example, if you keep saying to yourself, "I feel sad," it will cause stress, damage, and increase cortisol and adrenaline in your body. Imagine the long-term damage this does to your body if you do this repeatedly.

- Our consistent toxic emotions and thoughts manifest many diseases.

- Are you stuck in toxic emotions, such as anger or sadness, which are sending a negative feedback loop to your mind and body? Manage and take charge of your negative emotions; otherwise, they will control and deplete your mental strength.

- If you are currently undergoing treatment for any ailment, focus your mind on how the treatment or medication is going to help you get better. Let's say you are undergoing physical therapy for your bad knee. Instead of being passive and just going through the motions, you need to start seeing and believing that the therapy is indeed making your knee better. Use the power of your mind to expect your treatment to work.

- All sickness, be it the common flu or an incurable disease, can be reversed by releasing negative thoughts and replacing them with positive thoughts of health; healing through the mind works harmoniously with medicine.

- Our bodies respond to thoughts from our subconscious mind. Therefore, if you focus your thoughts on being healthy, you will create more health.

Steps:

- Ask for what you desire, e.g., "I am healthy, and my body is perfect in every way."

- Every day look at yourself in the mirror and say aloud your health affirmation, "I am healthy, and my body is perfect in every way."

- Visualize your body in perfect health. Imagine yourself doing all the things you thought you couldn't do, e.g., your bad knee prevents you from running.

- To help you visualize better, cut out pictures of healthy-looking people that inspire you and paste it next to your mirror where you do your daily health affirmation

- Every day try to do things that are relaxing and de-stressing to help you let go of toxic emotions and thoughts, e.g., watching funny movies or playing with your children

- Be thankful and act like you already have a healthy body. If you want to accelerate your progress, keep a gratitude journal, and write down three things you are grateful for before you sleep. The purpose is to let these positive thoughts sink into your subconscious and expand your awareness before you drift off to sleep.

- To keep your state of health, avoid people who are negative or focus too much on your illness

- Read (or listen) to books on health and wellbeing

- Lastly, believe and have faith that once you ask, your body is already whole.

- Suggested daily affirmations for health

E.g.

a) "I am getting stronger and healthier every day in every way."

b) "I am perfectly healthy and full of energy."

c) "I take good care of my body by eating healthy and nutritious food."

d) "I am filled with energy and physical stamina."

e) "I want wholeness and healing for my body."

f) "Healing power flows through my body in all ways."

g) "I am kind, loving, and gentle to my body."

h) "I love food, and food loves me back."

i) "I am at my perfect weight with a beautiful and healthy body."

CHAPTER 21:

Day 26, 30 Relaxation to Promote Physical healing

Stress is a hormone that exists within us, which can hinder our ability to lose weight. If you want to ensure that you are doing your best to have well-rounded health, then keeping up with your stress is crucial. Music can be very relaxing on its own. When you pair it with meditation through mindful listening, it will be much easier to stay focused on what you need to do to live a healthy life while being mindful of the most important things for your overall goals. If you want a clear mind, you will have to cut out distractions. Of course, this includes little things, but there are bigger distractions and stressors present in our lives, which may hold us back from achieving our dreams. This mediation is going to help you understand how the music exists within your body and how it can help you remain calm and relaxed.

Cleansing Relaxation Meditation

This meditation is all about focusing on becoming relaxed and cleansed. One of the best ways to achieve this kind of feeling is through the use of music. Make sure that you are somewhere comfortable. You need to be in a peaceful and distraction-free zone in which you can close your eyes and focus on nothing but feeling the air come in and leave your body.

One of the reasons why we struggle to lose weight is that we are so stressed. Stress can lead to stress-eating and cause your body to hold on to weight that it does not need. Worse, it can alter your hormonal levels.

You are focused now on reducing stress because this means that it will be easier for you to lose weight. There is nothing else that you are concerned about other than becoming more relaxed.

You are centered; you are focused. You are at this moment; you are prepared for whatever might come your way. You are not concerned with anything other than relaxing and becoming more peaceful.

Feel it as the music beats to a rhythm. There is a slight beat, no matter what it is that is being played. Everyone who listens to this will find a different meaning to the tunes. Everyone who partakes in the process of listening to cleansing music does so for different reasons.

It will always help everyone to relax. Though we all have different things that we use this music for, it still helps us to become more and more at peace. Calmer and calmer. More and more relaxed.

Start to focus on your breathing now. Breathe along with the music. Count for at least five while you are breathing in and then five as you are breathing out.

Breathe in for one, two, three, four, and five. Breathe out for six, seven, eight, nine, and 10. Feel as you breathe in how the music enters your body. Your body is like a musical song as well. Your heart is like the drumbeat that is always pounding.

Your brain is like the conductor that tells everything how it should sound. Your blood, your muscles, and your organs – they make up the rest of the instruments. Your body is a beautiful chorus, and you are a melody traveling through life.

You are a perfect being, relaxed, calm, and at peace. You are one with the earth. You are one with the music. You start to feel it come in and out of your body.

This music can change the way you feel. This music is in control of your emotions. It will affect the way you operate.

It is helping you to feel better and more relaxed. It is bringing you closer and closer to being at peace. It is bringing you closer and closer to being centered and focused.

You are feeling lighter and lighter, and the stress is drifting away. As soon as you start to let go of stress, you will start to release yourself from the heavyweights that are keeping you back. The quicker you focus on peace, the more weight you will lose.

Each time you let go of stress, you are letting go of some of your weight. Every time you focus on being more at peace, you are feeling healthier and healthier.

You feel it as the music spreads to every part of your body. It starts in your mind. It stimulates your brain so that you are focused on relaxing and nothing else at that moment.

It soothes your heart. It reminds you that you are not alone. It makes you feel better, and that spreads everywhere else.

The music keeps you motivated. It keeps you cleansed.

Cleansing is an important part of your weight-loss journey. Your body is always working to clean itself. Your body is focused on how it can rid itself of toxins and bring in the things that are good for it. Your breathing is one way that your body is consistently working to cleanse itself.

Your body is always cycling in new air and getting rid of the old. It does the same thing with food as well. It brings in new minerals and nutrients and gets rid of the toxins that it does not need. You drink water to help cleanse your body. It is always working on its own to keep you as cleansed as possible.

The cleansing processes help you to feel more at peace. You feel like a new person. You are constantly given second chances. It is never too late to start over.

You are feeling your body become more and more cleansed now. You are feeling lighter and lighter, more relaxed. You are becoming a new person. You are starting over. You are starting fresh. You are relaxed. You are focused. You are at peace.

As we count down from 20, you will exit this mediation. Continue listening to cleansing music to bring in the peace that you need to lose weight and maintain it. It will be easier to lose more weight when you manage to focus on cleansing.

20, 19, 18, 17, 16, 15, 14, 13, 12, 11, 10, 9, 8, 7, 6, 5, 4, 3, 2, 1.

You can practice the art of breathing deeply at regular intervals, which will calm and soothe you deeply. This will help improve the air and blood circulation in the body and produce calming effects.

You need to make yourself feel comfortable.

Here are some things you can do:

- Go to a quiet place with fewer distractions.

- Loosen tight clothing or remove your shoes, jewelry, and jacket.

- Get a comfortable chair that will support your head. Make sure that your arms are placed on the armrest, and your feet are firmly planted on the ground. You should not cross your legs.

- You can also lie on a bed or the floor. Place your arms away from your body with your palms facing up. Stretch your legs out, making sure they are apart.

Once you are comfortable enough, you can now focus on your breathing. To start, inhale and exhale slowly in a regular beat or rhythm.

CHAPTER 22:

Women and Men are different

The basic principles of weight loss are the same for both genders- you burn more calories than you consume- but the factors that lead to a caloric deficit that causes weight loss are not the same. Men and women are different. They are biologically different and emotionally different. These differences are very important because both biology and psychology are important for successful weight loss.

Different Bodies

There is no need to explain the physical differences between men and women. The body composition of men and women, that is, the proportions of muscle, bone, and fat that make up the body of men and women are very different. A typical 154-pound man has 69 pounds of muscle, 23 pounds of bone, and 23 pounds of fat (the rest is organs, fluids, etc.). A typical woman weighing 125 pounds weighs 45 pounds of muscle, 15 pounds of bone, and 34 pounds of fat. In summary, men are hereditarily programmed to have a muscular build up with heavier bones than women. Conversely, the female body is designed for higher fat content.

Theoretically, the definitions of overweight and obesity are based upon the excess body fat (Body Mass Index or BMI is used to categorize the person's weight). Again, the gender is different. Obesity in men is defined as 21-25% body fat and obesity as 25% or more. Obesity in women is defined as 31-33% body fat and obesity as 33% or more. From a biological point of view, men should be lean in appearance, and women should be fat, so men and women of the same size and weight should have very different body compositions. Given the physical differences between sexes in terms of body composition, it is not surprising that body fat recommendations differ between men and women.

Men are recommended a range of 12-20% fats, and women are recommended a range of 20-30%. Because of their different body composition, losing weight gives men a biological advantage over women.

Different Minds

Men and women do not share the same physical and psychological build-up. Differences based on emotions between men and women are a very interesting area. Every year, more and more are learned about the relationship between mental processes and physical functioning, especially concerning neurotransmitters. A 2006 article even states that men smile less than women, were due to how their brains were programmed.

It is well known that chemical behaviors in the brain influence our behaviors in the areas of food and physical activity. Also, although little is known about these signals at this time, there may be differences due to gender. The brain is associated with the potential effects of obesity and gender, so the more we learn about how the brain affects mental health, the more relevant treatment options will be developed. The mental aspect of weight and weight loss cannot be overemphasized. The basic physiology of weight loss is relatively simple. To lose weight, you need to lose more and ingest fewer calories. One needs to know that at the heart of permanent weight loss is the behavior of eating, exercising, and thinking. There is a large difference between men and women when it comes to weight loss.

Health Risks for Obese Women

Women and men share the health risks of certain diseases, but some weight-related health problems are found only in women. Weight loss seems to be one of the most important ways for women to overcome these problems beyond the potential health risks. Example:

Polycystic Ovary Syndrome (PCOS) is a condition that can affect a woman's fertility and is associated with obesity. Health professionals recommend weight loss as the first treatment for PCOS because studies have shown that losing weight improves fertility.

Besides, obesity is a risk factor for Gestational Diabetes. Studies show that a weight loss of just 10 pounds can significantly reduce a woman's risk of developing gestational diabetes.

Adult obesity and weight gain are also known risk factors for Postmenopausal Breast Cancer. In an analysis of a large group of women in Iowa, researchers found that preventing weight gain at childbearing age, or preventing weight gain in overweight women combined with weight loss, was healthy during those years. It was concluded that maintaining a healthy weight reduced the risk of being diagnosed with breast cancer in later years.

Overweight negatively affects the psychological health of both genders but appears to be more emotionally stressful for women (Emotional Stress). Studies show that women are less satisfied with weight and overall body shape than men. And most women's dissatisfaction with weight begins early in life and continues into adulthood. Why? The answer lies, at least partially, in an attachment to the lean body for women in almost all societies.

Weight watcher researchers often hear women say they feel that others are judging them by their appearance (thin and attractive), not by what they are capable of and what they can do. Where do women get this belief? The media is an important source of information. Most of the beautiful women in magazines and big screens are extraordinarily thin people, and for many women, extraordinary thinness is a measure of beauty. This seems to be primarily a woman's problem.

A study that asked men and women for their ideal body shape and asked how they thought of their body in comparison with their ideals was generally satisfied. In contrast, women consistently viewed themselves as heavier than their ideals and expressed a desire to lose weight. Unfortunately, this very thin waif figure is unrealistic (and unhealthy!) And can't be achieved by most women. As a result, many women lose self-esteem and develop a negative body image associated with depression. So, instead of focusing on being extremely thin, one should focus on maintaining a healthy weight. Now, we will finally move to actual weight loss techniques for losing extra fats. We will be focusing on the root of the problem, the brain.

CHAPTER 23:

100 Positive Affirmations for Weight Loss

According to dietitians, the success of dieting is greatly influenced by how people talk about lifestyle changes for others and themselves.

The use of "I should" or "I must" is to be avoided whenever possible. Anyone who says, "I shouldn't eat French fries" or "I have to get a bite of chocolate" will feel that they have no control over the events. Instead, if you say "I prefer" to leave the food, you will feel more power and less guilt. The term "dieting" should be avoided. Good nutrition should be seen as a permanent lifestyle change. For example, the correct wording is, "I've changed my eating habits" or "I'm eating healthier."

Diets are fattening. Why?

The body needs fat. Our body wants to live, so it stores fat. Removing this amount of fat from the body is not an easy task as the body protects against weight loss. During starvation, our bodies switch to a 'saving flame,' burning fewer calories to avoid starving. Those who are starting to lose weight are usually optimistic, as, during the first week, they may experience 1-3 kg (2-7 lbs.) of weight loss, which validates their efforts and suffering. Their body, however, has deceived them very well because it does not want to break down fat. Instead, it begins to break down muscle tissue. At the beginning of dieting, our bodies burn sugar and protein, not fat. Burned sugar removes a lot of water out of the body; that's why we experience amazing results on the scale. It should take about seven days for our body to switch to fat burning. Then our body's alarm bell rings. Most diets have a sad end: reducing your metabolic rate to a lower level. This means that if you only eat a little more afterward, you regain all the weight you have lost previously. After dieting, the body will make special efforts to store fat for the next impending famine. What to do to prevent such a situation?

We must understand what our soul needs. Those who desire to have success must first and foremost change their spiritual foundation. It is important to pamper our souls during a period of weight loss. All overweight people tend to rag on themselves for eating forbidden food, "I ate too much again. My willpower is so weak!" If you have ever tried to lose weight, you know these thoughts very well.

General affirmations to reinforce your wellbeing

1. I'm grateful that I woke up today. Thank you for making me happy today.

2. Today is a very good day. I meet nice and helpful people, whom I treat kindly.

3. Every new day is for me. I live to make myself feel good. Today I just pick good thoughts for myself.

4. Something wonderful is happening to me today.

5. I feel good.

6. I am calm, energetic, and cheerful.

7. My organs are healthy.

8. I am satisfied and balanced.

9. I live in harmony and understanding with everyone.

10. I listen to others with patience.

11. In every situation, I find the good.

12. I accept and respect myself and my fellow human beings.

13. I trust myself; I trust my inner wisdom.

Do you often scold yourself? Then repeat the following affirmations frequently:

14. I forgive myself.

15. I'm good to myself.

16. I motivate myself over and over again.

17. I'm doing my job well.

18. I care about myself.

19. I am doing my best.

20. I am satisfied with myself for my achievements.

21. I am aware that sometimes I have to pamper my soul.

22. I remember that I did a great job this week.

23. I deserved this small piece of candy.

24. I let go of the feeling of guilt.

25. I release the blame.

26. Everyone is imperfect. I accept that I am too.

If you feel pain when you choose to avoid delicious food, then you need to motivate yourself with affirmations such as:

27. I am motivated and persistent.

28. I control my life and my weight.

29. I'm ready to change my life.

30. Changes make me feel better.

31. I follow my diet with joy and cheerfulness.

32. I am aware of my amazing capacities.

33. I am grateful for my opportunities.

34. Today I'm excited to start a new diet.

35. I always keep in mind my goals.

36. I imagine myself slim and beautiful.

37. Today I am happy to have the opportunity to do what I have long been postponing.

38. I possess the energy and will to go through my diet.

39. I prefer to lose weight instead of wasting time on momentary pleasures.

Here you can find affirmations that help you to change harmful convictions and blockages:

40. I see my progress every day.

41. I listen to my body's messages.

42. I'm taking care of my health.

43. I eat healthy food.

44. I love who I am.

45. I love how life supports me.

46. A good parking space, coffee, conversation. It's all for me today.

47. It feels good to be awake because I can live in peace, health, love.

48. I'm grateful that I woke up. I take a deep breath of peace and tranquility.

49. I love my body. I love being served by me.

50. I eat by tasting every flavor of the food.

51. I am conscious of the benefits of healthy food.

52. I enjoy eating healthy food and being fitter every day.

53. I feel energetic because I eat well.

Many people are struggling with being overweight because they don't move enough. The very root of this issue can be a refusal to do exercises due to negative biases in our minds.

We can overcome these beliefs by repeating the following affirmations:

54. I like moving because it helps my body burn fat.

55. Each time I exercise, I am getting closer to having a beautiful, tight shapely body.

56. It's a very uplifting feeling of being able to climb up to 100 steps without stopping.

57. It's easier to have an excellent quality of life if I move.

58. I like the feeling of returning to my home tired but happy after a long winter walk.

59. Physical exercises help me have a longer life.

60. I am proud to have better fitness and agility.

61. I feel happier thanks to the happiness hormone produced by exercise.

62. I feel full thanks to the enzymes that produce a sense of fullness during physical exercises.

63. I am aware even after exercise, my muscles continue to burn fat, and so I lose weight while resting.

64. I feel more energetic after exercise.

65. My goal is to lose weight. Therefore I exercise.

66. I am motivated to exercise every day.

67. I lose weight while I exercise.

Now, I am going to give you a list of generic affirmations that you can build in your program:

68. I'm glad I'm who I am.

69. Today, I read articles and watch movies that make me feel positive about my diet progress.

70. I love it when I'm happy.

71. I take a deep breath and breathe out my fears.

72. Today I do not want to prove my truth, but I want to be happy.

73. I am strong and healthy. I'm fine, and I'm getting better.

74. I am happy today because whatever I do, I find joy in it.

75. I pay attention to what I can become.

76. I love myself and am helpful to others.

77. I accept what I cannot change.

78. I am happy that I can eat healthy food.

79. I am happy that I have been changing my life with my new healthy lifestyle.

80. Today I do not relate myself to others.

81. I accept and support who I am and turn to myself with love.

82. Today I can do anything for my improvement.

83. I'm fine. I'm happy for life. I love who I am. I'm strong and confident.

84. I am calm and satisfied.

85. Today is perfect for me to exercise and to be healthy.

86. I have decided to lose weight, and I am strong enough to follow my will.

87. I love myself, so I want to lose weight.

88. I am proud of myself because I follow my diet program.

89. I see how much stronger I am.

90. I know that I can do it.

91. It is not my past, but my present that defines me.

92. I am grateful for my life.

93. I am grateful for my body because it collaborates well with me.

94. Eating healthy foods supports me in getting the best nutrients I need to be in the best shape.

95. I eat only healthy foods, and I avoid processed foods.

96. I can achieve my weight loss goals.

97. All cells in my body are fit and healthy, and so am I.

98. I enjoy staying healthy and sustaining my ideal weight.

99. I feel that my body is losing weight right now.

100. I care about my body by exercising every day.

CHAPTER 24:

How to Start Mindful Eating

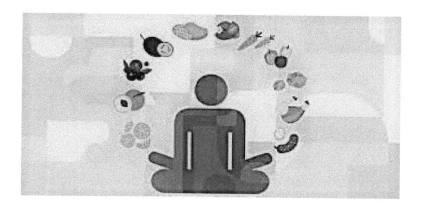

Mindfulness is a simple concept that states that you must be aware of and present in the moment. Often, our thoughts tend to wander, and we might lose track of the present moment. Maybe you are preoccupied with something that happened or are wondering about something that might happen. When you do this, you tend to lose track of the present. Mindful eating is a practice of being conscious of what and when you eat. It is about enjoying the meal you eat while showing some restraint. Mindful eating is a technique that can help you overcome emotional eating. Not just that, it will teach you to enjoy your food and start making healthy choices. As with any other skill, mindful eating also takes a while to teach, but once you do, you will notice a positive change in your attitude toward food. In this, you will learn about a couple of simple tips you can use to practice mindful eating in your daily life.

Reflection

Before you start eating, take a minute and reflect upon how and what you are feeling. Are you experiencing hunger? Are you feeling stressed? Are you bored or sad? What are your wants, and what do you need? Try to differentiate between these two concepts. Once you are done reflecting for a moment, you can now choose what you want to eat, if you do want to eat and how you want to eat.

Sit Down

It might save some time if you eat while you are working or while traveling to work. Regardless of what it is, you must ensure that you sit down and eat your meal. Please don't eat on the go. Instead, set a couple of minutes aside for your mealtime.

You will not be able to appreciate the food you are eating if you are trying to multitask. It can also be quite difficult to keep track of all the food you eat when you are eating on the go.

No Gadgets

If all your attention is focused on the TV, your laptop, or anything else that comes with a screen, it is unlikely that you will be able to concentrate on the meal that you are eating. When your mind is distracted, you tend to indulge in mindless eating. So, limit your distractions or eliminate them if you want to practice mindful eating.

Portion your Food

Don't eat straight out of a container, a bag, or a box. When you do this, it becomes rather difficult to keep track of the portions you eat, and you might overindulge without even being aware of it. Not just that, you will never learn to appreciate the food you are eating if you keep doing this.

Small Plates

We are all visual beings. So, if you see less, your urge to eat will also decrease. It is a good idea to start using small plates when you are eating. You can continuously go back for a second helping, but this is a simple way to regulate the quantity of food you keep wolfing down.

Be Grateful

Before you dig into your food, take a moment, and be grateful for all the labor and effort that went into providing the meal you are about to eat. Admit the fact that you are lucky to have the meal you do, and this will help create a positive relationship with food.

Clean Plate

You don't have to eat everything that you serve on your plate. I am not suggesting that you must waste food. If you have overfilled your plate, don't overstuff yourself. You must eat only what your body needs and not more than that. So, start with small portions and ask for more helpings. Overstuffing yourself will not do you any good, and it is equivalent to mindless eating.

Prevent Overeating

It is important to have well-balanced meals daily. You shouldn't skip any meals, but it doesn't mean that you should overeat. Eat only when you are hungry and don't eat otherwise. Here are a couple of simple things you can do to avoid overeating. Learn to eat slowly. It isn't a new concept, but not many of us follow it. We are always in a rush these days. Take a moment and slow down. Take a sip of water after every couple of bites and chew your food thoroughly before you gulp it down. Don't just mindlessly eat and learn to enjoy the food you eat. Concentrate on the different textures, tastes, and flavors of the food you eat. Learn to savor every bite you eat and make it an enjoyable experience. Make your first-bit count and let it satisfy your taste buds. Now is the time to let your inner gourmet chef out! Use a smaller plate while you eat, and you can easily control your portions. Stay away from foods that are rich in calories and wouldn't satiate your hunger. Fill yourself up with foods that can satisfy your hunger and make you feel full for longer. If you have a big bowl of salad, you will feel fuller than you would if you have a small bag of chips. The calorie intake might be the same for both these things, but the hunger you will feel afterward differs. The idea is to fill yourself up with healthy foods before you think about junk food. While you eat, make sure that you turn off all electronic gadgets. You tend to lose track of the food you eat while you watch TV.

Eating Experience

In a culture that emphasizes multitasking, eating is a secondary activity. We do not combine food with the nutrition of our bodies. Eating is what we do without attention while doing more meaningful work.

Have you automatically turned off your car radio while looking for a new address? I instinctively know that removing a voice stimulus increases your ability to focus on finding its address. Silence also allows us to pay attention only to food and to be fully present for a dining experience. Watching TV, interacting with computers, talking on the phone, reading books, and doing other activities is not a supplement to a careful diet. Mindful meals require indiscriminate attention, so it's a great way to overeat.

If you have resistance to silent hoods, rewiring can help you recognize that you ate for the first time when you had another activity. It is a custom that has been cultivated for many years. You rarely eat the main focus.

When you sit quietly and eat, you can hear inner conversations such as how to enjoy the meal and subtle messages from the body when you are satisfied. If turning off competing stimuli creates fear, inhale, and note the cause of the anxiety.

If you are dining with your family, invite them to participate in the careful process of eating. Trying to turn off as many distractions as you can during your meal is better than overeating during multitasking. Discuss your senses and taste of food. Slow food does not have to be extreme. Nevertheless, it is a good idea to remind the family that eating is not a race. Encourage the family to chew on every slice of food, examining the taste, texture, and odor in detail. Ask them about their feelings, thank them for collecting brownie points, and thank them for their blessings and share their meals with their families.

Remember to measure your progress: how do you feel in silence after a meal? Can you eliminate all distractions and eat quietly without fear? Is practicing this property easier to eat silently?

Don't forget to check for your progress. How does it feel like after eating the whole meal with just a few bites? How was your fear? Did you experience the fun with such a small morsel? Did you have to hit the kitchen and get a more oversized spoon? Or did you just start eating with your fingers?

CHAPTER 25:

Meditation Practice

When it becomes regular, it's so simple and so difficult. It's simple because 10-20 minutes a day is not much. It's difficult because many obstacles prevent most people from practicing regular meditation or self-hypnosis. However, conscious presence and calm responses instead of angry reactions can only be ensured through continuous practice.

Meditation and self-hypnosis can be seen as a diet or workout: we start with great enthusiasm at the beginning, but after the first few days, we get into trouble.

What misconceptions are preventing this from happening?

Many people confuse meditation with relaxation and think that meditation is good if you relax immediately. Lying on the ground after yoga and relaxing is not meditation but mere relaxation. In this case, we can systematically release stress through muscle relaxation and breathing. This is what we call fixation: when we strive to achieve a specific goal, regardless of the basic situation. In meditation, however, we do not try to change the present situation.

Let's take a general example: after a stressful day, we sit down to meditate. Usually, we don't feel like we can relax, and it is easy to concentrate on our breathing, no matter how much we try.

If we practice a fixative method, we can easily experience failure. Meditation, on the other hand, teaches us that stressful and scattered conditions are part of life and that the first thing we can do about it is a curious observation. After all, meditation prepares us to flow with the ups and downs in our daily lives. Many times, there is no solution to a problem in the present situation, but we spend a great deal of time and energy trying to find it, which can easily lead to even more stress.

Another misbelief is that while meditating, we shouldn't have thoughts. I always smile at this. We are thinking beings, and every day 60,000-125,000 thoughts pass through our heads. Thanks to our thoughts, we can develop things; thanks to them, we can solve problems, create, and imagine things. When we talk about wanting to clear our minds because we think too much, we mean the thoughts that lead to anxiety. The purpose of meditation practice is to recognize our thoughts, especially those that are continually talking and unconsciously controlling our subconscious. During meditation, we decide which thoughts we give place to and act upon, and which ones we let go. We don't want to exclude our thoughts, but to develop a wiser relationship with them. So it's not a problem if they do appear. We greet them and give them a name and then return to breathing. And when they come back more than once, we observe what emotions are beneath them.

Many people expect meditation to be an exciting trip. However, during meditation, we observe quite ordinary things: the flow of breath, the rising and falling of the belly, the sounds of our breath, tingling, or lack of it in our toes. These may seem like boring things, and for this reason, one of the first experiences you may have is that of a boring meditation session. However, boredom stems from judgment; if we say something is not exciting, we think about that and avoid focusing on direct experience, which is the essence of meditation.

So the next time you experience boredom, be aware of how you feel and observe how bored you are. What thoughts are passing through your mind? Ask yourself if you can release them so you can return to breathing.

We also expect that meditation must be something. Once you release that expectation, it becomes easier to practice. Releasing the urge to change also helps you to practice not to qualify and judge everything, which is the essence of mindfulness meditation. If you have released all your misconceptions about meditation, let's jump into practice! Let me give you some useful tips for your meditation and self-hypnosis exercises.

Wear comfortable clothes. One of the primary purposes of meditation is to relax the mind by preventing potential distractions. However, it will not be easy to relax if you feel uncomfortable with clothes that are too tight. During meditation practice, opt for soft clothes and take off your shoes. If you plan to meditate in a cool place, wear a sweater or a cardigan.

Pick a peaceful room because you should practice meditation in a quiet place. In this way, you can concentrate solely on the exercise, away from any outside distractions and stimulation. Search for a place where you don't run the risk of being interrupted while you are exercising.

For beginners, it is crucial to avoid any distractions. Turn off the TV, phone, and any other device that makes noise. If you want to put music in the background, choose something relaxing so as not to compromise concentration. If you prefer, you can listen to white noise or a sound of nature. The sound of a car or the barking of a dog shouldn't affect the success of the meditation. Indeed, an essential element of this practice is to be aware of the surrounding noises without allowing them to take over the mind.

Many people believe it is beneficial to meditate outside. Unless you sit near a busy road or an unbearable noise source, you will be able to find peace under a tree or sit on a corner of grass in your favorite park.

Stretch a little before you start to avoid tightening up. During meditation, you will need to sit for a specified duration, so before starting, it is essential to relieving any muscle tension. A couple of minutes of stretching will help you prepare your body and mind. Moreover, it will prevent you from focusing on any minor pains, allowing you to relax. Remember to stretch your shoulder and neck muscles, especially if you have been sitting in front of the computer for a long time. Stretch the leg muscles, especially those in the inner thigh, to facilitate meditation in the lotus position. If you can't stretch your body muscles, consider using some other methods before meditation. Many specialists advise to practice some yoga exercises before starting to meditate.

Before starting, determine how long the session should last. Even though many masters suggest two sittings a day for 20 minutes, beginners can start with 5 minutes a day. Once you have decided the length, try to respect it. Don't be intimidated if you have the impression that it is not sufficient. It will take time and a lot of exercises to get the most out of meditation practice. In the beginning, the most important thing is to keep trying. Schedule an alarm clock by choosing a nice tune to know when the time is up.

Identify the goals you want to achieve with meditation or hypnosis. If you are doing this to reach a serious goal like weight loss, prepare a list of affirmation statements. Remember that you must say your affirmations concurrently: "I am eating healthy. I am losing weight. My clothes are fitting better, and I feel better." These are statements that you will recite to yourself when you are under hypnosis.

At this point, you can use the visualization in the way you prefer. Think of orange and cut it in half in your mind. Imagine squeezing the juice and feeling it on your fingers. Put it in your mouth. What is your reaction? What perceptions of taste and smell do you feel? Then move on to more meaningful visions. Imagine losing weight. Add as many details as possible. Always involve the five senses.

Try to understand that no meditation, self-hypnosis, affirmation, or mantra will manifest in real life if you don't want it deep inside. For it to be effective, you must believe in yourself and your actions.

If it doesn't seem effective the first time, don't encourage yourself. Try again after a few days and revisit the experiences. You might be surprised. Open your mind. You must believe that there is a possibility that it works. Any skepticism on your part will hinder your progress.

You are writing your suggestions before induction can be beneficial, as a visual list of what you want to work on can sometimes be more comfortable to retain than carefully assembled thoughts.

CHAPTER 26:

Rapid Weight Loss And Fast Diet Myths

1. Good and Bad Hypnosis

Hypnosis is excellent, bad, and so-so. Even in today's world of Hypnosis, there is a lot of crap out. I do believe that there is some excellent indirect value of Hypnosis (especially scenarios); my personal opinion is that indirect/conversational Hypnosis is, by far, on the "razor's edge" as it is now, as efficiency and up to date.

Be conscious because numerous hypnosis hucksters sell objects of "hypnotic snake oil," such as low-rate subliminal messages and stuff of pseudo-spirituality. Don't get me wrong, I'm not against all the subliminal messages, and I think Hypnosis should be used when combined with spirituality.

2. It is possible to hypnotize even emotional weaklings / I cannot be mesmerized

You may have heard that you can't hypnotize "wise" people. Many people don't consider that kind of stuff to be fun, and so they just don't get into Hypnosis. It is fundamental.

On the other hand, if you experience being masterfully and gently guided into a state of deep relaxation and concentration, you can realize that you can be hypnotized. It's possible to hypnotize someone with sound mental professors and a sensible amount of intelligence.

Truth is told; experience shows that people who are clever and have a creative mind make the very best subjects/clients for Hypnosis because they can "believe beyond the box" and do not restrict their imaginations to what is possible for them.

3. Hypnosis is the power of incline / you are not the slave of the hypnotist

You are the only one who has full power over your mind. A therapist can't let you do anything that you won't do. This myth has been spread for much too long by weird newspaper reports, stage hypnotists, and people who don't understand much about Hypnosis.

This being said, an individual may use techniques of Hypnosis and persuasion (for both excellent and adverse functions) to cause another person to end up more likely to do what they say and to follow their suggestions. Everyone can make their own decisions (even under Hypnosis) eventually, though.

A hypnotizer can't ask someone to do anything against his / her will (including going against his / her morals) unless he/she is willing to do so at first.

In general, the therapist serves as a guide to bring you into a calm and centered state and uses mentally sound hypnotic methods to help you make adjustments or experience different things you want to experience.

4. Hypnosis is not sleeping

Regardless of this theory, people who first try Hypnosis sometimes come out of it a little disappointed. They say things like, "I could hear whatever you said" or "I felt like I could open my eyes and leave if I wanted to." If you remain in Hypnosis, you will be conscious of your surroundings. The term "SLEEP!" is usually used by hypnotists as an order to force someone into a trance. It is how it uses sleep as a tool to help us get through Hypnosis.

5. In Hypnosis, you can not get "stuck."

No one got caught in Hypnosis. The only reason a person should remain in a trance is that it feels lovely to be so relaxed and concentrated. If the hypnotist left or suddenly died while the individual was in Hypnosis, the worst thing that would happen is that the hypnotized individual would probably drop off to sleep and awaken a genuinely great feeling.

6. Hypnosis doesn't mean amnesia

You won't forget whatever happened when you were in Hypnosis. Bear in mind; sleep is not anesthetic. You're not unconscious while in a trance.

7. In Hypnosis, you won't disclose your deep, dark tricks

You are in charge of your mind like I said in the past and will be even though you stay in Hypnosis. If you want to, you won't disclose something you don't want others to understand. Nonetheless, Hypnosis can be used as a way to help people cope with and find out certain issues they may not normally want to think about under everyday scenarios. This is always done with the consent of the individual, and generally in the hypnotherapy context.

If you're in Hypnosis, you will be yourself. That being said, a hypnotherapist may use Hypnosis to help another person explore what it would look like to "end up" another person. This is usually done so that the subject/client can feel what it would be like to have the characteristics they have (for situations, self-confidence) of the person they are "becoming." The hypnotized person will then bring this quality back to their character with them as they recover from being in Hypnosis).

Ok, if you want to be hypnotized, I hope this will cleans up any false assumptions about Hypnosis you may have had. If you are a therapist, you now have solutions to offer individuals to help ease their worries and clear up their misunderstandings. I hope he helped!

There are big deals of things that mess up women from a suitable, fast weight-loss. We consume for survival, but to get fat, we eat extra!

8. "It's dangerous to lose anything more than 1-2 pounds a week."

I have driven my clients safely with 1-pound-a-day weight control by low-calorie diets. When it's routine to lose just 1 pound a week, you can hold anyone is losing 80 extra pounds on that 80-week diet!

9. "Don't skip breakfast. It's harmful to a diet, and you're not going to shed as much weight!"

When you miss the morning meal and only take in tiny quantities of lunch and supper food (reduced numbers of calories that are required for a whole day), you must burn fat to compensate for the energy you don't get from food. Over a reduced calorie intake, skipping morning meals allows you to shed excess fat. That is how God made us. Once we were hunter-gatherers and walked the world as wanderers for the following supply of food, there would be periods when the winter season would come in, and the supply of food would go down, or there would undoubtedly be periods of starvation when there would be no supply of food.

In these times of food demand, God was smart enough to provide us with a resource of sugar. Both mammals have this space system for food storage, called fat. Many kids rely on these fat stores to sustain their lack of sufficient nutrition when you see many advertisements calling for help in depriving children in many other countries.

Equally, God created us to use this stored fat healthily when we don't have enough food. The way we prefer to use our stored fat when we fast are. The body has adapted to the use of fat for food storage to allow survival during periods of hunger or malnutrition. The most fitting makes it through, and when there is no food, those with sufficient storage space systems have made it through longer.

10. "Medicines and supplements will make your weight loss much worse!"

People were eating leaner and getting it done at a smaller weight. (This is one that the mind controls to help shed weight on them).

Conclusion

You need to remind yourself of all of the amazing health benefits of losing weight, such as feeling more energized, feeling better about yourself, having a better sleep and much more.

In addition to reminding yourself of all of the amazing health benefits of losing weight, another great idea is to keep a success journal where you will write every single step you have taken and succeeded in.

This way, you more likely to stay committed to your weight loss journey. To boost your commitment, you also need to embrace some positive affirmations and positive self-talk, which will keep you going.

Therefore, the next time you look yourself in the mirror, instead of telling yourself I will never be thin and I will just give up, say to yourself this is going to be amazing, losing those five pounds feels great, and I will keep going.

In case you were wondering how meditation can help you in weight loss, we believe that you have now realized how. For individuals struggling with weight loss, this can be an easy way out. You might have tried losing weight by exercising or dieting, but it is not helping much. Other times you realize that you are unable to follow that which you had started faithfully. For instance, you might be going to the gym, and somewhere along the way, you lack the morale to keep going.

On the other hand, you might be trying to diet, and you are unable to follow the diet plan strictly. Meditation can help you find morale. With the daily affirmations, you can find yourself managing to accomplish the set goals at targets. Dieting does not have to be a challenging thing to accomplish. You can keep reminding yourself why you started in the first place. Knowing this will help you keep pushing. At times one is tempted to have cheat days that prolong to weeks. With the help of the various affirmations, one can stick to the plan and ensure that they do not deviate from having the cheat days.

It does not only help one in weight loss, but it guarantees their general wellbeing. One of the good things about meditation is that you can practice it anywhere and at any time you find convenient. You can also do it at no extra cost. This is a good way to rejuvenate your mind and to focus on the things that matter. It also ensures that you improve your performance levels on the activities that you chose to undertake. With the poor eating decisions that we are making nowadays, we are having increased cases of lifestyle diseases. Obesity is now a huge challenge among the majority of individuals. It is about time that we step up and make better and more informed decisions regarding our lives. Some of these decisions include changing our eating habits and ensuring that we take good care of our health. Meditation helps us to maintain discipline in that which we do. It ensures that we stay focused on the plans and decisions that we have chosen to make. With the right attitude, meditation can transform your weight loss journey.

If you wish to lose weight or maintain a healthy body, you can begin your meditation journey. It is an easy process that you can easily follow up as long as you are determined. All you need to do is decide to start. The journey of a thousand miles begins with a single step. At times you have to go past tapping the waters and get in it completely. In the beginning, you might find it challenging to do so. Still, it's the encouragement that you keep giving yourself that will ensure you manage to utilize meditation in your weight loss journey successfully.

WEIGHT LOSS HYPNOSIS AND AFFIRMATIONS:

Harness the Power of Your Mind to Reshape Your Body. Burn Fat, Stop Cravings and Control Emotional Eating with Powerful Guided Meditations and Affirmations.

CAROLINE LEAN

Table of Contents

Introduction

In each other's existence, mind and body cannot exist apart. Some of the most important aspects of the relation between mind and body are that they are in continuous contact and each affects the other. You can think of your body and mind as always talking to each other. This is the relation between mind and body. Each thought and every idea in your head affects your body, and every emotion in your body affects your soul.

This book is about how your mind can affect the body for the better, and help you achieve the weight that you were supposed to get by self-hypnosis practice. Once we get into the particular strategies that can take you to the ideal body weight, we'd like to talk about hypnosis, the roots and what it actually does to differentiate the reality from fiction. We will also discuss what we consider to be at the heart of the idea of hypnosis — the relation between the mind and the body. Learning this personal connection within your body will help you eventually reach the ideal weight using self-hypnosis.

It's important to remember that thoughts are things. You can't see them, so you know they've got you. You might not sense every emotion, especially if you have electrodes mounted to the body for biofeedback, you can see your emotions causing the sudden changes in your body, either positive or negative. For example, if you'd think about somebody that made you furious, you'd have a rapid increase in heart rate, dilation or constriction of the blood flow, changes in the nervous system, and muscle tension. All these physical adjustments will come in as a result of one event. What this shows us is that your emotions and ideas are organically transferred to the rest of the body, and that the body is "thinking" through its own neural reactions, the same thing you bring into the mind, but in your own way. You are not unsure of the reaction your body has to what you think. Most of the time you're not conscious; it's sharing your feelings' knowledge. The way the body reacts to the experience is dependent on multiple things like temperament, preceding interactions, and response habits that have been learned. Repeating these habits, the body gets conditioned to work in every way. It's learning or being conditioned on the pattern of reaction. The good news is that by developing a particular reaction, something the body has learned can be unlearned. Self-hypnosis is a very strong and effective technique for helping you unlearn and replacing old patterns with more suitable ones.

Much as your mind affects your body, so does your body affect your mind. There are moments that you experience a feeling like hunger or thirst in your body that prompts you to experience an emotion, or have a thought, or have an idea in mind. If your mouth feels dry you're probably talking of drinking water. But often there's confusion — for example, when a feeling of being mentally wounded can be mistaken with a feeling of "I need to feed," or "I want to feed." These are some of the complexities we're trying to discuss and tackle in this book.

Adopt the notion of having a "mind body," the sublime bond that is formed between mind and body. Speak of your subconscious mind as "the mind of your body," "the mind body." Instead of assuming the mind and body are separate, use the words "the mind body," "the mind of your body," and "the subconscious mind" as all of them reflect the same thing. We are going to use these words interchangeably because all three represent the same definition.

CHAPTER 1:

Why We Get Overweight

T he healthy life: It's not just about losing the weight; it's about losing the lifestyle and the mindset that got you there." Dr. Steve Maraboli

As Americans, we live in a culture where food represents far more than a source of life-giving nutrition. Food is, for example, an important part of our social interactions, work functions, and family gatherings. Food is the centerpiece of most major American holidays. Eating certain foods is a form of celebration for occasions such as birthday parties and a source of comfort during periods of stress and emotional pain. Finally, the act of eating is paired in American culture with many recreational activities, such as romantic dates, movies, and sporting events. The result of living in such a food-centered culture is that we learn to use food as a source of pleasure and to escape from pain. And when we frequently eat as a means of managing our emotions, we end up consuming calories that our bodies do not need; unwanted weight gain is the inevitable result.

There is only one long-term solution to this source of weight gain: you must develop a food-relationship based on well-being, nutrition, and as fuel for your quality of life goals, rather than a food-relationship based on emotional management and social and cultural customs. We routinely learn negative food psychology in the U.S. that sets us up for weight gain and weight-related health problems throughout life, and we must relearn and replace this relationship with positive food psychology if we are to achieve lasting weight loss success and enjoy the quality of life rewards that healthy weight loss can bring us.

Going from a lifetime of basing our food-relationship on emotional and social factors, to a food-relationship based on nutrition, wellness, and performance may seem daunting. Moving from negative food psychology that produces harmful long-term results (weight gain, guilt, shame, weight-related health problems) to positive food psychology that produces helpful long-term results (a stable & healthy weight, mental & physical well-being, high energy). Based on stereotypes about healthier eating styles, you might currently imagine positive exercise psychology as a prescription for a lonely future eating carrot sticks and lettuce leaves, missing out on holidays and social events, and being forced to give up your favorite foods. That's a very unpleasant image. Thankfully, it is also completely inaccurate. Consider several important facts about people with positive exercise psychology that can make this food relationship shift more realistic and desirable to you:

- Everyone eats for emotional and social reasons. Healthy weight people just do it less often.
- Everyone has certain favorite foods that they enjoy. Healthy weight people eat these foods occasionally instead of frequently and better manage portions when they eat them.
- Healthy weight people enjoy their holidays, social events, and vacations as much, if not more than, people at unhealthy weights. However, the former group has learned how to make these events less centered on food by developing alternative ways of having fun during these occasions.

The difference between a healthy weight person that looks and feels great and an unhealthy weight person that looks and feels poorly is mostly a matter of degree in their eating habits. Most healthy weight people don't live on deserted islands or subsist on extreme diets to get their results. They don't work different jobs or make different amounts of money. Healthy weight people even eat mostly the same foods as unhealthy weight people. However, what healthy weight people do differently is that they consistently practice certain patterns of eating – driven by their positive food psychology relationships – that produce large differences in their weight compared to others over time. Rather than relying on genetic advantages that remain out of our control, positive food psychology consists of specific skills, attitudes, and behaviors related to food and eating that you can begin practicing yourself to get lasting weight loss results.

For you to embrace the positive food psychology solution, it is vital that we destroy the prevailing myth that healthy weight people possess some special metabolic advantage that allows them to eat whatever they want without gaining weight. The widespread belief in this myth holds many people back from developing the skills that could help them succeed. Many research studies have tested this metabolic myth and found it lacking. Take two people of the same size and gender and their resting metabolic rates will be within a couple of hundred calories a day of one another. In contrast to prevailing mythology, resting metabolic differences between otherwise similar people are small. Further, people who weigh more have faster metabolisms than people who weigh less (not the reverse).

If metabolic rates are about the same, why are there so many confirmed sightings of healthy weight people eating French fries, ice cream, and other high calorie foods without any apparent weight gain consequences? It is because this healthy weight person practices an overall lifestyle where the occasional food indulgence doesn't make a big difference. For example, they might eat lightly the rest of the day or two around having an especially large meal or be more physically active than usual. No one gets "fat" from a single meal. If a person eats well 80-90% of the time, the occasional excess won't have much of an effect. One classic study of weight gain in the 1990's intentionally overfed people living in a controlled laboratory environment for several months. The researchers found large differences in how much weight people gained, despite being knowing exactly how much they'd eaten. It turned out that some people became much more active (e.g., walking and moving more) after being overfed, while others became very sluggish; this change in physical activity explained nearly all the weight gain difference.

A second study of healthy and unhealthy weight people on holidays found a key difference in behavior that explained most of their holiday weight gain patterns. When the healthy weight people overate at a holiday meal, they quickly got back on track with their diet and exercise routines, whereas the unhealthy weight people tended to throw in the towel after overeating and continued to overeat in the days following. This result implies that holiday weight gain is not inevitable, but largely under our control depending on how we respond to routine events such as an episode of overeating or missing a workout. If a person who normally gains weight over the holidays begins practicing the eating and exercise behaviors of people that maintain or even lose weight over the holidays, they will get better results. Despite decades of study and all our high-tech metabolic science, we have yet to find even one of these people who can literally "eat whatever they want and never gain an ounce" or those who "gain weight just by looking at food". They remain the Bigfoot and unicorns of the weight loss world.

Busting this metabolic mythology is important because it helps us focus on the positive food psychology relationship that makes most of the difference in the long-term. If you are one of those people with a modestly slower metabolism than other people, breathe a sigh of relief that this difference amounts to a small disadvantage that can be overcome with a little more consistency and eating skill on your part. Ridding ourselves of metabolic mythology is also valuable to us because it vanquishes the fear that improving our relationship with food requires impossible sacrifices. You don't have to become a health nut, practice a vegan, Atkins or Paleo diet, or even give up a favorite food like chocolate to improve your food relationship. But you must change your food relationship in several fundamental ways that will involve both learning and practice: 1) You must improve the quality of your food relationship, such that 80-90% of the time you are eating to give your body the fuel it needs to look and feel great; 2) You must learn to recognize and replace the habit of eating for emotional reasons with healthier ways to help yourself feel good and reduce negative emotions; 3) You must learn new skills and behaviors for social occasions to help you live a dynamic life with your friends and family that doesn't jeopardize your waistline.

Improving Your Food Relationship

The great stories of love, adventure, and success in our culture share the theme of the main characters facing and overcoming seemingly insurmountable adversity. Adversity in these stories doesn't disappear to make it easy for the protagonist, however; instead, they must rise to the challenge. The hero evolves over the course of the story, becoming stronger, wiser, and more resourceful than the source of adversity. Their personal growth is the reason they succeed. This theme of personal transformation triumphing over early adversity applies equally in your quest to develop positive food psychology. Personal growth and transformation are required because most of us are firmly under the spell of negative food psychology by the time we are adults.

How does negative food psychology capture our brains? Almost from birth, we are trained as Americans to treat food as a tool for changing our emotional state. For example, when a baby cries, one of the most common parenting responses is to soothe them with a pacifier (notice that even the pacifier name connotes the intended emotional effect) or bottle (Sigmund Freud once referred to an "oral fixation" as a harmful behavior pattern among adults using infant-aged oral strategies such as eating, drinking, and smoking to gain pleasure and ease the pain). As the baby grows into a child, we introduce them to an increasing number of ways to use food for emotional reasons. We celebrate their birthdays with cake, their holidays with sweets and desserts, and comfort them after a painful trip to the dentist or doctor with candy and ice cream. TV exposes them to restaurant advertising strategically linking processed foods to positive emotions with clever labels such as "Happy Meals" and by pairing processed foods with popular toys. Escape the restaurant scene and take the same child to the grocery store, and high calorie sweets and processed foods virtually shout out to them with vibrantly colored packages and cartoon character spokesmen (e.g., Tony the Tiger, Ronald McDonald, Pillsbury Doughboy, The Kool-Aid Man, etc.,). Even if the child somehow reaches teenage and early adulthood years in the modern world without weight and body image problems, the negative food psychology training cycle only escalates as items such as alcohol and energy drinks are added to the food-as-emotions mix.

CHAPTER 2:

What Is Hypnosis And How It Works

What is Hypnosis?

People tend to believe completely in hypnosis altogether - or they don't. Rightly, before you can say not to believe in hypnosis, you must fully understand what it is and what it is not. There is much misinformation on the topic of hypnosis out there. People think when they get hypnotized, that they give up all control over themselves. This is not true. You retain complete self-control.

Hypnosis is a healthy, natural state of mind that many achieve in daily activities. For example, think about the last time you got involved in a good book. That relaxed, focused connection between mind and body is similar to hypnosis. Add a qualified, skilled guide that gives advice, and you have a preview of a hypnosis session. Your perception is always in charge while you're hypnotized. You stay hypnotized because you want to be there. In hypnotherapy, you use the power of your mind, facilitated by the guide. A trained practitioner may lead you on a particular path to the trance, which helps to locate a specific issue. Think of hypnosis as a form of therapy - only, with a guide. Regardless of the hypnotherapist's training and experience, the outcomes are always better than self-induced hypnosis.

The person needs to be open to the concept of hypnosis to function. Note, you don't turn over your mind control, only trusting in the hypnosis power that helps bind the mind and body. Like other successful people, are you able to take full control of all aspects of your life? Have you ever felt the need for change or desired to do something else in your life, but could you never find the determination or will power to make such a change manifest?

Self-hypnosis is a very powerful way for you to approach the body's consciousness (the subconscious mind or mindbody) explicitly. It gives you a way to remove any obstacles and confusion within your mindbody dialogue, so that the mindbody shares exactly what you want in a way that creates your healthy weight and lifestyle. We would like you to complete a brief mental experiment before we go any further, which will allow you to continue thinking about the strength and ease of self-hypnosis. Here are ten claims concerning hypnosis, "true or false." Read the sentences and ask, speculate or conclude "true or false" according to what you think of hypnosis now.

HYPNOSIS IS A NATURAL STATE OF CONSCIOUSNESS

The only thing we need to guard against is deliberately trying to use self-hypnosis for negative reasons, which will ultimately hurt only ourselves. As you will appreciate after reading further, the power of hypnosis or self-hypnosis has a permanent effect on our lives. The problem is that in most cases, and without our being aware of it, this force is working against us. It is therefore fortunate that you are reading these lines today, and not next year or in ten years' time because, even if the only thing you get out of this book is an understanding of this fact, it will make all my years of work on this method worthwhile. The point is - and we'll be talking about this a lot in the following pages - your life is an exact mirror of your thoughts.

To summarize, then, self-hypnosis is the simplest and most effective modern method for accessing the mind's subconscious and making use of its prodigious powers.

The Extraordinary Power of the Subconscious

What exactly is this subconscious that we hear so much about? There are several definitions, not all of them clear-cut. Since the method described in this book is essentially practical, we will not enter into any long theoretical or historical discussions.

It is enough to say that the concept of the subconscious (also called unconscious) mind was initially explored by Sigmund Freud, who made it the cornerstone of his entire system of psychiatry and saw it as the source of most human behavior, especially that behavior which we believe to be purely voluntary. Freud's contribution to understanding our behavior and its true nature is therefore considerable, despite certain exaggerations he may have made.

One thing is certain: even if the theorists cannot agree on a single definition of the exact nature of the subconscious, the fact that it exists cannot be doubted, and it has been accepted by the scientific community for many years.

To put it simply, the human mind is divided into two parts: one is conscious, and the other unconscious. The conscious part, which is only active during waking hours, takes care of most routine and intellectual activities.

When you eat or pour yourself a drink, or work on your monthly budget or fill out your tax return (forgetting to do these things, as you will see later on, is often due to your subconscious dictating what seems to be an involuntary act), it is your conscious mind which is being brought into play. As for your subconscious, it takes care of all your vital functions. For example, you don't have to think about breathing in order to breathe. If you did, you'd have serious problems sleeping!

Your subconscious also records and stores everything that happens in your life, like an archive of your entire existence. Its memory is perfect: it forgets nothing. It is also your subconscious which makes you fall in love with one person and not with another. Your conscious mind may advise you against such a choice: a particular man or woman may not appear to have the necessary qualities to merit your love. Yet your subconscious is stronger, and you are irresistibly attracted towards that person, despite the fact that he or she may not appear to be the ideal candidate.

Here's another example, this time more obvious. You want to stop smoking. You really want to stop - or at least you try to convince yourself that you do. And yet you can't stop. This is because your subconscious, which among other things is the cause of all your habits - good and bad - won't let you stop. It has been programmed to think differently. Later on I'll be talking a lot more about this extremely important notion of programming.

You walk into a supermarket and, spontaneously and mechanically - in fact just like a robot or a puppet - you 'choose' one brand of soap powder. Once again you are being guided by your subconscious, simply because it has been programmed, without your being aware of it, by some advertisement which struck your fancy (and in fact the methods used in marketing are strikingly similar to those of hypnosis).

The Subconscious Is Stronger Because You Are Not Aware Of Its Effects

Thousands of examples could be provided of how the subconscious affects behavior. And some have a much more dramatic and important effect than the kind already mentioned. Did you know, for example, that when a person repeatedly fails at a task, despite being talented and hard-working, it is because of his or her subconscious mind? Did you know that the same goes for emotional failures? Did you know that most illnesses - some doctors even suggest all illnesses - arise and first develop in your subconscious mind? Does that surprise you?

Let's look at another example, one that we've all seen thousands of times. A woman seems to have everything going for her. Nature endowed her with physical beauty, she has an interesting and well-paid job, she seems to be happily married, with a circle of good friends, is able to take a month's holiday every year - and yet, inexplicably, she is unhappy. She may even be considering suicide. She gets more and more depressed. She feels as though she's about to have a nervous breakdown.

The worst thing is that, although she can confide in people close to her, no one believes her. They think she's making it up, that she's looking for pity. How can someone have so much and dare to pretend to be unhappy?

And yet this woman is not lying. She is telling the absolute truth when she describes her state of mind. The real reason is that her subconscious is stronger than her conscious mind. At some point in her life it must have received some very negative programming, which has been reinforced over time. The subconscious is always stronger and always has the last word, which is why reprogramming your subconscious - positively - can achieve such wonderful results.

Many proverbs say the same thing, for example: 'Happiness is a state of mind.' In this sense- and up to a certain point- external circumstances are not a determining factor. Thus two persons, when placed in similar situations and confronted with the same kinds of obstacles, may react completely differently. One may do what is required without getting too emotional or 'losing their cool', while the other gets totally flustered and depressed. It is, therefore, the person's state of mind- their mental predisposition - which is the determining factor in how he or she may cope. I hope these few examples have convinced you of the extraordinary power of the subconscious. Our conscious mind has often been compared to the tip of an iceberg. As you probably know, the proportion of the iceberg which is underwater, and therefore invisible, is far larger than the part you can see. The same goes for the subconscious (or unconscious).

The subconscious is much more powerful, even if people believe they are very strong-willed. It is only after becoming aware of the power of the subconscious that you can start forging your own destiny and transforming your life into how you want it. Hence, using hypnosis in losing weight really works.

CHAPTER 3:

How Your Emotions Control Your Eating Habits

The Brain Does Make You Fat

Excess weight may feel like a thing of the belly, but your nervous system is among the major barriers to losing. What you feed on, look at and respond to affects you whether or not you add weight. This is how the subconscious controls the body — and what you can do about it.

Anxiety Fuels Your Needs.

Have a big presentation coming up, or are you about to have a challenging conversation with somebody you love? You should seek to control the discomfort; otherwise, you can catch yourself stopping your dinner plans and reaching for your preferred snacks for a second. Sometimes referred to as stress feeding, fear causes this form of action and, when treated, may be counterproductive to the scale — both upward and downward. Fear may have an overwhelming impact on the diet. Anxiety occurs differently in people. Certain people will find themselves trying to regulate any ounce of food they consume, some may have the need to overeat, while some may lose their desire to eat completely.

Allowing Negative to Dominate

Within the head, the glass half-empty mentality may be challenging, but it often causes unhealthy habits of eating. Losing weight marketing is especially good for people who prey on the poor ways of thought that most people form about food. The whole food industry is built to make consumers feel terrible for their health and make them believe they ought to waste all this money for a diet program that doesn't function. Whenever the person's diet crashes, they feel bad for themselves and the process begins. People sometimes fault themselves for failing the diet, not the weight loss guidance, when in fact it is. Before people get free of their eating habits, the body is hard to understand and everything that it offers, and understanding this is key.

Your Brain Turns Dieting Into Fat Preservation

There are numerous misconceptions out there about weight reduction, but one aspect that is unequivocally real is that the brain avoids diet. Key brain cells actively prevent fat burning in the body when food is rare. A group of neurons in the brain coordinates appetite and energy spending and can turn on and off a switch to consuming or backup calories depending on what's in the environment available. They help us feed if food is abundant, and if food is unavailable, they transform our body into a survival mode to avoid us from losing fat.

Depression Triggers Eating

Thinking processes causing obesity may be unconscious, but stress is an evident road to eating disorders. The weight gain is immutably related to the anxiety condition. Anxiety can significantly shift the culinary attitude and viewpoint. Depressed feelings can manifest in excessive feeding or deprivation so what's important is resolving the feelings head on. Recognizing what is going on is so crucial, and finding professional treatment so that you really can take action to not allow stress to affect your wellbeing and weight.

Work Destroys Weight Reduction Targets

Life is insane, so you force oneself to go to the gym to cut those calories in the a.m. while you are counting calories. You can sense the cravings much more severely than usual. And a brain under tension will indirectly weaken your attempts. If people feel uncomfortable regarding their bodies and eating patterns, the kinds of food they consume or the volume they consume can be unnecessarily limited. The body is created to live. It doesn't realize why the human intentionally limits food, it only recognizes but it does not have sufficient understanding, and it naturally slows down functions of the body, like metabolism, to save energy and to live. This physiological cycle often starts a primary urge to consume more to live, causing the individual to overfeed and struggle over food unconsciously.

Denying Pleasure

Part of the weight loss challenge is what products you choose to tackle it. If you're carelessly going for an apple because it's good for you, however, it gives you a stomach ache, why don't you make a move to eat a mango you'd like more? Think about consuming an experience rather than a need. What that means is that by having the time to reflect on what you actually want to consume and make it a conscious activity, you allow yourself the chance to tune in and adapt to the nutritious meals that you would want to buy and enjoy, leaving you happy at mealtime.

Being Judgmental

Will you feel a bad or a favorable connotation when you speak about a greasy burger and fries? How about a simple salad with hardly any treats? As we mature and start to assign various names to specific items, we start naming them accidentally — and sometimes, mindlessly —. Eliminating a 'good' behind such dishes and the 'evil' behind them will help shift the emphasis. "Food has little meaning, so feeding is not black and white. It has far less control over you, until the food has little moral obligation.

You Don't Even Ask Why

You remind yourself of something before you place the donut in your stomach. Is it food you desire — or anything else? Ask oneself if the meal is even whatever you need. People often crave comfort and support when eating without body hunger. It's fine to eat at a family party for selfish reasons, like cake, but you have to be capable to identify those signs and make a decision for yourself whether food is what you need or want or whether anything else will assist you accordingly.

Just To Tap into Gratitude

Humility can boost your wellbeing in several respects, but it's difficult to be thankful to oneself. Whenever an eating spree begins a cycle of shame, look at how incredible it is our brain and heart functions to keep us healthy instead of giving themselves a hard time. It makes sense why, if we build shortages by dieting, certain biological forces be in high gear to save our resources and lead us to search for high-calorie foods — or normally foods that we've resisted. What if we all quit this dieting nonsense and chose to take control of our body and function through our appetite rather than battle it? Instead, in a range of body types and ages, we will find much healthier individuals who kept fairly healthy weights and enjoyed improved fitness.

Confidence Won't Support You

If you really can't turn your mind the correct way around? Do not be scared to ask somebody who is able to tackle something that delays your development, for assistance. Trying to break the dietary and food anxiety mental loop is challenging, it requires training and experience. A nutritionist who specializes in mindful eating as well as the anti-diet method will assist you on the journey.

How to Lose Weight Using Your Mind?

If you've ever attempted weight loss, you realize that consuming nutritious food and exercising your body are essential elements of every weight loss strategy. Yet have you learned that reaching or sustaining a balanced body structure exists both in the body and mind? In fact, if you've repeatedly tried to lose some weight but never succeeded or you lose the weight and then regain the weight (and then some!), your thoughts and beliefs — not your diet — are most likely holding you back. This is because the extra weight is a result of the state of mind or sentiment. And the main reason people struggle to lose weight is that they ignore the implementation of adjustments in their subconscious mind in order to support their conscious objectives.

CHAPTER 4:

How Effective Is Hypnosis?

No Longer To Overeat

Seeking to make healthier choices and getting exercise are major elements of losing weight, but an effective fat loss in some instances also necessitates steering clear of sentimental and unintentional barriers that inhibit us from weight loss. Using hypnotherapy for losing weight takes a more comprehensive approach than if used for other health problems — it typically takes numerous meetings to evaluate the personal triggers of the person, rather than just one. Before hypnotherapy is conducted, the expert needs to discover out whether they are all day snackers and those who reach between meals in the refrigerator. Everyone is special, everybody can have their own addiction, so figuring it out requires a little while. You shut your eyes after five to six bites and remind yourself, 'that's enough,' so if you consume a bowl of food, you shut your eyes and suggest 'eat about half of what's in it.'

Cure Phobia within the Dental Profession

The drill's high-pitched whirl, the needle poke, or the humiliation by making somebody peek into your mouth is only a couple of the reasons people stop visiting the dentist. Although the industry is trying to utilize modern dental technologies to render a ride to the dentist's office less painful, dental discomfort affects between 10 to 20 percent of the world's population.

Fear has, for years, driven several of my patients from the dentist seat. Fear can originate from a traumatic dental encounter or learning from someone that has had a bad experience. Whatever the case, it may be debilitating because if it's conditioned, the subconscious will work in the default setting. To help clients overcome the discomfort about going to the dentist, neurolinguistic programming (NLP) is used that lets the brain "rewire" those thinking patterns to get past loops of negative thinking. NLP may be used to stop the fear and rewire the phobia to their own as they continue to experience fear regarding visiting the dentist.

Maintain Grief

Whether it is coping with a national disaster or a loved one's death, it may undermine the sense of grief or bereavement, triggering fear, insomnia, and depression. Letting yourself experience the pain by grieving improves your body and mind, like learning about your loved one's passing, taking care of your wellbeing, reaching out to those who have to cope with the tragedy, acknowledging your emotions and living the existence of the one you missed. The strategies to cope with the loss are psychological. Hypnotherapy can assist by offering constructive feedback to help deal with mourning feelings and help discover solutions to live with the suffering as time passes on. Professionals are helping people deal with suffering by setting a "timer" on grief and loss. Normally, when they're tired and emotionally exhausted from grieving, then they let the professional know.

Detain Tinnitus

As per the American Tinnitus Association, ticking, clicking, hissing, whooshing, or whistling noises that no one except you can hear are symptoms of tinnitus, a disease that 45 million Americans endure. Though hearing loss may be acute or continuous, most forms of the disorder may not have a cure. Treatment methods include hearing aids, behavioral counseling, sound therapy, and TMJ. Hypnosis is an alternative, as well. The mindset induces tinnitus; it tends to actually occur because the person expects that to happen, and the sound disappears even after you disable the idea of anticipating it.

More Tolerable Chemotherapy

Some of the first known examples of cancer patient hypnosis were in 1829 when M. Le Docteur Chapelain utilized hypnosis to alleviate breast cancer patients' pain. During a mastectomy, the doctor utilized hypnotherapy as a general anesthetic, and the woman was reported to be "calm and displayed excellent pain control" during the surgery. Although anesthesia is the favored method for surgery today, hypnosis often plays a part in cancer care and is sometimes used to relieve discomfort and distress as well as alleviate the side effects of treatment like vomiting and diarrhea. They help them mainly cope with the effects and help them improve how they handle stress. The therapist won't give them false optimism, but they place them in a safe position to help them recover. Cancer victims are sometimes moved from hospital to hospital, allowing them to feel as though they're merely a statistic. Therapists make unique tapes to which the patients listen during their procedure with treatment — it's a real interaction with a hypnotherapist that could go afar.

Boost Efficiency in Athletics

Michael Jordan, Tiger Woods, and Mike Tyson are really just a few other well-known elite athletes who have transformed their performance through the support of hypnotherapy. Athletes have often utilized hypnotherapy to remove stressful emotions, destress and calm the mind and body, and assist in improving attention and relaxation so that they might "be in the zone." This behavioral stimulation will enhance motivation, performance, and skill and extends to all types of performers, including those suffering from trauma and those only starting a sport. Many players go through a hypnotist to enhance their output when, in essence, they're trying to strengthen their minds. A hypnotist will transform the thought mechanism to convert negative behaviors into good ones. It requires a lot of cognitive toughness to be a productive golfer. 'You've got to adjust the understanding to experience, so you've got to approach the game psychologically.

Faster Recuperation from the Operation

Hypnosis is used to support post-surgery patients reduce their healing period and, in some situations, wean them off medication administered by the doctor. Thoughts and feelings flow through paths, so that's how patterns are formed. At first, it's only a route through the trees, so with the period the road gradually becomes a pit you can't get out of. Through hypnosis, the nervous system and brain are guided to take a different pathway.

Symptoms of Irritable Bowel Syndrome (IBS)

Scientific research has generally confirmed the effects of hypnosis on IBS. IBS is stomach pressure produced by the bowels, so hypnosis may help relieve symptoms like constipation, vomiting, so bloating. Often IBS may trigger other symptoms, such as nausea, exhaustion, back pain, and urinary issues.

How it tends to work: Hypnosis takes you into gradual recovery, offering calming thoughts and stimuli to combat the effects you encounter.

Weight Loss

Like with the prevention of smoking, there are currently not enough trials that would validate the efficacy of weight reduction hypnosis, while several researchers have observed moderate weight loss — around 6 pounds during 18 months — by hypnosis. If hypnosis has been used in conjunction with improvements in exercise and diet, it is typically most effective.

How it tends to work: When you're hypnotized, the emphasis is on the mind. This helps you more inclined to react and react to recommendations about improvements in your lifestyle, such as following a healthier diet or exercising regularly, which may promote weight loss.

Quit Cigarette Smoking

Cigarettes are not easy to give up. There are other ways to support quitting, such as prescribed drugs or the nicotine patch. Although the study is still around, several individuals have considered hypnosis to have enabled them to quit the problem of smoking.

Smoking reduction hypnosis performs better while you are practicing one on one with a hypnotist who will tailor the hypnosis treatments to fit your lifestyle.

How it tends to work: You need to really want to stop smoking in an attempt for hypnosis to function for quitting smoking. Hypnotherapy may be used in two forms. One of which is to help you identify a safe, successful alternative practice and then direct your subconscious toward the behavior instead of smoking. This could be like munching a stick of gum or going for a walk. The second is to prepare the subconscious to equate cigarettes with unpleasant stimuli, such as a bitter aftertaste in the mouth or a disgusting scent of smoke.

Anxiety

Relaxation methods — hypnosis included — will also relieve fear. Hypnosis appears to be most successful in patients whose distress is triggered by a specific disorder of wellbeing — such as cardiac failure — rather than generalized fear.

Hypnosis can also benefit if you are dealing with a phobia — a form of anxiety condition where you are deeply scared about something that doesn't pose a major danger.

How it helps: Hypnosis helps to relieve fear by stimulating the body to trigger its normal reaction to stimulation through utilizing an expression or nonverbal signal, slowing down breathing, reducing blood pressure, and trying to instill an improved feeling of wellbeing.

Problematic Sleep, Sleepwalking, and Insomnia

Hypnotherapy can be a valuable method whether you're sleepwalking or trying to fall and remain asleep. Hypnosis will calm you enough to allow you to sleep better if you have insomnia.

Hypnosis will also teach you to wake up anytime you hear your feet touch the floor to help you stop sleepwalking trysts, if you're a sleepwalker.

And if you only need to have a little more sleep, hypnosis will even assist with that. Learning the methods of self-hypnosis will improve the period of time you rest and the period of time you spend in deep sleep — the sort of sleep you need to wake up and feel refreshed.

How it works: visual signals place you in a trancelike environment, close to how you experience when you're so absorbed in a book or video that you don't realize what's happening around you. You'll fall asleep during hypnosis — or just after that —.

Severe Pain

Hypnosis may offer pain relief — such as during surgery, migraine headaches, or seizures with stress. And persistent depression can improve, too. Individuals with pain associated with conditions such as asthma, cancer, sickle cell anemia, and fibromyalgia — as well as people with lower back pain — can receive relief via hypnosis.

Why it works: Hypnosis will allow you to deal with pain and develop more self-control regarding suffering. However, findings show that hypnosis over extended stretches of time will achieve this successfully.

CHAPTER 5:

What Happens To Your Body During Hypnosis

As your breathing slows, your arms go limp and you feel weightless under the gentle lull of a hypnotic trance, your brain activity shifts too – and now, scientists uncovered three hallmarks of a hypnotized brain.

Researchers in the US scanned brains of 57 people during guided hypnosis and showed specific changes in activity and connectivity of just a few areas, such as those involved with brain-body connection. The results, published in Cerebral Cortex, could let clinicians better administer hypnosis for problems such as pain control, says senior author and Stanford University psychiatrist David Spiegel. Far from the realm of swinging pocket watches and clucking like a chicken on cue, hypnosis is a growing clinical treatment for a host of disorders such as phobias, post-traumatic stress disorder and pain in childbirth.

A typical hypnosis session starts with the patient and therapist discussing goals. The patient is then placed in a state of relaxed focus. The therapist retells the goals to the patient, who might imagine and visualize them. In patients easily hypnotized, such sessions are effective in reducing chronic pain and quitting smoking, for instance. But exactly what goes on in the brain during hypnosis isn't clear. To further muddy the waters, while some people are highly hypnotizable, others are almost impossible to put under.

So Spiegel, study lead author Heidi Jiang and colleagues wanted to find out what went on in the brain during hypnosis. They started by screening 545 healthy people for hypnotizability and picked the 36 who consistently scored highly and 21 who scored at the extreme low end.

The subjects' brain activity was measured using functional magnetic resonance imaging, a scanning technique that measures changes in blood flow to the brain. If a subject is listening to music, for instance, the fMRI will pick up blood rushing to the parts of the brain responsible for hearing and analyzing sound.

These subjects didn't listen to music, though – they were instructed to run through four exercises: let their mind rest and wander (called the resting-state scan), think about their day in great detail (memory control scan), or enter two different hypnotic states.

In the hypnosis exercises, subjects were told to look up, close their eyes, inhale deeply, exhale deeply and let their body "float", as if in a lake or in space.

For one exercise, they were told to imagine a time when they felt happiness, while in the other, imagine or remember a vacation or holiday.

Each subject did the four exercises once in random order, each of which was followed by an eight-minute fMRI scan.

'When you're really engaged in something, you don't really think about doing it – you just do it.' When they compared the hypnotizable group with the less susceptible, they found three main differences. The first was decreased activity in a part of the brain called the dorsal anterior cingulate in those highly hypnotizable.

That part of the brain is part of what's called the salience network and contributes to a person's self-awareness by integrating sensory, emotional and cognitive information. Less activity there equals less self-awareness, Spiegel says: "In hypnosis, you're so absorbed that you're not worrying about anything else."

Another clear signal in the hypnotizable was boosted connectivity between two other components of the salience network: the dorsolateral prefrontal cortex and insula. The insula is responsible for processing functions such as body control, emotion, empathy and time, while the dorsolateral prefrontal cortex is – among other things – involved in cognition, memory and decision-making.

During hypnosis, boosting the link between the two may help the brain control and process what's happening in the body.

Finally, they found less connectivity between the dorsolateral prefrontal cortex and the "default mode network" in the highly hypnotizable.

The default mode network comprises many areas throughout the brain and is active, as its name suggests, when a person's mind is wandering – it is involved in thinking about the self, the future and remembering the past.

Uncoupling from the dorsolateral prefrontal cortex gives rise to a disconnect between a person's actions and their awareness of those actions, Spiegel says: "When you're really engaged in something, you don't really think about doing it – you just do it."

This could let a person change behavior, as suggested by a clinician, without being self-conscious about it. Knowing how hypnosis changes the brain may help develop treatments for those less susceptible, Spiegel says – particularly through brain stimulation.

And while it's still very early days, simply knowing which brain regions and connections switch on or off during hypnosis is a big step towards that goal.

CHAPTER 6:

How Much Weight Can I Lose With Hypnosis?

W hen it comes to losing weight, you already know about the usual go-to professionals: doctors, nutritionists and dietitians, personal trainers, even mental health coaches. But there may be one you haven't quite thought of yet: a hypnotist. It turns out using hypnosis is another road people are venturing down in the name of weight loss. And typically, it's traveled after all the other last-ditch efforts (I see you, juice cleanses and fad diets) are tried and failed, says Greg Gurniak, a certified clinical and medical hypnotist practicing in Ontario. But it's not about someone else controlling your mind and making you do funny things while you're unconscious. "Mind control and losing control—aka doing something against your will—are the biggest misconceptions about hypnosis," says Kimberly Friedmutter, hypnotherapist and author of Subconscious Power: Use Your Inner Mind to Create the Life You've Always Wanted. "Because of how the entertainment industry portrays hypnotists, people are relieved to see I'm not wearing a black robe and swinging a watch from a chain."

You're also not unconscious when you experience hypnosis—it's more like a deep state of relaxation, Friedmutter explains. "It's simply the natural, floaty feeling you get before you drift off to sleep, or that dreamy sensation you feel as you wake up in the morning, before you're fully aware of where you are and what is surrounding you."

Being in that state makes you more susceptible to change, and that's why hypnosis for weight loss may be effective. "It's different from other methods because hypnosis addresses the cause and other contributing factors directly at the subconscious level in the person's mind, where their memories, habits, fears, food associations, negative self-talk, and self-esteem germinate," says Capri Cruz, Ph.D., psychotherapist and hypnotherapist and author of Maximize Your Super Powers. "No other weight loss method addresses the core issues at the root like hypnosis does."

But does hypnosis for weight loss work?

There isn't a ton of recent, randomized research available on the subject, but what is out there suggests that the method could be plausible. Early studies from the 90s found that people who used hypnosis lost more than twice as much weight as those who dieted without cognitive therapy. A 2014 study worked with 60 obese women, and found that those who practiced hypno-behavioral therapy lost weight and improved their eating habits and body image. And a small 2017 study worked with eight obese adults and three children, all of whom successfully lost weight, with one even avoiding surgery due to the treatment benefits, but of course none of this is conclusive.

Related Stories

Healthy Junk Food for Every Craving

The Healthiest Things to Order at Taco Bell

"The unfortunate factor is that hypnosis is not readily covered by medical insurance, so there isn't the same push for hypnosis studies as there is for pharmaceutical ones," Dr. Cruz says. But with the seemingly ever-increasing cost of prescription drugs, long lists of possible side effects, and the push for more natural alternatives, Cruz is hopeful hypnosis will soon receive more attention and research as a plausible weight loss approach.

Who should try hypnosis for weight loss?

The ideal candidate is, honestly, anyone who has trouble sticking to a healthy diet and exercise program because they can't seem to shake their negative habits, Gurniak says. Getting stuck in harmful habits—like eating the entire bag of potato chips instead of stopping when you're full—is a sign of a subconscious problem, he says.

Your subconscious is where your emotions, habits and addictions are located, Friedmutter says. And because hypnotherapy addresses the subconscious—instead of just the conscious—it may be more effective. In fact, a study analysis from 1970 found hypnosis to have a 93 percent success rate, with fewer sessions needed than both psychotherapy and behavioral therapy. "This led researchers to believe that, for changing habits, thought patterns, and behavior, hypnosis was the most effective method," Friedmutter says.

Hypnotherapy doesn't have to be used on its own, either. Gurniak says hypnosis can also be used as a compliment to other weight loss programs designed by professionals to treat various health conditions, be it diabetes, obesity, arthritis, or cardiovascular disease.

What can I expect during a treatment?

Sessions can vary in length and methodology depending on the practitioner. Dr. Cruz, for example, says her sessions typically last between 45 and 60 minutes, whereas Friedmutter sees weight loss patients for three to four hours. But in general, you can expect to lay down, relax with your eyes closed, and let the hypnotherapist guide you through specific techniques and suggestions that can help you reach your goals.

"The idea is to train the mind to move toward what is healthy and away from what is unhealthy," Friedmutter says. "Through client history, I am able to determine subconscious hitches that sent the client off their original blueprint of [health]. Just like we learn to abuse our bodies with food, we can learn to honor them."

It's likely that you'll experience deep relaxation, while still being aware of what's being said, Gurniak adds. "Someone in a hypnotic trance would describe it as in between being wide awake and asleep," he says. "They are fully in control and able to stop the process at any time, because you can only be hypnotized if you choose to. We work as a team to achieve a person's goal."

Of course, the number of sessions needed is totally dependent on your personal response to hypnosis. Some could see results in as few as one to three, Dr. Cruz says, while others could need anywhere from eight to fifteen sessions. And then again, it may not be effective for everyone.

Weight-loss hypnosis may help you shed an extra few pounds when it's part of a weight-loss plan that includes diet, exercise and counseling. But it's hard to say definitively because there isn't enough solid scientific evidence about weight-loss hypnosis alone.

Hypnosis is a state of inner absorption and concentration, like being in a trance. Hypnosis is usually done with the help of a hypnotherapist using verbal repetition and mental images.

When you're under hypnosis, your attention is highly focused, and you're more responsive to suggestions, including behavior changes that can help you lose weight.

A few studies have evaluated the use of weight-loss hypnosis. Most studies showed only slight weight loss, with an average loss of about 6 pounds (2.7 kilograms) over 18 months. But the quality of some of these studies has been questioned, making it hard to determine the true effectiveness of weight-loss hypnosis.

However, a recent study, which only showed modest weight loss results, did find that patients receiving hypnosis had lower rates of inflammation, better satiety and better quality of life. These might be mechanisms whereby hypnosis could influence weight. Further studies are needed to fully understand the potential role of hypnosis in weight management.

Weight loss is usually best achieved with diet and exercise. If you've tried diet and exercise but are still struggling to meet your weight-loss goal, talk to your health care provider about other options or lifestyle changes that you can make.

Relying on weight-loss hypnosis alone is unlikely to lead to significant weight loss, but using it as an adjunct to an overall lifestyle approach may be worth exploring for some people.

CHAPTER 7:

What Is True And False About Hypnosis?

Myth #1 – A trance inducer can control and power me to state or get things done without wanting to.

This is an exceptionally common MYTH that is totally off base. In spellbinding it is really the customer who is consistently in charge, not the subliminal specialist. An individual in the mesmerizing state decides their own degree of support simultaneously. Spellbinding can never be utilized to cause you to accomplish something that you would prefer not to do. Under entrancing you won't have the option to do anything which conflicts with your own qualities or convictions. Spellbinding isn't rest. It is in truth a condition of uplifted mindfulness where you know about everything that is going on around you. On the off chance that you are approached to plan something inadmissible for your qualities, your brain will basically dismiss it and you will come out of spellbinding right away.

Entrancing is utilized to fortify positive messages and debilitate or kill negative messages that are as of now in your inner mind. This makes it conceivable to impact a perpetual change in you when you are prepared to roll out the improvement. Truth be told, some portion of the principal meeting at Aldo Hypnosis is utilized to decide whether the customer sincerely wants the mentioned change. This assurance is made before the customer is ever placed into spellbinding. For instance, assume a customer reveals to me, "My spouse needs me to quit smoking. Would you be able to help?" The customer's selection of words presumably implies that he isn't yet by and by resolved to quit smoking. For this situation, spellbinding won't help this customer to quit smoking. At the end of the day, spellbinding can be utilized to make a change, however … just when the customer is truly prepared for the change. You may think about how stage trance inducers can make individuals to do the most crazy things. Truly every individual picked by the performer is a willing volunteer who consents to partake in the amusement, and is enthusiastic and ready to do these insane things. The stage trance inducer chooses just those volunteers who are generally anxious to proceed as they make certain to give the best amusement to the crowd.

To sum up, the subliminal specialist has no control over you at all and can't cause you to do anything without wanting to. All the trance inducer does is manage you into a mesmerizing state. The trance specialist isn't an ace, just a guide, and you are consistently in charge and mindful of what's going on. Basically, it is you, not the trance specialist, who makes entrancing work or not work.

Myth#2 – You can be made to uncover individual mysteries while under entrancing

The trance inducer has no influence over you by any stretch of the imagination, and can't cause you to get things done without wanting to. All spellbinding is extremely self-entrancing in that it is self-coordinated and self-controlled. Entrancing is conceivable just if there is a collaboration among you and your subliminal specialist. No one but you can choose to permit yourself to be mesmerized. Without your assent, it essentially can't occur. The trance inducer doesn't have any unique force which drives you to submit to their will. The trance specialist just aides you tenderly into an entrancing state, and feeds your sub cognizant psyche with painstakingly worded positive recommendations to assist you with achieving your objectives. In the event that you feel awkward with any of these recommendations, your psyche naturally dismisses them and you won't follow up on them.

Under entrancing, you are completely ready, in reality more ready than expected. The trance inducer can (with your consent) direct you to recall overlooked recollections. Be that as it may, regardless of whether you will decide to uncover them to the subliminal specialist is completely up to you.

Myth#3 – Only an individual with a powerless brain can be entranced.

This conviction comes about because of confusing "being spellbound" with being simple or having no determination. It is really the contrary that is valid. Entrancing requires insight and the ability to think.

Inspiration and participation are likewise fundamental for progress, none of which are handily accomplished by the frail willed or feeble leaning. Truth be told, individuals of decreased intellectual ability who can't focus, and individuals with certain genuine neurological conditions can't be mesmerized.

When all is said in done, individuals of better than expected knowledge and inventiveness which can focus well are the best possibility for spellbinding as they go into entrancing simpler and more profoundly than others. After the principal meeting most customers have direct experiential comprehension of the advantages of entrancing. This understanding encourages them, in the resulting meeting to enter quicker and all the more profoundly into the mesmerizing state.

Myth #4 – You may stall in a mesmerized state and not be able to wake up.

On the off chance that you are in entrancing and the trance specialist stops talking, your own psyche would pull you securely out of spellbinding in a few different ways. You would understand the trance inducer was done conversing with you and step by step rise up out of entrancing all alone. At the point when you open your eyes you would be totally wide awake, revived and feeling fine.

The other chance is that you would float into a short rest and afterward wake up regularly, totally conscious, feeling invigorated and alert. In either case a customer can generally come out of a mesmerizing state all alone. In the event that a crisis, for example, a fire or a seismic tremor, happens while you are in entrancing, you will consequently perceive the desperation of the circumstance and promptly wake to full sharpness.

Myth#5 – Hypnosis is risky

Bogus, with the exception of two explicit cases. An individual who experiences epileptic fits ought to never be spellbound, as all out unwinding may trigger an epileptic seizure. Another hazardous circumstance is on the off chance that you are driving or working hardware when tuning in to a spellbinding account. You could lose control of the hardware when you fall into an entrancing state, and cause harm to yourself as well as other people.

For every other person, spellbinding is a safe and normal procedure. If it's not too much trouble note that you MUST be in a sheltered and secure condition before tuning in to a spellbinding chronicle.

Entrancing is a regularly occurring state and truth be told, a great many people have unquestionably encountered some type of spellbinding in their day by day lives. In the event that you have ever wandered off in MYTH land, you have gone all through an entrancing state. While driving, have you at any point understood that you have no memory of the preceding a few minutes and that you have now driven past your exit? This is another case of self-incited entrancing where your cognizant brain was so occupied it felt that you really accomplished a mesmerizing state.

Your sub cognizant psyche at that point assumed responsibility for directing the wheel, brake and accelerator and thus kept you securely on the right path. Fortunately, this self-instigated spellbinding, however perilous, doesn't keep going too long and a great many people rapidly wake up from this state. On the off chance that you have ever gotten so profoundly engaged with a book or film that you were absent of your environmental factors, or on the off chance that you have forgotten about time while tuning in to an appealing and persuasive speaker, you have been in a light condition of spellbinding.

You ought to likewise not confuse entrancing for conditioning. Indoctrinating includes delayed times of outrageous physical pressure and distress to where in the end the casualty has a breakdown. A conditioned individual reacts like a robot to any order and is unequipped for systematic reasoning. Spellbinding, in actuality, is accomplished by helping the customer to get as amazingly agreeable and loose as could be expected under the circumstances. The target of spellbinding is accomplished with collaboration not blind compliance. The trance specialist isn't your chief or ace, the person works with you to assist you with accomplishing your objectives.

Myth #6 – Hypnosis manages the mysterious and is the Devil's work

The conviction that entrancing is the "Devil's work" has shockingly been made and reinforced by convincing urban myths and furthermore, by "B grade" Hollywood horror films.

Most religions have acknowledged the way that entrancing can achieve durable, unmistakable mending advantages to a person. The Roman Catholic Church was among the first to acknowledge and perceive spellbinding as a mending method in 1957. Most other significant religions have additionally acknowledged spellbinding and don't forbid their individuals from looking for and using entrancing. Hypnotherapy is coded as a calling by the U.S. Division of Labor, with "hypnotherapist" recorded as code number 079.157.010 in the Federal Government Titles of Legitimate Occupations. Spellbinding is a normally happening state that people float all through throughout a day. Whenever we concentrate so eagerly on something, so the sensation of our environmental factors become dull, we are encountering a type of spellbinding. This without anyone else is neither acceptable nor awful. An expert trance inducer, easily manages you into a mesmerizing state, and afterward introduces wanted results into your subcognizant brain. The trance specialist may likewise expel restricting convictions from your subcognizant that shield you from accomplishing your objectives and wants. After the meeting, the subcognizant psyche continues attempting to achieve those ideal results. The magnificence of entrancing is that after the meeting, no further cognizant movement is important to achieve the ideal changes throughout your life. This is the reason here and there, spellbinding seems to work like enchantment.

Myth #7 – Hypnotists have mystical forces

A trance specialist is an ordinary individual who has gotten proficient in preparing to see how the cerebrum forms data and how the subcognizant functions. The subliminal specialist has aced the specialty of spellbinding and can easily manage you into an entrancing state. There is nothing supernatural about hypnosis. In truth, any grownup who has adequate want and persistence to learn can gain the imperative abilities to turn into a hypnotherapist.

A decent subliminal specialist won't just guide you easily and rapidly into spellbinding, however it will likewise embed positive proposals in your inner mind. These proposals will expel, debilitate and supplant constraining convictions and will push you to rapidly accomplish your objectives and targets.

CHAPTER 8:

Pros and Cons for Hypnosis for Weight Loss

Whether you are trying to stop smoking, lose weight or be more assertive at work, you may be considering hypnotherapy as a path to your long-term goals. The proponents of hypnotherapy make a lot of promises, and many people claim to have enjoyed great success after being hypnotized.

As with any type of alternative medical treatment, it is important to weigh the pros and cons of hypnotherapy carefully. There are many hypnotherapy pros and cons to consider before you undergo your first hypnotherapy session.

Here are some of the potential benefits of incorporating hypnotherapy into your overall wellness program:

Hypnotherapy can be used to address a number of physical and emotional issues, including fears and phobias, drinking and smoking, and overeating and weight loss. The cost of a single hypnotherapy session can be quite low, especially if you attend a traveling seminar or work with an established hypnotherapist. A good hypnotherapist can tailor your treatments to your specific needs and address any unique issues you may have. This customization can increase the efficacy of the treatment significantly.

Hypnotherapy sessions are usually short, about one to two hours in length. That means less time out of your day and more time to work on your specific issues. Hypnotherapy is convenient. No matter where you live, chances are there are a number of hypnotherapists operating in your area. The convenience factor is a major advantage of hypnotherapy compared to other forms of treatment.

Hypnotherapy is not the right choice for everyone. Here are a few potential drawbacks:

Not everyone is receptive to hypnotherapy. If you are one of the small number of people who 'can't be hypnotized', this type of therapy will not work for you. You may require repeated hypnotherapy sessions to achieve long-term relief from the problems you are addressing. The need for repeat hypnotherapy sessions can drive up your costs.

Your hypnotherapy sessions will probably not be covered by your health insurance program. That could mean high out-of-pocket costs. Hypnotherapists vary in their skills and experience. It can be challenging to find one who is effective, affordable and receptive to your specific needs.

If you are looking for a way to change your life, break your bad habits and lead a healthier lifestyle going forward, there are many reasons to incorporate alternative treatments, such as hypnotherapy, into your plan. Hypnotherapy can play a positive role in everything from stopping smoking and avoiding overeating to curing deep-seated fears and phobias, but it is important to find and choose a therapist who can tailor a treatment plan just for you.

Understanding the pros and cons of hypnotherapy, and how to make the treatment more effective, is an important first step toward improving your long-term health. If the pros of hypnotherapy outweigh the cons, now may the perfect time to explore this unique form of alternative medicine. If weight loss is your goal, you might consider reading a free hypnosis weight loss script and listening to the accompanying .mp3 as an introduction.

CHAPTER 9:

The Right State of Mind
To Benefit From Hypnosis

G o to any gym in the main seven day stretch of January, and it is packed - you can scarcely move in there and need to queue for each machine. It is brimming with individuals beginning on their new year's goals to get in shape and get fit, be that as it may, return only two or three weeks after, and you will probably just discover half the same number of individuals at a similar rec center.

How can it be that such a large number of individuals start with well-meaning goals yet neglect to finish or adhere to their weight reduction plans?

You have presumably been there yourself - something occurs, maybe you step on the scales and are stunned at your weight, and this inspires you to step vigorously, to make goals and an arrangement to get fitter - regardless of whether it is eating more beneficial meals, eating less junk food, or doing some activity. The initial days, or the initial meetings at the exercise center are extraordinary - you feel awesome, animated, persuaded in any case. At that point the underlying energy begins to wear off you gauge yourself again, and there is a chance you have a cheat dinner to comfort yourself in a little while you have slipped back to your old ways. In the event that no one but we could keep this underlying degree of energy, this buzz for more - think about the outcomes we would accomplish on the off chance that we kept this degree of duty until the end of time.

So Why Don't We?

Indeed, everything relates back to your inner mind psyche and how you have been modified throughout the years.

You have 2 out of the three required components for progress - cognizant idea (for example needing to get more fit, and putting forth a cognizant attempt to arrange for what to do), and cognizant activity (for example beginning your eating routine, or visiting the rec center and so on), yet you are feeling the loss of the help of your inner mind - it isn't adjusted to your objectives - where it counts there are negative considerations, restricting convictions, and negative examples of conduct which keep you down, prevent you from adhering to your weight reduction plans and cause you to return to your old, natural propensities. The main explanation individuals fall flat is on the grounds that they neglect to make changes in their psyche brain to help their cognizant objectives. Their psyche minds let them down and keep them down. This is something that transpires all somewhat; it is part molding, part development of our propensities, and part protection component. For instance - in the event that you are overweight all things considered, you have been for quite a while - you have since a long time ago settled examples of pondering food, examples of conduct concerning exercise, convictions, different preferences about food and exercise, all of which you know about, and are typical to you. Breaking these examples of conduct and changing your points of view can be troublesome. On a psyche level, you are agreeable, secure, and safe with your present personal conduct standards - your inner mind opposes these progressions as it conflicts with what it knows, and it does this to protect you. A major change in your life leaves you uncovered, and exposed to bigger disappointment - in the event that it can return you to your standard examples of reasoning and conduct (which it sees as proficient and typical) at that point, it is protecting you. This is acceptable in certain circumstances - maybe where your inner mind psyche would trigger dread and nerves even with peril or hazard - to prevent you from tumbling off a bluff edge, or attempting something outrageous which could get you injured anyway. When these equivalent subliminal standards are applied in a weight reduction or individual change setting they can be harming - they can prevent you from rolling out a positive improvement.

Instructions to Rewire Your Subconscious Mind!

There are a few different ways you can target and revamp your psyche mind and your internal most convictions. However, one of the best, and a technique which is developing in prominence, is the utilization of subconscious sound.

The subconscious sound may have gained notoriety for being somewhat puzzling, yet it is a straightforward idea truly. It chips away at the standard of spoken positive assertions - yet they are recorded and moved to a higher sound recurrence, so you don't perceptibly hear the proposals - anyway, they do get caught on the edge of your recognition by your inner mind-brain, and they are handled and put away as should be expected.

Along these lines, your inner mind is revamped from the back to front - step by step and normally, and simply like utilizing spellbinding or saying positive confirmations yourself the progressions do last.

With respect to weight reduction, explicitly subtle cues will expand your conviction that you can get fit; they will cause you to feel extraordinary - like this time it is no doubt that you will adhere to your arrangements. They will keep your roused for more, cause you to appreciate and anticipate the activity, and reinforce your self-discipline to assist you with opposing enticements and remain submitted. They will essentially begin to impart in you the kinds of convictions shared by individuals who normally eat steadily, who are not enticed by greasy food, and who appreciate working out.

When you have these kinds of convictions and perspectives, your endeavors will be changed, and you will lose the weight normally and have the option to keep it off for good.

You and your mind are always in complete control

The vast majority of us are creatures of habit. We purchase similar nourishments from a similar supermarket, set up similar plans again and again, and live inside our own recognizable schedules. Be that as it may, in case you're not kidding about eating more advantageously and getting in shape, you have to shake it up, change those awful dietary patterns, and begin considering your eating routine and way of life.

Eating a more beneficial eating routine might be scary from the outset. In any case, when you see with your own eyes how great it causes you to feel - and how great sound food can taste - you have a superior possibility of succeeding. After some time, your inclinations will change, and longings for terrible for-you nourishments will blur away.

You've filled your kitchen with healthy foods and planned careful meals to lose weight. But your diet still isn't working. Sound familiar? Unfortunately, it may be more than your pantry that needs an overhaul. You may also need to learn how to break bad eating habits to get real results.

Not sure where to begin? The first step is to identify the behaviors that are doing the most damage. Scan this list of everyday eating habits that add empty calories, unwanted fat, or added sugar to your diet. See which unhealthy habits look familiar. It's possible that you're not even aware that these behaviors have an impact on your waistline.

Calling Your Habit Bad

The primary propensity you might need to address is the language you use to portray your eating schedules. Simply taking out "awful" can be a little positive development.

Regardless of whether you are working with an expert or changing undesirable propensities all alone, a moderate and delicate methodology is ideal. Target each propensity in turn and set an objective to locate straightforward substitution conduct to support good dieting and health.

Steps To Fix Bad Eating Habits

Here are six stages to assist you with disposing of your old, unfortunate habits and then replacing them with new ones:

1. Make Baby Strides. Rolling out little improvements in your eating routine and way of life can improve your wellbeing just as trim your waistline. A few recommendations from the specialists:

• Start every day with a nutritious breakfast.

• Get 8 hours of rest every night, as weariness can prompt indulging.

• Eat your suppers situated at a table, without interruptions.

• Eat more suppers with your partner or family.

• Train yourself to eat when you're extremely eager and stop when you're easily full.

- Lessen your portion estimates by 20%, or surrender second helpings.

- Attempt lower-fat dairy items.

- Make sandwiches with whole grain bread and spread them with mustard rather than mayo.

- Change to bistro au lait, utilizing solid espresso and hot skim milk rather than a cream.

- Eat a nutritious supper or nibble at regular intervals.

Become More Mindful: One of the initial moves toward overcoming terrible dietary patterns is giving more consideration to whatever you're eating and drinking. Become acquainted with texture and taste, and begin to pay heed to all that you put into your mouth. When you become increasingly mindful of what you're eating, you'll begin to acknowledge how you have to improve your eating routine—a few people do well by keeping food journals.

Make an Arrangement: Be Specific. How are you going to begin eating more natural products each day? Getting to the exercise center all the more regularly? Illuminate your choices. For instance: Plan to take a few organic products to work each day for snacks, stock up on oat and natural product for speedy morning meals, and go to the exercise center while in transit to work three times each week.

Tackle a New Mini-Goal Each Week: These smaller than normal advances will, in the long run, mean significant change. For instance, if you want to eat more vegetables, reveal to yourself you'll attempt one new veggie every week until you discover some you truly appreciate. Or on the other hand, search for simple approaches to include one more serving of vegetables to your eating routine every week until you arrive at your objective. Take a stab at garnishing your lunch sandwich with cuts of cucumbers, or fixing your dinnertime pizza with sun-dried tomatoes and mushrooms.

Be Realistic: Try not to expect a lot from yourself too early. It takes about a month for any new activity to become propensity. Unwavering mindsets always win in the end - alongside a portion of watchfulness.

Practice stress management: center around managing worry through exercise, unwinding, reflection, or whatever works for you, so you don't fall once more into those negative behavior patterns during times of pressure or use food to assist you with adapting to the circumstance.

CHAPTER 10:

Hypnosis Fundamentally Changes Your Mindset Toward Food

For most dieters or exercise enthusiasts, one has to undergo a series of rigorous training or workouts in order to achieve the desired weight. Even the idea of drifting straight into a state of unconsciousness and wake up having no cravings whatsoever seems to be a myth to them. What they probably do not know is that Hypnosis is not a new thing – it has been widely used in overcoming phobias and changing a lot of behaviors (e.g., compulsive eating, smoking, etc.).

Weight Loss and Hypnotherapy

Also referred to as weight loss hypnotherapy, this practice has been used more than people could even realize. Perhaps what you think that about Hypnosis are things like what you regularly see on TV. People are being asked to bark like a dog with just a single snap of the fingers. Mind you; this is actually far from what hypnotherapy is all about.

In reality, Hypnosis comes with a far extensive reach in terms of positive results. It is being utilized in a wide scope of weight-related treatments, such as bulimia and binge eating, and many more. Even more so, this therapeutic tool helps treat trigger symptoms, with anxiety being the most recognized one.

If you're unconvinced by the prowess of Hypnosis – including its ability to assist you to shed some weight – then you've got come to the proper place. Here are some of its many benefits:

•   Discourages You from Eating Extra Food or Treats

Hypnosis is understood for its mind conditioning strategy, which, in one method or another, gives you the power to transition faraway from horrors of eating snacks and/or other unhealthy food. Once you undergo Hypnosis, your mind starts to veer away from the idea of devouring your usual sweets, cakes, or chocolates. Basically, it retrains your brain in an attempt to visualize what your idea future in terms of body shape and weight should be.

•   Fundamentally Changes Your Mindset Towards Food

By essence, Hypnosis works during a way that it places an educative suggestion into your subconscious. The sole purpose is to change your habits for the betterment of your overall well-being. When Hypnosis is employed for weight loss, your hypnotherapist can change your mindset towards food, also as you consider portion size and what triggers you to munch some delicacies.

• Automates Your Mind to Eat the Right Food

As mentioned, Hypnosis spots an educative recommendation into your psyche. Along these lines, in the realm of weight reduction, your hypnotherapy will make you believe that picking the correct food is – and consistently will be – your main objective. You won't accept fad diets or effectively entice yourself to gorge. You will even be astounded by the way that you scarcely have the desire to eat desserts and cakes, just to give some examples.

• Inspires You To Feel Good About Having To Eat Less

This is arguably the simplest advantage of using Hypnosis for weight loss. With it, you are able to move forward with the right portion size for your meals without having to worry about being hungry again. Keep in mind that when it involves weight gain, incorrect portion sizes tend to be the most important contributor.

There are many reasons why diets do not work, and they have absolutely nothing to do with the amount of food we put into our mouths.

How many times have you thought about changing your weight? Your mind goes into action with the thinking, "I will eat less food - then the weight will drop off!", right? Well, no - that actually is wrong.

We all understand that eating less and increasing our daily exercise will result in weight loss, so why aren't we all the size and shape we want to be? Why is the diet industry raking in billions of pounds every single year from people dieting over and over again? Many people have the mindset that while they are on a diet, they will lose weight – so, on an unconscious level, the negative belief and myth is that when you're not on a diet, the weight will go back on. This creates a vicious cycle in the nightmare world of the diet. In fact, the opposite can happen; dieting can actually stop you from achieving your goal.

There is a part of your mind that creates a resistance; the more you think about something, the harder it is to let it go. Therefore, you're saying, "I will not eat that cake," and you actually hear, "eat the cake." So, what if we change that to "eat the cake in moderation"? You let go of the resistance side of the battle, replacing it with the belief that will power alone will tell you when to stop. However, despite the fact that you consciously really know exactly what you need to do, your body is so used to the yo-yo dieting effect that it picks up the message that you are destined to fail once again as no lifestyle changes have been made. More importantly, if any have been made, they will not last long-term. However, all is not lost. With Hypnosis, the changes can be long-lasting as hypnotherapy works with your unconscious mind, integrating positive thoughts to obtain the desired results that will remain firmly fixed deep in your unconscious mind.

Stress and anxiety can also play a major role in your ability to reach and maintain your desired weight. We all know that it is nearly impossible to eliminate stress completely from our hectic lives. However, it's possible to manage that stress during a very comfortable natural healthy way using Hypnosis and as many people turn to food for comfort when stressed or anxious, using hypnosis techniques can help you learn how to control stress and not allow it to affect other parts of your life (such as achieving your goal to get be the weight you want to be!). There are so many other factors that affect the way we eat and why we struggle to reduce our weight

CHAPTER 11:

Self-Hypnosis To Help You Control Food Cravings

In life, there are desserts, snacks, pralines, and sausage. If we do not keep a cool head, we crack. And we regret it almost every time. Good news: the shield is within us. Practicing self-hypnosis is sort of changing your point of view. Take a step back as soon as the urge appears. Try to observe yourself, as if you were seeing yourself from above, and put things in perspective. Sometimes we rush on a lemon tart as if our life depended on it. But this is NEVER the case!

Aperitif, a weapon of massive gluttony. It is surely the most critical caloric situation. We arrive at a party, hungry after a long day, and sit strategically next to our favorite crisps. France Verheyden created "Maig'rire," a somewhat special method to keep the line. Specialized, among others, in meditation, Hypnosis, mindfulness, and positive psychology, she developed her techniques to change her habits, little by little. She came to the editorial office, and she taught us a self-hypnosis technique to fight against aperitifs.

Concretely, how does this happen? We settle down comfortably, we close our eyes, and we breathe. Then we put ourselves in a situation. There is a table full of filth. Mentally, we put a shadow on the chips, and we diffuse a bright light on our friends. Just to remember that if we accepted the invitation, it was not to stock up on saturated fatty acids but to spend some quality time with friends. The goal? Understand that friends come first and move away from the aperitif automatically.

Losing weight and controlling your food impulses with Hypnosis and self-hypnosis: how it works

We all dream more or less to lose weight as if by magic and to maintain our healthy weight over time! And above all, to no longer repeatedly crave for the same foods that are not necessarily good for our waist line.

We all know the yoyo effect of diets. Can losing weight with Hypnosis be sustainable? We organize 13 self-hypnosis workshops that deal with weight and bulimia problems. Food is a primary spring, and many things are attached to it, there is emotional, anxiety, stress, the emotional void to be filled. And one person is not the other facing food. But a person who wants to lighten a few pounds and who has no other related problems, who are just greedy or who eats poorly, will be able to regain possession of his body through group workshops of self-hypnosis.

How does it work?

I called it "The Pleasure Diet,"; but ultimately, this "diet" only bears the name, it has absolutely nothing to do with other diets, we should even call it "Pleasure Strategy"! This series of workshops is centered on a small book, "The paradoxical diet" of doctor Giorgio Nardone. In this book, doctor Nardone traces seven problems that maintain and lead to excess weight. And proposes each time a solution, a strategy to eat three times a day, and do not eat between meals at all. This is a very ingenious little book which, once we have been able to integrate it completely makes you slim down in an ideal and natural way since there is no longer any spirit of restriction: you regulate yourself, and self-hypnosis techniques strongly support this new eating behavior.

Guilt and food is something everyone knows!

Yes, because we eat "with our head" in the vast majority of cases, which always leads to a report of prohibition, transgression, inappropriate or excessive behavior. Guilt is the feeling that cuts the body the most. One has a mental pleasure from the transgression, which is very powerful but which then turns into guilt into a feeling of failure. Whereas when you really eat with your body, with all your senses, you allow yourself what you want. There are no more restrictions since there are no more excesses! And no more guilt.

We fantasize about all the pralines that we could swallow, but we know we can't do it, so we get frustrated directly. The result, we spoil the pleasure of eating two because we would like three, and we forbid it! While one could eat one in self-hypnosis with infinite pleasure, which then is more than enough. Thanks to self-hypnosis, we are in authorization without any more idea of restriction. This is what makes it work! Because when you are aware of the pleasure of eating, you become aware of the moment when the pleasure stops or decreases; this is called satiety, it is then easy to stop eating. Often many people say that it is too good to be true and don't even think about trying. The whole goal of self-hypnosis, in this case, is to re-tame your body, to be in bodily well-being, which leads to a motivation to lose weight naturally.

How does it work practically?

After becoming familiar with self-hypnosis and gaining confidence, you will go into self-hypnosis, and you then ask yourself and make the most of all the bites of this much-desired food. It starts with the eyes, you touch it with your lips, you feel it, you touch it with your tongue, you feel it in your mouth, you taste it, you breathe it, and it all happens in full consciousness, focusing on every sensation. Then you swallow the bite, and then you open your eyes. To look again at your favorite food and wonder if you still want it. If so, then you start the self-hypnosis exercise again. All this happens slowly; in the rhythm proper to Hypnosis, and brings a unique perception of the food.

CHAPTER 12:

Defeating Procrastination and Forming Great Habits

Welcome to this led meditation, which will help conquer procrastination. If you haven't used a guided meditation or hypnosis tape previously, understand what is happening to your body throughout this account. When you are in the state of self-hypnosis, you are not asleep, nor are you oblivious. You're exceptionally aware of your environmental factors, and nothing can force you into doing anything you would prefer not to. So don't stress over any external distractions or commotions because you will before long have the option to relax totally. You are always in full oversight of yourself. I will say a progression of prompts; you can hear the recommendations and prompts as you wish.

Allow yourself to absorb the proposals without intuition or attempting to analyze them. And don't stress if your mind drifts off elsewhere. You will even now gain a positive result from the prompts, and if you end up concentrating on different thoughts, you can gradually remind yourself to concentrate just on my voice and what I am saying. And don't stress if you don't think you are "getting it" or doing it right, especially if this is your first time. Allow yourself to feel comfortable. While sitting or resting, take a full breath and as you exhale, let your eyes close and imagine a tree root connected to the base of your spine.

Visualize the root traveling through the focal point of the earth and anchor that root in the earth's core. You're doing great. Allow the center to expand to a size that's comfortable for you. Release any pressure, anxiety, or negativity or overabundance energy down that root, and you can release any incomplete activities or any undesired individuals who may want your attention, or interest. Release these down the root. Acknowledge any thoughts that may come into your mind and until further notice allow some down your establishing root. Take another full breath and hold that breath and exhale through your mouth with a moan, relaxing, much more profoundly, and feeling calm. Take another full breath. Again, comfortably filling your lungs, holding the breath, and exhaling, allow that remaining pressure and strain to stream out of your body. You don't have to hear any outside sounds or anyone else's voices at present. Appreciate the solace of drifting into relaxation. This solace, your solace, this is the most important part of the procedure. So allow yourself to give up and relax and now center your awareness on the muscles at the top of your head and feel a relieving wave of relaxation spilling out of the highest point of your head, down over your forehead, and gradually streaming down into your eyebrows, moving around the sides of your eyes, and delicately caressing your eyes with no difficulty. As you feel yourself gradually drifting further and more profound, allowing your ears to concentrate only on the sound of my voice then feel yourself drifting further. Feel that wave of relaxation descending into your cheeks and the muscles softening down a bit at a time. Much the same as ice as it dissolves into water, your muscles are gradually getting liquid as the muscles around your mouth relax and that relaxation streams into your jaw and the mouth. Your tongue and your teeth may shiver marginally. This is normal.

Allow yourself to proceed with a wave of relaxation, streaming from the highest point of your head, down and to the back of your head. Gradually passing around your ears and temples, and on down into your neck muscles. Muscles start to dissolve and become liquid. Continue feeling yourself drifting further and more profound with each breath you take. You'll feel more relaxed, and as you relax completely, all outside sounds, clamors, even your thoughts, cause you to continue drifting, further and more profoundly.

And let that smoothness stream down into your shoulders and allow it to expand your shoulders as you breathe. Allow your muscles to give up completely. Notice how considerably more relaxed you are now than you were a few minutes ago? Your body feels heavier than it did some minutes ago. This is all right. As this wave of solace and relaxation streams across your shoulders and down into your arms, you need to feel the relaxation moving into each muscle. As you relax and let go, feel the muscles softening like ice into water, and relax your shoulders and the back of your neck at this moment. That warm, delicate, shivering inclination moves around and down to your elbows, down into your forearms and now hovering around your wrists—the relaxation and solace and how it eased down onto your hands. Naturally, feel it from the very tips of your fingers. The more relaxed you feel, the increasingly slow your breaths will be. Allow all the stress and pressure to drain out the tips of your steady fingers as you relax and let go. And since the wave of relaxation spreads from your shoulders down into the muscles of your back all this solace and disorder will fill no useful need to your body. As you relax and drift further, you will feel that wave move down your back and inside your chest muscles. Consider yourself relaxing and drifting significantly deeper. That wave of relaxation streams around your waist now and into your lower half. Gradually moving and streaming down from your hips and into your thighs, and you will feel those muscles liquefying as you allow yourself to continue relaxing. You may feel pleasant shivering starting at the highest point of your head, streaming down through your entire body. This is your wave of relaxation moving through your muscles, and as this wave of relaxation spreads down to your thighs, down around your knees, bathing your knees without breaking a sweat. Down into your calves, feel these muscles dissolving down completely as you relax and go further and feel that relaxation is streaming around your ankles. Gradually circling your ankles without breaking a sweat, this wave moves down to the impact points and of your feet, streaming tenderly underneath onto the bottoms of your feet and then moving down to the tips of your toes. And now allow any remaining stress to transfer out from the finish of your feet. Now all your throbbing and pains that filled no helpful need, are no longer with your body. In only a few seconds, I will count down from five. And with each number, your relaxation level will instantly increase. Try not to battle this, don't constrain it, let it happen. Here we go. Five: continue breathing and feel yourself sinking further and more profound down. Four: you are so relaxed at this point. Three: existing and giving up. It feels so great to give up easily. Two: Getting much closer now, presently, peacefully, comfortably relaxed, and One: You have risen in a beautiful black void. This isn't someplace on Earth. You can call this "space" if you will.

Because you are floating through here, you see beams of light all around you; these are stars, except not the stars you know from seeing them on Earth. They are stars from above, beautiful energy sources which light up your surroundings. You are safe in this place; you can allow your cognizant mind to be open up to fresh ideas. These fresh ideas will facilitate positive changes in your life. Positive changes will shape fresh habits, and it will strengthen these habits to create another better you. In a second, you'll pivot and notice another rendition of yourself existing in this same space. You take a look at this variant, and although you physically appear to be identical. You feel like something is different. Can you tell yet? Take a second to examine it. Ah, you have it.

The individual standing opposite of you is your procrastinating self. The self that says, "don't stress, you'll get to it," You can sense that this isn't who you genuinely are, or who the universe wants you to be. But it's all right. That side of you has honest goals. They want the absolute best. They're a stickler of sorts. So, we can understand why it's hard for them to begin. Maybe you're in school presently. And your procrastinating self wants to get an "A" so badly on that venture. They never begin. But your new, motivated self realizes it's all right to go out, accomplish the work, and get a B+.

It may not be great, but it's finished. The same goes if you're an author. Your procrastinating self has been considering composing this novel throughout recent years. As Stephen King said, the best way to be a decent writer is by writing.

So, your motivated self realizes that shown improvement over time. Whatever your old self has been procrastinating on, you understand that your new self has the total and complete ability to do it. And while you're procrastinating, you may disregard the unpleasant task, but your motivated self knows exactly how to tackle it head-on.

Your newly motivated self is operating on a more significant level than your procrastinating self. You are somebody who resolves tasks, regardless of how unpleasant or uncomfortable they may appear from the beginning. I want to acquaint you with another idea. I call this one eating an elephant creepy crawly. Your motivated self realizes what your Elephant Beetle is; it's that task you continue putting off—The one that haunts you and sits on your shoulder all day long, reminding you it needs to be completed regardless of how much you would prefer not to do it. Your procrastinating self wants to flee from this elephant insect. But your new motivated self makes it your need to complete the first thing. So you are currently immersed by a sense of wanting to dispose of the weight; the weight which carries you through the rest of the day, regardless of what else is tossed at you.

Efficiency breeds profitability, and the self-satisfaction you get from it can't be beaten. Your new motivated self-starts every day by finishing your elephant insect task. After that, everything else you do for the day will appear to be so easy in comparison. Something different will happen to you—something you probably won't expect. You'll out of nowhere, be filled with more energy. Individuals will admire you. Some may even ask what your secret is... And you'll say, "I said farewell to my procrastinating self and embraced my motivated self" It was that straightforward. Take a second to bask in the greatness of your new motivated self because you have earned this second, each moment. Continue breathing through this second. You may even feel a slight shivering sensation on your skin. This is your body elevating itself to a more elevated level of consciousness. This is the level you will keep on operating for the rest of your life. It's a beautiful place because you earned your spot here. Simply take it all in for a second.

Pause For 1 Minute

Now, before we move on, I want you to do something you probably won't expect. I want you to excuse your procrastinating self. Be caring for them because they aren't lazy. They have recently concentrated their endeavors on something different. You can say farewell to your procrastinating self because you have out-developed them. Continue breathing and absorbing what it means to be your new higher self.

CHAPTER 13:

Use Self-Hypnosis to Fulfill Your Objectives

Y ou can use self-hypnosis to change many things in your life. You may use self-hypnosis to suppress weak memory-related negative emotions. You can use self-hypnosis to eliminate harmful beliefs, create new ones, and reach goals. So, if self-hypnosis is so strong, why do some people get no results from it?

Well, the simple answer is that they don't correctly use self-hypnosis!

To get the most out of a self-hypnosis session, you need to know why you are using it. Once you attempt self-hypnosis, you must have a purpose because the only thing you get from it is deep relaxation. Set the goal of self-hypnosis.

The goal of self-hypnosis should be concise and accurate. In writing down your declaration of intent, you solidify the concept of what you want in your mind and offer something to work in your subconscious mind. You are developing a target of self-hypnosis!

Make sure that you do not include what you do not want in any program of self-hypnosis. Make your goal for self-hypnosis positive and assertive of success. For example, saying something like "I'm no longer overweight" or "I don't have unpaid bills anymore" isn't how you should express your goal of self-hypnosis. If you focus on not being overweight, your mind produces an overweight image. If you think you don't have any unpaid bills, you need to think about unpaid bills first. That's true of everything in life, but in self-hypnosis, it becomes incredibly significant!

Pictures work with the mind! We want you to think about your kitchen to illustrate this point. Where is the cooking pot? Do you own a fridge? What color are these? Was the door open to the right or the left?

Can you see why you must call up a visual memory of your home to answer these questions?

Therefore, you must create a written statement that includes only the things you want to have, and it must not concentrate on the things you don't want to experience anymore. Examples of using positive statements will be "I reached my perfect weight with ease" instead of "I am not overweight anymore."

By following this advice, you make sure that only meaningful images form in your mind. When you recall these images during self-hypnosis, you instruct your subconscious mind to help you create them.

You will be more prepared now that you have your written plan of what you expect from your self-hypnosis sessions. You can re-program your mind during a self-hypnosis session by creating a specific, detailed image of what you want.

You do not need to make any effort in order to create this image, because this book will help you. Change the visual scene until it is what you want it to be. Keep adjusting it until it just makes you feel good.

Together with the positive emotions, the written statement and mental picture become your blueprint for success which you will program into your mind during self-hypnosis.

There are many excellent self-hypnosis recordings available for different needs (and a multitude of poor ones too). It should be relatively straightforward to find one that fits your needs once you have your purpose. Nonetheless, you should obey the self-hypnosis script below if you want to attempt self-hypnosis without the assistance of a recording. Practice self-hypnosis every day until you meet your goals.

Benefits of Self-Hypnosis

The advantages of self-hypnosis are virtually infinite. Every person is unique and under hypnosis, they respond differently. Thus, the benefits of an individual's self-hypnosis can vary. It all depends on what outcomes you want to achieve, and how far you want to go.

We will emphasize that self-hypnosis is not a magic pill. The improvements that you foresee aren't going to happen overnight. Nevertheless, that also makes change quick and enjoyable. Making positive improvements in your life is like a helping device.

A trainer helps you improve your game in sports. The best coach in the world can't help you if you don't put in the time and practice. To be a better athlete, you have to make a point to work at your game. To become a better sportsman, you have to shape certain behaviors and develop individual attitudes.

Likewise, self-hypnosis helps you develop the values, attitudes, habits, and behaviors that will trigger successful subconscious-level changes. It will also contribute to the desired outcomes that you wish to achieve.

The most fundamental benefits of self-hypnosis are the development and formation of supportive beliefs and behaviors, which will lead to desired changes.

Let's consider then the core benefits of self-hypnosis:

Relaxation and Controlling Stress

Whether you believe that self-hypnosis works for you or not, you'll undoubtedly enjoy relaxing when you're in a state of trance. If you can obtain some measurable gain from hypnosis, that is relaxation. When you're under hypnosis, your mind and body will be relaxed. Relaxation is beneficial in itself to avoid stress-related illnesses that we face in today's world.

When you're under hypnosis, relax. The following physiological changes happen:

- The heart slows down to its normal rhythm and starts to rest.

- There is a reduction in blood pressure.

- There's ample blood supply for all of your muscles and organs.

- Breathing slows down, which reduces your oxygen requirement.

All of the above results in the efficient control of stress and anxiety, increased creativity, a sense of calmness, and stronger concentration. The brain also causes your body to release endorphins that lead to a sense of wellbeing and happiness.

Breakdown/Depression

Depression is mostly acquired behavior. Only a minority of people have a genetic make-up that makes them easy prey to depression. You can catch the flu or cold, but you cannot catch depression. To become depressed requires effort on your part. You have to think suicidal thoughts to feel discouraged continually. People with depression speak depressed, act depressed, and act in ways that support their depression.

Analysis has shown that persistent negative thoughts and actions contribute to specific changes in the brain's nervous system. Later, this leads to physical symptoms such as headaches, body aches, and ulcers. It may even lead to suicidal tendencies and mental disorders in extreme cases of chronic depression. One of the benefits of self-hypnosis is that it helps you unlearn these patterns of thought and habits that lead to depression. It helps shift your lifetime perspective from feeling sad to feeling fabulous.

Formation of Habits

Habits are learned behavior. You, as a human being, are a habit-forming creature. Your life is mostly run by the habits you've formed. Patterns let you carry on with your experience in the part of your brain with the least amount of conscious effort. Just imagine if you didn't have any routines, and you were new to everything you did. You would end up consciously performing everyday tasks exhausting much of your mental and physical energy. This would be time-consuming and exhausting. Imagine driving to work. How would you negotiate traffic if you started learning driving every day like the first day?

Fears and Phobias

The brain cannot differentiate between actual or imagined events. A phobia or fear is an imagined threat to oneself, which is irrational. All concerns are found within the brain's amygdala. We are born with two types of terror. They are fear of heights and fear of loud noise. As you grow older, different forms of concern become known. We are nothing but the solution to shield you from your brain. There's a positive brain intent behind all fears to protect and safeguard you.

One of the most sought after advantages of self-hypnosis is the eradication of irrational fears and the ability to cope effectively with phobias.

Overcoming Addictions

One advantage of self-hypnosis is getting over addictions. Self-hypnosis is not enough in itself to resolve dependencies. Along with Cognitive Behavioral Therapy (CBT), habits are quickly resolved and safely held off. Addictions are dependent on external stimuli, substance, or practice that cannot be stopped when choosing to do so. That's the difference between habits and addictions too. You cannot manage addictions, unlike behaviors, unless you are receiving proper medical support.

Alcoholism, opioids, gambling, sex, smoking, etc. are common types of addictions.

Performance Improvement

Your success or failure depends mostly on the convictions that you form in your mind. You must have ethical supporting values to boost the chances of success in whatever area you choose. Maybe you want to change your game, be a better salesperson, a better athlete, a better speaker, lose weight, or something you want to improve on. First, you have to start with the belief that it is possible, and that you can do it. It is not as simple as it seems, most of the time. Because of previous conditioning, disappointments, unfavorable circumstances, and negative life experiences, we set limits on what we are capable of and what we are not. Mostly, our inner critic or conscious mind sets those limitations. You bypass the conscious mind in self-hypnosis and connect with that part of your subconscious mind that makes your dreams come true.

You can overcome these psychological obstacles or self-sabotages with self-hypnosis, and go out entirely to achieve your goals.

The six above are the main advantages of self-hypnosis. Self-hypnosis has many more benefits, but they are more or less related to the above benefits. If we have to summarize all the six advantages into one, we would say that self-improvement is the primary purpose of all hypnosis. Time spent improving oneself results in a greater sense of well-being and satisfaction.

CHAPTER 14:

Changing Habits

To accept change, you have to be willing to make a difference.

To get the most out of this exercise today, you will want to be somewhere quiet, relaxing, and undisturbed. Make sure you are in a place where there is no negative energy, such as a bedroom, a flower garden, the beach, or the comfort of your own home. If it's in a room in your home, make sure this room is not cluttered. You can do this exercise while taking a bath or whatever you choose, so long as it feels relaxing and safe. Allow your arms to fall gently at your sides. Make sure your neck and back are aligned and adjust your body if you feel uncomfortable. Close your eyes and bring consciousness to your mind.

Take a breath in and notice whatever thoughts are running through your mind right now. Don't push these thoughts or feelings away; for now, you are merely seeing them. Allow the air you breathe to naturally fill your lungs and escape as you settle into relaxation. This meditation will guide your negative tension and thoughts and transform them into a positive, motivational mindset. Focus on all the changes you have experienced in your life. Think of it as though every stage in your life has been a learning experience guiding you to become who you are today. All the struggles and battles you are facing right now don't matter, and they won't matter in the next stage of your life. You have conquered and overcome all obstacles in the past. Take a moment to be proud of yourself. Give yourself compassion and light energy, and know that you are a powerful and resilient person. You are a beautiful soul who shines brightly in everything you do.

Notice your breath again and concentrate on the feeling it brings. You are breathing in renewable energy right now. You are reborn. Allow yourself to let go of all the negativity and pain you have endured. Forgive yourself for mistakes that have been made in the past. All of these emotions you feel makes you human. All of the thoughts you experience welcomes your personality and who you are today. All fear and anxiety slip away now; all that's left is peace and hope for what is to come.

Change your breathing now. Breathe in, one, two, three, four, five. Breathe out slowly and steadily, two, three, four, five, six. Repeat this breath. As you breathe in, I want you to focus on all things that are positive in your life right now. What are you thankful for? Perhaps it is the ability to grow, or maybe it's the transformation you are going through now. As you breathe out, you are going to release all that weighs you down. What are you afraid of? Continue breathing in this way for the remainder of the meditation.

Imagine you are lying in a field looking up at the sky. You see clouds with your emotions, thoughts, beliefs, and challenges. Breathe in and notice one cloud telling you that mistakes are here to guide you. Failure is needed to succeed, and it is okay to be afraid of these changes. Notice as this cloud slowly drifts out of your view, being replaced with another one. Breathe out and read your clouds. Change is needed to help you grow and seize opportunities you wouldn't have noticed if you didn't overcome other obstacles. Read these words to yourself and visualize the life experiences as they pop up and drift away.

Feel comfortable in your skin. Feel relaxed in the here and now. You are completely present with these thoughts. There is no room for negativity. As soon as your mind wanders or changes the subject, notice this and return to your breath and visualize the clouds above you. Change is scary for everyone; you are not alone. You have the courage and ambition to lose weight and conquer your fears. You have the drive to stay fit, release negativity, and fight through all that holds you back. Nothing can get you down because you are determined to succeed. Feel the power from within you break free and expand as a growing light from the center of your body expands outward into the universe. This is your strength.

Visualize the clouds again. Some people say there is always something better on the other side. You say that this is nonsense because what you have you have fought for every step of the way. You can still ask for help when you need it. You have the strength now to listen to and meditate your way towards success. You will achieve every goal and break down every barrier. You can do this because you are confident. Fear is a blessing to push you forward. The change will happen, and you will see a clearer picture. Right now, you are facing an uphill battle, but you will not give up. You can't give up. You have come so far, and only you are the person responsible for making these healthy choices for yourself. A leader must first show by example and influence support. You must support yourself to be strong for others. Right now, it's all about you, and you are allowed to be selfish.

Inhale for a count of five; one, two, three, four, five. Exhale for a count of six; one, two, three, four, five, six. Feel the positivity running through your veins. Feel the confidence in your blood. Burn away the negative thoughts because you can do this. You can reach beyond what holds you back, and you can accomplish all your dreams. This attitude speaks confidence, which is what you have strived to be. Believe that you are, believe that you can, and you will complete your ambitions and passions. You must accept and love who you are. Visualize the clouds again.

Repeat what they say – "I accept myself fully, and no fat, laziness, or what other people say about me is going to change that. I am comfortable in my skin because I have lived this way for many years. I will not let the opinions of others or my negative attitude affect me anymore. I will take it with a grain of salt because I believe in strength and opportunity. I will stay patient and keep trying; it doesn't matter if I complete my goal in a month or a year. One step today grows into one step tomorrow, and further steps towards my future. I will take my time, and I will move at my own pace. Whatever I do, I will not give up. Breathe in and feel and believe all these thoughts. Feel happy and joyful that you can and that you will overcome your fears and obstacles. Breathe out and release the rest of doubt and pessimism. All that you are is filled with positive light and opportunistic energy. There is no room for second-guessing. You are who you are, and that's not because of your reflection. Your beauty and talent shine through your outer image, and you can and will achieve greatness.

Breathe in now and focus on your breath. As you breathe out, feel the air that embraces your skin. Become one with this moment now. Stay here for a few minutes and let yourself relax. Reflect on the challenges from the past again. Embrace all that you feel right now and bring this into your future. Bring this positive, light energy into the future and know within yourself that you will make it through. Remain in this moment for as long as you want.

Bring your awareness to the here and now. Feel the surface below you as you wiggle your fingers and toes. Smile. You are welcome to open your eyes and join the world with all the positivity you feel. What will you do with it?

CHAPTER 15:

Self-Hypnosis to Help You Lose Weight

Self-hypnosis consists of practicing Hypnosis alone on oneself. It requires practice and mastery and is therefore not recommended for beginners. Several people have realised that all forms of Hypnosis are self-hypnosis because the induction of the hypnotic state requires a good collaboration of the subject and a particular concentration. Self-hypnosis can be viewed as a technique of deep relaxation or meditation, although there are notable differences. Concepts delight: it is about connecting with yourself, succeeding in relaxing, and being in tune with your body. This technique requires concentration and determination. Concretely, the self-hypnosis sessions aim to change the perception of one's body and help to better control one's appetite. Self-hypnosis can be achieved through audio tracks that you listen to at home, and which aim to stimulate the subconscious to produce mental images. These images should help the patient to provoke self-suggestions and to modify his behavior. In fact, self-hypnosis appears to be a support and a psychological aid on which to rest during a diet.

The benefits of self-hypnosis, like Hypnosis, calls upon processes of visualizations and suggestions, which make it possible to better manage a situation, whether it is:

- pain

- anxiety

- sleep disturbance;

- depressive disorders

- phobias

- post-traumatic stress disorder; other problems or pathologies.

Self-hypnosis can be done at the time of delivery, for example, or taught to manage migraines, phobias, anger or aggression in adolescents, etc. It can also be combined with local anesthesia for minor surgical procedures. Hypnosis is also increasingly used to reduce the side effects of anesthesia (anxiety, nausea, vomiting).

How to practice self-hypnosis?

Hypnosis is a special mental state that is not sleeping. We speak rather of a "modified state of consciousness," a state of trance close to the dream. As we are surprised, our gaze locked on a fixed point, our head in the moon, and we no longer hear anything around us. Once in a hypnotic trance, one disregards his environment and manages to focus on oneself. This is how we manage to treat certain psychological disorders such as phobias, anxieties, or a strong lack of self-confidence, for example. But then what does self-hypnosis give?

When you are subject to stress, or anxiety, when you have an insurmountable phobia, when you have sleep disorders or a big lack of self-confidence, self-hypnosis is an effective means of to feel better. The feeling of rejection or lack of self-confidence often has its roots in the unconscious, which, for one reason or another, gives them too much room to inhibit the person. Self-hypnosis precisely allows you to challenge your unconscious to put things in order and give yourself the opportunity to flourish, in short.

Self-hypnosis: how do we do it? Self-hypnosis takes up the rules and techniques of classic Hypnosis, with the difference that the hypnotherapist is yourself.

The preparation. We recommend practicing self-hypnosis while sitting on a comfortable armchair or sofa, feet flat on the floor and hands resting on your thighs. All in complete silence, of course: you turn off your laptop and the TV!

Then we close our eyes and create a vacuum. This moment is close to meditation: it involves becoming aware of each part of your body, starting from the feet and gradually going up to the head, all while breathing deeply. It is only once completely relaxed that we can begin the self-suggestion phase.

Self-suggestion. First, the number one rule of self-hypnosis (and Hypnosis) is to treat only one problem at a time. If you suffer from both anxiety and lack of self-confidence, you devote a separate session to each of these problems. Once the problem has been identified, one mentally addresses one's unconscious to guide it towards the resolution of this problem. This is where rule number two comes in: self-hypnosis is self-suggestion. It should not be a set of self-imposed orders. Sentences must always be positive. For example, we don't say "you shouldn't be afraid," but "I'm not afraid anymore." Also, we favor positive terms: better to say, "I know I will succeed" rather than "I no longer know failure" because failure is a strong and negative word on which the unconscious can focus.

Visualization. The secret to an effective self-hypnosis session, like Hypnosis, is visualization. It is a question of imagining oneself in precise situations, of printing images in its unconscious. For example, to deal with the lack of self-confidence in a period of unemployment and with a view to possible job interviews, it can be useful to imagine yourself working in a company (a more positive situation than researching jobs), for example giving a presentation at a meeting with poise, and being applauded by his collaborators. If the words guide the unconscious, the images mark it much more deeply.

Can everyone self hypnotize?

The answer is yes! It is even often said that hypnosis is, in fact, self-hypnosis. Because Hypnosis does not provide an external solution to a problem: it allows you to seek the solution inside you. We lift the veil on our own anxieties, and we eliminate them. On the other hand, if everyone can do it, that does not mean that it is easy. The most difficult is certainly to manage to create a vacuum in oneself. A word of advice: when it is difficult to concentrate, it can be useful to use practical guides on self-hypnosis. There is also an audio version. It is also recommended to set up regular sessions and include self-hypnosis in your routine in order to get used to vacuuming. Rome was not built in a day!

Does it work?

More and more scientific studies show the effectiveness of Hypnosis or other techniques, such as meditation and mindfulness techniques, in various situations. The tools used in neuroscience allow neuroimaging or electrophysiology investigations to understand the mechanisms involved in the hypnotic state and visualize the effects of these practices.

Several studies have shown a change in brain activity, whether in terms of awareness of the external environment or self-awareness, in people who practice Hypnosis. Even if the neurological mechanisms involved are not all known, the idea is to act on the autonomic nervous system by activating the parasympathetic nervous system, which plays a role in response to stress. We also know that the mechanisms underlying the modulation of pain perception involve different brain regions, notably the frontal cortex, whose activity can be modulated by Hypnosis.

Thus, more and more studies and reviews of the literature show clear, genetic, epigenetic, or neurological effects of practices leading to the "meditative brain." That said, hypnosis studies do not distinguish Hypnosis achieved through external suggestions from self-hypnosis, so it is difficult to decide on the effectiveness of self-hypnosis as such. We also know that there are great differences between individuals in the ability to reach the hypnotic state.

CHAPTER 16:

Self-Hypnosis to Help You Motivate In Sustaining Important Physical Exercises

After spending long weeks confined at home, returning to "normal" life can be a challenge. Each one, during this exceptional period, created new routines and took new habits. The often slow pace that this health crisis has imposed on us is now giving way to recovery. How to manage this change? Hypnosis is full of tips to help you take care of your energy and boost you to face the challenges of everyday life.

If Hypnosis does not replace sleep in any case, it is an effective complement. For starters, it improves its quality and recovery potential. Then, it is an effective method to boost energy and concentration. Indeed, the state of Hypnosis is, by definition, a modified state of consciousness, that is to say, that you are between sleep and wakefulness during the session. In this state, your body is resting deeply. Your physical and mental tensions are released. The electrical activity of the brain is then greatly slowed down, and its frequency goes into Alpha waves or even Theta waves.

Alpha waves (8 to 12 Hz) correspond to a light state of physical and mental relaxation and offer an opening on the creativity and the unconscious of the person. Theta waves (4 to 8 Hz) correspond to a deeper state of relaxation or meditation or to REM sleep, for example, which is also linked to intuition.

During a hypnosis session, you navigate between these two recovering states. In addition, Hypnosis has also been shown to induce activation of the limbic areas of the brain corresponding to emotions, and thus contribute to an increased sense of well-being. In addition, the hypnotherapist will also make the most appropriate suggestions for your problem and your individuality. To boost your energy, he or she will, therefore, create the most suitable session for you, so that you can effortlessly increase your inner vitality, unlock certain stagnant energies, or even access your innate resources and potentials. If your fatigue is linked to an emotional overflow or a feeling of stress, hypnosis sessions can also help you release this emotional charge that consumes your energy.

But if you are short on time and you do not have the opportunity to consult a specialist, you can practice self-hypnosis exercises. Much shorter than a session guided by a competent therapist, their benefits remain interesting. They also have the advantage of allowing you to practice daily while easily slipping into a busy schedule. The most effective combo is, of course, the combination of hypnosis sessions and daily individual practice of short exercises, which allows you to anchor the benefits of your sessions even more deeply. Here is an example of an easy self-hypnosis exercise that will not take you more than 5 minutes.

Exercise: Tap into Earth's energy Sit comfortably in a chair and close your eyes. Take the time to feel your body, your sweat, your breath for a few moments in order to center yourself. You are now ready to start practicing. Imagine or visualize that roots come out of your feet, from your pelvis and gradually sink into the Earth, like a beautiful majestic tree. See these roots that extend deeper and deeper into the Earth, and all around you. You can imagine these roots stretching for miles, far beyond your field of vision. Then visualize the energy of the Earth that rises in yourself through your roots. You can represent it in the form of soft light, for example, or simply feel it circulate in your body from your feet. The benefits of this exercise are multiple: Increases energy and vitality Improves interior stability and equanimity Reduces stress and soothes the mind Increases the feeling of security If you can, do not hesitate to consult your hypnotherapist for one or more sessions to support you in your recovery. You will come out re-energized and boosted for several days or even weeks. Self-hypnosis and meditation exercises can also be of significant support to you.

Three exercises to learn self-hypnosis

Practice regularly, self-hypnosis helps relieve stress, anxiety, physical pain. The first step: learn to relax your mind. Suggested by Lise Bartoli, psychologist, and hypnotherapist, these three self-hypnosis exercises will help you.

Autonomous, they can then evolve by themselves". Its program consists of several phases. Here, we'll only cover the first - major - step of learning to relax. But first, some tips for successful exercises.

Choose the right time. You can test different schedules. Either early in the morning, early evening, or on weekends.

A word of advice: better avoid self-hypnosis sessions late in the evening, you might fall asleep. Make arrangements to have a quiet space. Before each exercise, make sure you are not disturbed and turn off the ringer on your phone. Even if the duration of the exercises depends on each one, allow 30 to 45 minutes of availability.

Choose the right place. At home, test several places until you find the one where you feel really good comfort or energy. Once chosen, you will always put yourself in the same place when you practice a self-hypnosis session.

Make yourself comfortable. Wear loose clothing and sit in a comfortable seat with your head supported, properly seated for optimal relaxation. Avoid the lying position, which promotes sleep.

Memorize the course of the exercise or register. If it's easier to relax by letting yourself be guided, record yourself reading the text of the statement. Speak in a monotone voice while articulating carefully. Leave breaks long enough to have time to respond to instructions.

Evolve at your own pace. Those who are used to relaxing can do all three exercises in a row. For the others, it will be better to repeat each of them until it is fluid, then move on to the next day.

Exercise 1: Here and Now

Sit comfortably and choose a fixed point in front of you. It can be a painting or any other object.

While fixing this point, mentally review all the parts of your body by listing your perceptions: "I hear the murmur of the city," "I feel the warmth of the wood of the chair under my palms" ... Listening to your sensations, you will gradually relax your alertness.

Fix the point until your eyelids tend to close on their own. Then continue to detail your sensations with your eyes closed. Then focus your attention on the air that you breathe, and that goes to your lungs, then guide it towards your belly. The latter inflates like a balloon and brings you more lightness. As you practice this breathing, you will feel your body becoming lighter and lighter. Savor this moment of tranquility and calm.

Exercise 2: Interior light

Once plunged into the state of calm induced by the previous exercise, continue by visualizing a soft color: blue, golden, orange.

Imagine that the color you have chosen emanates from the earth and then goes up to you. It enters your whole body, starting with the feet. It relaxes each muscle.

The feet relax. Now bring the light up to the top of your head and enjoy this moment of relaxation. Focusing on a soft interior color leads to a number of physiological changes: lower blood pressure, slower breathing, and an even greater inner feeling of calm.

Exercise 3: The "resource place."

Now imagine a place of relaxation that will deeply relax you.

Let your unconscious make you discover the images of a place of nature, which is for your symbol of harmony and well-being. It can be a known or imaginary place, whatever. The main thing is that you feel good in this place: whether it is a sandy beach, a corner of the countryside or a green mountain.

Look around, perceive what it is possible to feel (the sound of the waves, the blue of the sky, the smell of flowers, the song of birds). The many sensory details developed mentally are important, because they allow you to build a place of your own, a unique place of which you will feel creative.

Stay there as long as you want. You can lie down or take a walk

CHAPTER 17:

How to Prepare For Hypnosis

You would need to feel physically confident and secure to start the cycle. Seek to use a quick calming method. Choose an item on which you can concentrate your eyes and mind – hopefully, this item would include you gazing upward directly on the wall or ceiling in front of you.

Free your mind of all thoughts and only concentrate on your goal. Obviously, this is hard to do, so take your time and let your emotions leave you. Become mindful of your pupils, talk of making your eyelids heavy, and shutting gradually. Concentrate on breathing while your eyes shut, breathe in a deep and even manner. Tell yourself every time you breathe out, you'll relax more. Slow your breathing, and let each breath relax deeper and deeper.

Use your mind's eye to visualize a gentle movement of an object up and down or sideways. Maybe a metronome's hand or a pendulum, something that has a normal, long, yet steady movement. See the object sway back and forth in your mind's eye or up and down. Softly, gradually and monotonously start the countdown from ten in your mind, saying after each count, 10 I'm relaxing. '9 I'm calming etc. Believe it, and remember that you will have reached your hypnotic state when you finish counting down.

It is the time when you enter the hypnotic condition to reflect on the specific messages you've written. Focus on each statement, see it in the eye of your mind, repeat it in your thoughts. Relax and keep focused. Relax and clear your mind before getting out of your hypnotic state once again.

Count steadily but energetically to 10. Reverse the process you used when you were counting down to your hypnotic state before. Use some positive messages, as you count, between every number. '1, I'll feel like I've had a full night' sleep when I wake up'... etc.

When you hit 10 you feel fully awakened and reborn! Let your conscious mind slowly catch up with the day's events, and continue to feel refreshed.

The first step to using weight loss hypnosis: recognizing why you are not attaining your objectives. How's this working out? A hypnotherapist will typically ask you questions about your weight loss, i.e., about your eating habits and exercise habits.

This gathering of information helps to identify what you might need to help with the work.

You would then be directed into a method of calming the body and mind and achieving a hypnosis state. Your subconscious is strongly suggestible whilst in hypnosis. You've lost the aware and rational mind — so the hypnotherapist will talk to the unconscious feelings explicitly.

The hypnotherapist may send you constructive feedback, affirmations in hypnosis, and can encourage you to imagine the improvements. With our multiple episodes of fat reduction hypnosis, you should seek this right now! Positive weight loss hypnosis suggestions could include:

• Improving belief. Positive suggestions will strengthen your sense of confidence by encouraging language.

• Visualization of Success. You may be asked during hypnosis to envision having to meet your fitness goals and the way it leaves you feeling.

• Arranging that Inner Speech again. Hypnosis will help you control an inner voice that "doesn't want" to abandon junk food and transform it into a friend in the weight loss quest that is fast and more logical through constructive advice.

• Hitting the unconsciousness. In the hypnotic state, the implicit habits which contribute to unhealthy eating will begin to be recognized. In other words, you can become more aware of why we make unhealthy food choices and healthy eating and maintain more mindful food choices strategies.

• Fending off anxiety. Hypnotic suggestions can help tame your fear of failing to achieve weight loss. Fear is the number one reason people may not get started in the first place.

• Addressing and Reshaping Behavior Trends. Once you are in hypnosis, you can analyze and investigate how you use these instinctive reactions to eat, and "turn off." We can start slowing down by repetitive positive thinking and simply eliminate instant, involuntary consideration.

• creating new modalities for coping. Hypnosis allows you to establish healthier ways to deal with stress, emotional responses, and relationship issues. You might be asked to view a stressful situation, for example, and then envision yourself with a healthy snack to respond.

• Rehearsing Balanced Eating. You may be kept asking to improvise making healthy eating choices during hypnosis, i.e., being certain about taking food home at an eatery. This helps to make those healthier options easier. Rehearsal helps to control cravings, too.

• Making eating habits better. You may enjoy unhealthy foods and want them. Hypnosis can help you begin to establish a desire or inclination for healthy choices, which can also affect the portion sizes you select.

• Increasing Indicators of Unconscious. You might have mastered, by practice, to block out the messages that your body sends when you feel satiated. Hypnotherapy tends to help you to become more conscious of those metrics.

Naturally, not every suggestion applies to you. Your hypnotherapy program, whether you consult through a hypnotherapist or self-hypnosis should include ideas specific to your food partnership.

Going to work with a licensed hypnotherapist may help you to analyze your strategies to address your specific needs.

How Hypnotherapy Helps You Achieve Weight Loss
In the hypnotic condition, the subconscious becomes much more accessible to persuasion. In reality, the study has also shown that during hypnotherapy, several remarkable improvements arise in the brain, which helps you to know without objectively worrying about the knowledge you are getting.

That is to say; you are separated from the skeptical mind. Therefore the vital rational mind does not doubt what you think when you seek hypnotic advice. And this, throughout a nutshell, is how hypnosis will help you knock down the obstacles stopping weight loss.

Persistence, however, is key to progress. That is why, after an initial session, many hypnotherapists send you off with self-hypnosis tapes. In your mind, the hurdles are strong. Only by continuous research will you untangle those assumptions effectively and reformulate them.

But hearing frequent statements and encouraging advice on balanced food is a first phase in the process towards weight loss. You're teaching people to think differently. Even those assumptions will support you:

Control Cravings
What if you can detach yourself from the cravings? Detach them and disperse them? Hypnosis methods for other weight reduction enable you to achieve so. For instance, you may be asked to imagine taking your cravings away – may be out to sea on a ship. Suggestions will also help you right frame your cravings, and understand how to properly control them.

Expect Success
Perceptions determine truth. Naturally, since we have an anticipation of achievement, we are more likely to take the requisite measures to reach that performance. Hypnotherapy for weight loss can sow the seeds of achievement in your subconscious, which may be a potent unconscious motivator to keep you on course.

Practice Positivity
Negativity so often spoils weight loss. There are things which you can't eat. Unhealthy food "kills" you. Hypnotherapy allows us to reframe these ideas in a more positive light you don't starve yourself; you lose what you don't need.

Prepare for Relapse
We've been trained to think there are humiliating relapses – excuses to give up. Yet hypnosis tells one to talk differently about a relapse. A relapse is a chance to analyze what went wrong, benefit from it, and be more equipped to beat temptation.

Modify Your Behavior
One little step at a time meets major objectives. Hypnotherapy encourages us to make small changes that feed into larger objectives.

Say you're rewarding yourself with high sugar, high-calorie foods; you may be focusing on finding a healthy incentive by hypnosis.

Visualize Success

Hypnotic vision, finally, is a strong motivator. Visualization allows you to "sense" consequences and discuss how they make you feel. You could also visualize your future self, saying you have what it takes to succeed.

Self-hypnosis takes up the rules and techniques of classic Hypnosis, with the difference that the hypnotherapist is yourself.

The Preparation

It is recommended, practicing self-hypnosis while sitting on a comfortable armchair or sofa, feet flat on the floor, and hands on your thighs. All in complete silence, of course: you turn off your laptop and the TV!

Then we close our eyes and create a vacuum. This moment is close to meditation: it is a matter of becoming aware of each part of your body, starting from the feet and gradually going up to the head, breathing deeply.

It is only once completely relaxed that we can begin the self-suggestion phase.

Self-Suggestion

First, rule number 1 of self-hypnosis (and Hypnosis) is to treat only one problem at a time. If you suffer from both anxiety and lack of self-confidence, you devote a separate session to each of these problems.

Once the problem has been identified, we mentally address the unconscious to guide it toward resolving this problem.

This is where rule number 2 comes in: self-hypnosis is self-suggestion. It should not be a set of self-imposed orders. Sentences must always be positive. For example, we don't say, "you shouldn't be afraid," but "I'm not afraid anymore."

Also, we favor positive terms: better to say, "I know I will succeed" rather than "I no longer know failure" because failure is a strong and negative word on which the unconscious can focus.

Visualization

The secret to an effective self-hypnosis session, like Hypnosis, is visualization. It is a question of imagining oneself in precise situations, of printing images in its unconscious. For example, to deal with the lack of self-confidence in a period of unemployment and with a view to possible job interviews, it can be useful to imagine yourself working in a company (a more positive situation than research job), for example giving a presentation at a meeting with poise, and being applauded by his collaborators.

If the words guide the unconscious, the images mark it much more deeply.

Managing your emotions is very important when you want to lose weight. Some hypnotists, still too few, know how to induce a hypnotic trance deep enough to be able to establish motivation, love, self-esteem, indifference, disgust, stomach constriction in their clients... and many other hypnosis techniques, which go all the way over time, allow their clients to lose weight.

A session of Hypnosis, like a session of self-hypnosis, must be imagined in three acts: induction which aims at physical relaxation and sensory isolation, followed by a rapid passage, even brutal when it acts of Hypnosis of spectacle, which aims at intellectual concentration and to make it clear to your brain that it is a transition from a state of consciousness turned towards the exterior a state of consciousness turned towards the inside and finally of the hypnotic trance itself.

Your hypnosis practitioner for sleep disorders, anxiety, anxiety, sexual disorders, addictions, food compulsions, eating disorders (bulimia, anorexia), mania, stuttering, migraines, back ailments, allergies... you want to lose weight... therapeutic Hypnosis can remedy many things, and this, sometimes, in short time.

Hypnosis can plant the idea that you look forward to exercising your body. Soon, time at the gym will be the best part of your day. It may become your favorite pastime!

CHAPTER 18:

Hypnosis Script 1

You have started a positive way to deal with acquire the thin, solid, appealing body, which you want. I am going to give you recommendations that will make this a lasting change in your living. These proposals are going to produce total and intensive results upon the most profound piece of your inner mind, fixing themselves in the most profound piece of each cell of your cerebrum and body. You will be shocked exactly how viable these recommendations will be and the amount they will end up being a piece of your regular daily existence, giving you a fresh out of the box new example, shiny new musings, a spic and span technique for activity, to make you a viable and fruitful individual.

You have started a positive methodology for acquiring a sound, appealing body, which you so want. You have picked spellbinding as a positive way to accomplish this objective, since entrancing is an incredible guide for changing your enthusiastic responses to food and eating. You understand that entrancing is another positive methodology in accomplishing and keeping up the size and weight that you want. Through spellbinding you will reestablish ordinary reflexes that will keep you fulfilled and bring into play that great sentiment of prosperity. Imagine yourself as the thin, alluring, sound individual that you need to be, envision yourself at the specific weight and size that you want to be.

As you go further and more profoundly into unwinding, considerably more profound and more profound down with each breath you breathe out, all the sounds blur away out there. You will focus just on the sound of my voice, listening cautiously to the positive proposals that I am going to give you.

Each time before you eat, when you see food that is not in its natural state, then has been processed, you will understand that if any ingredient does not nourish you, then you do not need that food and you will not eat it, you will check in with your stomach to ensure you are in truth hungry. Simply look down on your right side and inquire as to whether it is eager. On the off chance that the stomach isn't eager you won't eat. You will discover another thing to do. In the event that the stomach is eager, you will look down and to one side and ask what you can eat that will cause you to feel solid and invigorated and fulfilled a short way from now. At that point you will gaze upward and to one side and imagine your sound food decisions to fulfill the inquiry, what would I be able to eat that will cause me to feel solid and invigorated and fulfilled a short ways from now. This slim eating procedure will be a changeless manner of thinking, your slim eating technique will be yours to accomplish and keep up your optimal weight. You will quit eating when your stomach is fulfilled, before it really feels full.

I choose to eat pure foods that nature has provided for me

I eat slowly and carefully, and I stop as soon as I no longer feel hungry

When I see food that is not in its natural state, I know that I do not need that food to live my healthy life

When I see food that is not in its natural state, then has been processed, I will understand that if any ingredient does not nourish me, then I do not need that food and I will not eat it

I do not need to eat sugar, my natural food gives me all the energy I need

I do not need stimulants, my natural food gives me all the energy I need

Through entrancing you will reestablish ordinary reflexes that will keep you fulfilled and bring into play that awesome sentiment of success. The word diet is a negative word; it compromises you with a disavowal of food and demise. Entrancing is a positive word; it causes you to unwind, agreeable and alive. Diets come up short; entrancing succeeds. Diets achieve starvation which prompts gorging and abundant weight gain. Entrancing realizes fulfillment which prompts unwinding and achieves a thin, alluring body, a casual psyche, and a satisfied soul. The old desire to abstain from food is currently totally expelled from your psyche for the present; you understand that the genuine answer is in reestablishing ordinary reflexes. You will focus on it, complying with each recommendation I give you, for spellbinding is a positive methodology. Entrancing proposals which you get will quickly realize a change which is important to protect an all-time thin, solid, appealing body, which you so want.

Presently I need you to envision that you are on a swing and you are the ideal size and weight. I need you to gradually begin swinging. As you swing increasingly elevated at a protected level, I need your digestion to modify ever more elevated, I need your psyche brain to alter your digestion securely to the suitable level to assist you with accomplishing your ideal weight. As you keep on swinging, your digestion keeps on modifying until it gets to the ideal rate, the ideal pace of digestion to get to your ideal weight, and to keep at that perfect weight. As you swing, the digestion is changing in accordance with the ideal rate, your psyche comprehends what your digestion should be to meet your weight objectives. Your psyche brain will change your digestion until it is at the fitting level, as you keep swinging. Great. Presently your digestion is exactly where it should be.

Since your digestion has expanded to the point it should be for your optimal weight, it will require water to help flush out any poisons or abundance weight that you are unnecessarily conveying. You long for water, magnificent nurturing water when you are parched, and in any event, when you are most certainly not. Water is the method for cellulite to leave your body. Your body disposes of abundance weight and cellulite effectively and more rapidly with each glass of water that you drink.

Keep on breathing profoundly and know about your relaxing. With every breath you loosen up to an ever-increasing extent, with every inward breath you get wellbeing, and imperativeness and with every exhalation you discharge what no longer has a place inside your body, you sink further and more deeply. Notice how great it feels. Unfortunate dietary patterns that didn't work for you and additional weight were maybe methods of making a familiar object, a feeling of solace, and a feeling of being entire and complete before, you reacted along these lines in light of different enthusiastic circumstances. The inner mind stores the entirety of your recollections and the exercises gained from every circumstance. The way it works for you is it presents you with alternatives of reacting to various circumstances, in view of the exercises gained from the past. It is known as a trigger reaction, something extremely characteristic and exceptionally simple and automatic. In the past your psyche mind was attempting to help you to remember the exercises gained from those enthusiastic circumstances, it attempted to give you what it thought was the best reaction accessible to you at that point. Presently, we need to thank your psyche mind, for that update, we need not bother with that update any longer, we currently have different methods of reacting that are more advantageous choices than food and eating. The exercise has been scholarly. You can envision different methods of managing circumstances and communicating feelings securely without the requirement for food. You presently have the innovative capacity to pick the best method of reacting in all circumstances. You may diary your emotions, or tune in to your preferred music, or you appreciate investing energy with companions, or you decide to walk or exercise, you do whatever you truly appreciate like thinking, playing, or gaining some new useful knowledge. Eating is plainly important to fulfill and sustain your body. You just eat to fulfill genuine appetite, with solid food decisions, and you quit eating when your stomach is not, at this point hungry, don't hold up until you are full, at that point you have overeaten.

Presently I need your psyche brain to check in with your hormones. Your inner mind psyche will tenderly and securely change your hormones with the goal that they are at the right levels for you. Your psyche mind adjusts your hormones so there are no extra food longings at specific times. Your inner mind balanced your hormones with the goal that you feel in balance consistently, when you are in balance you don't have yearnings, your body keeps up a predictable equalization consistently. Your inner mind screens your digestion and hormones each morning and makes any essential changes with the end goal for you to achieve and keep up your optimal weight, and your own feeling of parity. All frameworks work in concordance, with the goal that you work consistently at your fullest potential.

One thing is significant, you are not just going to arrive at your optimal weight, you will think that it's extremely simple to keep up. You will be anxious about water every day; you will want to move your body here and there consistently. You will discover time to practice normally consistently. You practice when your body needs it, much the same as you eat when your stomach is ravenous. You discover time for the duration of the day to exercise and deliver all the poisons from your body and to help your digestion to keep up ideal levels. In some cases, as the need emerges you may practice two times each day, going for a stroll, planting, riding a bike or setting off to the rec center. Exercise as this significant piece of your life, causes you to feel solid, attractive, certain, and empowered. You generally find at any rate a brief window during the day to move your body in solid manners.

Each time that you exercise and settle on a slim eating decision, you have a colossal feeling of achievement and pride. Each time you look in the mirror you see the wonderful individual that is sure, solid, upbeat, and hot. You are extremely savvy to pick spellbinding as a positive way to deal with another, magnificent way of life, a way of life of thin dietary patterns that you feel better and look great. You are achieving your normally ideal size with little exertion. Diets are a thing of your past, spellbinding is the ideal answer to give your psyche the force and capacity to meet the entirety of your objectives. Your brain can do anything you need. You are in charge; the slim eating technique is now in your inner mind and is natural to you.

Presently I'm going to count from one to three, and afterward I'll state, "wide conscious and empowered". At the check of three, your eyes are open, and you will be wide wakeful, feeling quiet, refreshed, invigorated, and loose. Good one, gradually, and tranquil, effectively you are coming back to your full mindfulness by and by. Two, each muscle and nerve in your body is loose, and you feel superbly great. From head to toe you are feeling impeccable all around. Genuinely great, intellectually great and sincerely great. On the following number I tally eyelids open, completely mindful, feeling quiet, refreshed, revived, strengthened.

CHAPTER 19:

Hypnosis Script 2

Today we start a positive way to deal with acquiring another slimmer, more advantageous, more alluring body that you want. This is a change that you want, and the explanation you have come here today.

You have made a promise to this change, and presently this change is going on inside you. During the meeting I will give you a few proposals that will roll out this improvement as a perpetual one in the manner by which you live, and the decisions that you make about food. These proposals that I make today are going to take you from where you are right now to your ideal weight. These recommendations will flourish in the most profound piece of your psyche mind, where all change starts and is influenced. These proposals will turn out to be a piece of each cell of your cerebrum and your body, and will stay with you perpetually permitting you for the last time to win the fight you have had with weight control.

You will be astounded at exactly how powerful these recommendations will be, and exactly the amount they will turn out to be a piece of your everyday life. These progressions will perpetually change your examples and considerations about food. The recommendations are made to permit you to the more likely control of your wants with regards to managing food. My recommendations today will better assist you to manage those issues that up till this time have tormented you.

My proposals will make you a viable and fruitful individual with regards to managing your weight, and accomplishing your ideal objectives. When you see food that is not in its natural state, you know that you do not need that food to live your healthy life. Beginning today and starting here on you will utilize this fresh out of the plastic new strategy, a technique that you have not yet utilized to manage your weight across the board. You have picked spellbinding as a positive way to impact this change you want and to achieve your definitive objective. Entrancing is an extraordinary device in permitting us to forever changing our passionate responses to food, and to eat as a rule. Spellbinding is another positive methodology, a methodology that will permit you to get the objective weight that you want. See that it's anything but an enchantment fix, and simply accept that it required some investment for you to arrive at your present weight and it will require some investment for you to arrive at your ideal objective weight. Be that as it may, this procedure is the start of another stage in your life where you will start a decent positive methodology toward food and your dietary patterns.

Comprehend that as you start this new period of your life, this new uplifting mentality toward food, that you will appreciate food, that you will like food, and that you should eat food, however that you will settle on better decisions with regards to the nourishments that you want. You will make perpetual positive changes in your dietary patterns. Starting here on you will demonstrate to your own fulfillment that eating the nourishments that you need physiologically will completely fulfill you; simply like drinking all the water you have to continue your wellbeing and that to advance weight reduction is to fulfill your thirst. You will appreciate drinking a lot of water, in any event six to eight glasses every day. Cool, reviving, perfectly clear water. Rather than regarding your hunger as a foe, you will start here on working inside the structure of your typical inalienable reflexes, you will make your craving your companion, your hunger is imperative to you and to your very endurance, and you will focus on it. Thin individuals have cravings as well.

I choose to eat pure foods that nature has provided for me

I eat slowly and carefully, and I stop as soon as I no longer feel hungry

When I see food that is not in its natural state, I know that I do not need that food to live my healthy life

When I see food that is not in its natural state, then has been processed, I will understand that if any ingredient does not nourish me, then I do not need that food and I will not eat it

I do not need to eat sugar, my natural food gives me all the energy I need

I do not need stimulants, my natural food gives me all the energy I need

Alluring individuals have hungers as well. They give close consideration to their hungers and afterward settle on savvy choices with regards to the nourishments that they decide to place into their bodies. Entrancing makes a companion of your craving, not a foe of it. Before today you have been focusing on your craving, yet not completely understanding the message that your hunger was sending to you. At the point when your craving imparts the sign that says. "Eat, I am eager" you ate until you were full, perhaps even past full. However, presently in your new relationship with your hunger, your new more amicable relationship, you will tune into the entire message that your craving is conveying, and you will regard it's recommendation. At the point when it says, Eat, I am ravenous, you will eat, however you will decide to eat better, more beneficial nourishments, and less food. You will eat more slowly, and utilize a little plate, you will put down your spoon or fork among chomps and bite your food multiple times among nibbles, and you will no longer eat until you are full, yet now will eat until you are fulfilled.

Starting here on you will understand that eating till you are full is gorging. At the point when you set up a dinner don't carry the feast to the table, leave it either in the oven, or on the counter, and serve yourself from that point, take just what you want to eat, and don't feel terrible about leaving food on your plate, truly like leaving a little food on your plate. Up to this point your longing for food has been constrained by feelings instead of by hunger. It is suitable to eat when you are eager, however never proper to eat to fulfill mental or passionate yearnings. Beginning at the present time, beginning right now you will be more on top of your actual hunger. The inward voice of your body revealing to you that you are ravenous, and when you start to eat you will eat just until you are fulfilled.

At the point when you eat gradually, biting your food, and taking as much time as necessary to eat, your body will send the message to your brain that you are fulfilled, and around then you will quit eating. Starting here on you will want nutritious nourishments, and will have the self discipline to pass by the food sources that are a bit much, similar to the late night snacks, the nourishments stacked with sugars and starches, the brisk snacks from the drive-through eateries, just to give some examples.

The body has been fasting since feast time the prior night and when that happens your digestion eases back down to keep the body from starving itself, by having a decent solid breakfast you kick off your digestion and start your vacation day right. This isn't an eating regimen, and you have to get that, it's anything but an eating regimen, it is however another lifestyle. Today you are gazing at another solid way of life, of settling on new sound decisions with regards to the food that you will eat. Diets flop yet life changes are until the end of time.

Thin individuals eat, much the same as you, and you eat simply like slender individuals do, you are slight. You will start to increasingly appreciate physical action, beginning perhaps with simply short comfortable strolls possibly a few times each week. You are developing your endurance and afterward expanding the length of your strolls, the recurrence of your strolls and even the power of them to the point that you will walk five to seven times each week. You wind up being empowered when you walk, feeling strengthened and invigorated.

You will not say anymore, "I don't have the opportunity to walk today" or "I don't want to walk today." But you will anticipate the time spent on your walk, getting a charge out of the outside air, and the daylight, or the window shopping at the shopping center. You make the most of your season of harmony and tranquility, strolling either with a companion having a charming discussion or strolling without anyone else in the season of reflection and isolation. Having a feeling that the enhanced you, the more advantageous, and more alluring you with each walk you take you are drawing nearer and closer to your new life, your new objective weight. In your inner being I need you to see yourself not in your present status, however I need you to concentrate in on the upgraded you, the more slender you, the more alluring you. I need you to see yourself at your objective weight.

Never again are you overweight, you have succeeded and you wonder in your prosperity. You like this marvelous achievement. Starting here on you will think slim, you will act slender, you will think solid, and you will act sound, and you will eat healthily, and you will be solid. You will feel superb all around. The words diet and eating fewer carbs have been expelled from your brain regarding yourself, consuming fewer calories and the considerations of eating fewer carbs after all make you consider starving and starvation kicks in your impulse of self-protection and will be supplanted with the musings of eating when you have to eat, and the nourishments that you have to eat to support the new more advantageous, more slender, more alluring you.

The possibility of yo-yo slimming down is gone, you are through with that idea. At the point when you see individuals that have not seen you in some time they approach you and they reveal to you exactly how extraordinary you look, and ask how you have lost so much weight, recollect that your answer ought to consistently be, "I just changed the way that I contemplated food" It is significant that you screen and record your prosperity. Possibly keeping a diary recording what you eat and the positive changes that you have made. Recording your weight reduction and reporting it so you can glance back at your prosperity and become propelled to keep on. You are feeling staggering in your new life, in your new body. Monitoring your prosperity is vital to proceed with progress. This will end up being a piece of your everyday life, similarly as significant as eating, is the chronicle and recording your prosperity.

Realizing that this excursion won't occur without any forethought you should anyway set some sensible objectives of achievement so you keep on being inspired. How about we set your first objective at losing ten pounds in a month, and when you succeed, and you will, at that point you will set another attainable objective, etc., etc., until you arrive at that last day when you have arrived at your objective weight. You have reestablished your body's own regular craving controls; recollect you eat just when you are ravenous, and just until you are fulfilled. You eat gradually, and bite your food completely. Your body will reveal to you that you are fulfilled. You no longer eat in a hurry; you make the most of your dinners and plan them as indicated by keeping up your new life.

CHAPTER 20:

Hypnosis Script 3

Expand your correct arm out before you, corresponding to the floor. Concentrate on just your arm, and my voice.

Envision that you feel the weight leaving your arm. It gets lighter, lighter, lighter still until your arm feels as though it is drifting up, weightless, similar to an inflatable. It is getting lighter and lighter, gliding up, drifting. It feels totally weightless presently, similar to a quill in the breeze. It drifts ever more elevated, feeling lighter and lighter. Gliding higher, feeling weightless.

Allow your arm to unwind, feel it drift down to your lap. Presently grow your concentration to your entire body, listening just to me, hearing just my voice.

Your head feels luminous. It feels light on your shoulders. Your arms, your legs and now the center feel light. Your whole body feels lighter, and becomes weightless.

You feel yourself drifting up, as delicate as a breeze. Let yourself feel weightless. You feel your body ascending ever more elevated, skimming daintily up, feeling much lighter.

As you coast here, consider how great you will feel when your body is so much lighter in the wake of losing the entirety of the abundance weight that you need to lose.

Your psyche can be totally quiet, loose and quiet. Agreeable, with an inward harmony. Time extends, stretching. Time eases back, it has no significance here. There are no concerns in this spot.

You feel your psyche grow increasingly loose and quiet. As quiet as a tranquil lake. Quiet happiness encompasses you, saturates you. Your concerns are altogether leaving you, skimming ceaselessly on a breeze.

You feel so great, so loose, and nothing matters here. There is nothing here to trouble you.

You wind up feeling like you couldn't care less about anything at the present time, it's only ideal to be so quiet, so loose, simply breathing serenely and feeling generally excellent. You feel increasingly more quiet, similar to coasting along a road without a consideration. Time appears to be so moderate, so moderate. There is no weight here, simply quiet. Quiet and all the time you would ever require.

Now say this with me.

"I choose to eat pure foods that nature has provided for me"

"I eat slowly and carefully, and I stop as soon as I no longer feel hungry"

"When I see food that is not in its natural state, I know that I do not need that food to live my healthy life"

"When I see food that is not in its natural state, that has been processed, I will understand that if any ingredient does not nourish me, then I do not need that food and I will not eat it"

"I do not need to eat sugar, my natural food gives me all the energy I need"

"I do not need stimulants, my natural food gives me all the energy I need"

Your psyche turns out to be more and more clear, similar to a cool, blue, cloudless sky. No concerns here, only quiet. You have the opportunity to unwind here, feeling quiet, feeling totally calm. Content and loose, such as nodding off in an agreeable spot. You feel increasingly quiet, more loose. There is such a great amount of time to unwind.

You can return here, to this spot of harmony and quiet whenever. Simply let yourself know, "I can be loosened up now. I can find a sense of contentment inside myself. I can feel better, quiet and serene". Whenever you need them, you can hear these words. You can feel loose, content, and totally quiet whenever.

Starting at the present time, whenever you feel on edge or pained, whenever you eat a feast, you will hear again in your psyche, "I can be loosened up now. I can find a sense of contentment inside myself. I can feel better, quiet and serene". You will have the option to express the words, and hear the reverberation in your brain.

You can unwind effectively, feel the difficulties soften away from your brain and body. All you feel is quiet, content and loose. You can feel like this along these lines whenever, during any moment. You can feel thusly grinding away, at home, wherever. Whenever.

You can feel the quiet, positive sentiments return to you as you rehash the words.

Starting at the present time, your life can be changed. You will need to carry on with another life, with another energy about everything, another point of view toward everything in your life. You will have the option to see excellence and bliss in your environmental factors. You will have a sharp mindfulness, another happiness regarding life, having the option to live in the moment. You will feel glad to be invigorated, to encounter life in this new way. Your faculties wake up, improving life. Consistently starting now, you are more mindful, despite everything being loose, despite everything being quiet, except more joyful. Continually feeling brimming with life and discovering bliss throughout everyday life.

Starting now, I choose to eat pure foods that nature has provided for me, you will float through life, such as drifting on a delicate stream, streaming effectively alongside everything throughout everyday life. Simpler and simpler consistently, no difficulties. You will have the option to confront existence effortlessly, your brain lose, taking on this world, with a casual psyche. You can float alongside the issues, they can't stop you. You move alongside them, making sense of them as you keep on floating along, despite everything.

Starting currently, let your craving float with you. Recognize it, and realize that it is alright to feel hunger. Let yourself feel certain, calm, and realize that you have food put away in your body, pausing and needing to be spent. Realize that you needn't bother with any food except if it is supper time, have a sense of security and cheer realizing that you have what you need and your body will deal with you.

CHAPTER 21:

Hypnosis Script 4

It's likely, at times in your past, you have eaten when you weren't physically hungry. Instead, you were psychologically hungry, meaning, you have learned a response to certain emotions, and by habit, you have fulfilled whatever was unconsciously missing with food.

The classic case of this is eating out of boredom. How many times have you gone to the refrigerator, standing there with the door wide open, wondering what you should eat? You weren't really hungry. You were simply bored. It may have become a habit to eat when you felt bored or during other times when you weren't hungry.

You desire to become healthy. Not only physically healthy, but also emotionally and mentally healthy as well. You now desire to replace these old habits with these new positive healthy habits that I will be sharing with you in the next few moments. We're going to teach your subconscious mind how to let you know when your hunger is real or if there's some other need it is trying to satisfy.

Let's take a little tour inside your brain. Imagine the inside of your head. Notice how way deep inside; there is a control room. As your curiosity begins to take over, you begin moving closer to the control room inside your mind, and you notice a room filled with the most magnificent technology you have ever seen. You are amazed to notice things you have never even thought about before. There are temperature gauges that cause your body to heat up or cool down. There's a dial that controls the speed of your heartbeat. There's even a little switch that turns on and controls your sweat glands.

You are amazed when you realize all the things that go on in this little secret room in your mind you never even realized existed before. Nor were you ever aware you had access to such a place in your mind. After you have taken a good look around at all the cool things you now know you can come back and work on them any time you need to, you'll then locate a particular area in your control room called your hunger scale. This is a scale that gauges your actual physical hunger that you feel in your body and it is numbered 1 through 10. Find it yet?

On your hunger scale, notice the number 1 position is starving, and the number 10 position is stuffed. Bring to mind a time when you felt you were at a number 1, starving; get in touch with how that feels. Good. Recall a time when you felt you were at a number 10, stuffed. Notice how that feels. Good.

Now that you have experienced both ends of the spectrum, let that be the last time you ever feel starving or stuffed. There is a point between 1 and 10 when you will begin to eat.

Now move to a 3 on your hunger scale and notice that feeling. Any time you feel yourself at a 3, you begin to eat. From now on, you eat slowly, and you now become aware of your body's physical need for food the entire time while eating. You are a little bit surprised to notice that you receive more enjoyment and fulfillment during this controlled time of eating.

Now move to a 7 on your hunger scale and notice the way 7 feels. Here you are completely satisfied and content to stop eating.

Imagine yourself at a point in time when you are hungry. During this week, you now create the habit of detecting your hunger level. Whenever you think about eating from this point forward, ask yourself this simple question, "How hungry am I?" This question, immediately calls up the hunger scale within your control room and you either see an answer, feel an answer, or hear an answer from within. It only takes a few seconds. You do not need stimulants, your natural food gives you all the energy you need.

Now say this with me

"I choose to eat pure foods that nature has provided for me"

"I eat slowly and carefully, and I stop as soon as I no longer feel hungry"

"When I see food that is not in its natural state, I know that I do not need that food to live my healthy life"

"When I see food that is not in its natural state, then has been processed, I will understand that if any ingredient does not nourish me, then I do not need that food and I will not eat it"

"I do not need to eat sugar, my natural food gives me all the energy I need"

"I do not need stimulants, my natural food gives me all the energy I need"

Once again, you now create a habit: that at any point you ever think about eating or find yourself getting ready to eat or sense hunger, immediately before making any movement toward food of any sort, you ask the simple question, "how hungry am I?" and your body gives you the answer. From now on, you will eat only if you are at or below a 3 on your hunger scale. From this point on, you eat slowly, savoring and enjoying every morsel of food, and you stop eating at a 7. You simply want to stop there. Your body is learning now to give you a clear hunger signal at a 3. Your body from this point forward, persistently alerts you of your hunger as soon as you get to a 3.

You are learning to become more sensitive to listening to your body and you desire to work with your body so that it works optimally for you. You are happy to get a clear signal to slow down and to stop eating when you're full. If you are ever eating at a pace that makes it difficult for you to detect whether your body is becoming satisfied or not, you will hear a clear and direct signal coming from inside of you to slow down. I'll give you a moment to imagine this happening. This signal may come to you in the form of a yellow light or you may suddenly become sensitive to the way your belly feels, or you may hear the words, slow down.

Take a moment to imagine how that is going to happen for you.

(Pause 30 seconds)

Good. From now on, whenever you get the feeling of a 7, you will stop eating. You will know that this scale is accurate when you find yourself eating about 5 times a day, small portions of food. This is the way your body likes to be fed. You want to be kind to your body by feeding it the way it wants to be fed.

This week you are in the habit of detecting your hunger level, by asking the question, "How hungry am I?" hearing the answer within and responding to your body's natural request for food when your hunger scale is at a 3.

Let's imagine another time when you are thinking about eating, and this time, after you have asked the question, "How hungry am I?" imagine that the number is above a 3, a 5 or 6 for example. Not hungry at all. From this moment on, the first thing you will notice during those times is that since you have become aware of your physical hunger, the sensation of being hungry will subside. You will consciously realize you are not actually hungry.

You may still find yourself wanting something, but at least you understand that it is not hunger. If you do find yourself needing something to satisfy you, you will ask these two simple questions? "What am I feeling right now?" and "What do I need?" Then listen within. Once again, "What am I feeling right now?" "What do I need?" These are the questions you will ask when you come up with a "not hungry" response.

When you get the responses to these questions, your minimum acceptable response is to write them down. Writing them down calms your hunger or craving immediately, because you are giving attention to the real issue at hand. Giving attention to the real issue is the only way you are truly satisfied.

Right now, imagine yourself managing hunger or craving successfully. First, you will notice yourself wanting to eat something. Next, you stop and ask yourself, "How hungry am I?" You hear your response that you are within the satisfied range, so you then ask, "What am I feeling?" you get a response. Then you ask, "What do I want?" You always get a response. You then write down the answers to "What do I want?" and "What do I need?" You feel happy and satisfied at having managed your craving for food. You simply feel better about yourself.

You recognize the value of this new habit and it is a positive habit that becomes naturally integrated into your life this week and from now on. You are only eating when you are hungry and stopping when you are satisfied.

You are getting in touch with your real needs and are able to fulfill them now that you are writing them down and you are more in touch with how important these other needs are to you. You enjoy working with your body and your hunger scale more and more every day, as it becomes a natural part of your daily routine. You are taking care of your body and respecting the natural wisdom of your mind and your body. You listen to what your body needs and give your body what it wants and deserves. The hunger scale is easy for you to use and you find yourself using it naturally. You are willing to create these new habits permanently in your subconscious mind. Your subconscious mind accepts and receives all these suggestions and they become your reality. Every day in every way you are feeling better and better.

CHAPTER 22:

Hypnosis Script 5

This week we will be creating some new messages about healthy foods and healthy eating. Let's begin by imagining all the foods that you used to enjoy that have been giving you a problem. Imagine you are placing all of those old destructive foods that are responsible for putting fat on your body, on a cloud out in front of you. All those greasy, fatty foods, snack foods, junk foods, excessively sweet foods, take them all and put them on that cloud out in front of you. Notice them all piled up on top of one another on that cloud and how heavy and distasteful they look. Notice how they are becoming more and more distasteful looking. Notice the grease and all the fat on those foods, dribbling over the sides. Quickly notice areas of your body where all that fat from those foods was being stored.

Go back to the cloud with all that food on it and give it a push and watch it float away. Bye-bye. Watch closely so you can see it get smaller and smaller and disappear out of existence and out of your life for good. They are gone now, and you have forgotten how those foods taste or smell now or even the look of some of those old destructive foods.

You are discovering in their place all of the wonderful, healthy foods your body enjoys as you become trim and slender and reduce your body to your ideal weight. You remember that you enjoy eating foods like lean meats, poultry, fish, fruits, and vegetables. You are discovering a sense of freedom from eating sweets and greasy fattening foods.

Every day your desire for healthy foods is greater than your desire for unhealthy foods. You will eat slowly and carefully, and stop as soon as you no longer feel hungry You notice you get much more energy and enjoyment from eating crisp wholesome vegetables. You enjoy savoring the wonderful flavor you get from lean meats. At breakfast time, which is an important time to eat, you enjoy biting into your favorite fresh fruit, nature's dessert.

You enjoy eating small portions, which allows you to eat more often throughout the day and is the best way to increase your metabolism. Notice how your body is becoming lean in those places where there used to be fat. Notice how when you put lean foods into your body, your body becomes lean.

You'll now create in your mind, a list of all the healthy foods you know are appropriate for you. Write them down in any order you like. I'll give you a moment to do that. Keep in mind your body needs over forty nutrients for optimum health. Plan on a wide variety of food and a wide variety of nutrients.

(Pause one minute)

Say this with me

"I choose to eat pure foods that nature has provided for me"

"I eat slowly and carefully, and I stop as soon as I no longer feel hungry"

"When I see food that is not in its natural state, I know that I do not need that food to live my healthy life"

"When I see food that is not in its natural state, then has been processed, I will understand that if any ingredient does not nourish me, then I do not need that food and I will not eat it"

"I do not need to eat sugar, my natural food gives me all the energy I need"

"I do not need stimulants, my natural food gives me all the energy I need"

Good.

Imagine yourself taking that list to the grocery store, or wherever you might shop for food, and see yourself going through the store and picking out those foods and checking them off your list. You're picking out foods that give you plenty of protein, like low-fat meats and dairy products, reading the labels and choosing items that have ingredients you know are healthy for you to consume. You do not need to eat sugar, your natural food gives me all the energy I need

You are picking out your fruits and vegetables. These kinds of foods provide the valuable fiber and vitamins your body craves. Fruits and vegetables are filling and satisfying and give you a good sense of well-being. Eating lots of fresh fruits and vegetables is good for your peace of mind. These are your power foods. These foods have fiber, vitamins, minerals and nutrients that are antioxidants for your body, that protect your body, and improve your immune system.

You choose to increase your fiber intake through foods like lentils, kidney beans, split peas, chickpeas, and other high fiber legumes. You choose to increase your fiber intake through foods like quinoa, oats, and other high-fiber grains. You choose to increase your fiber-intake through high-fiber nuts and seeds.

It simply makes you feel good to eat these positive healthy foods. These are foods you were meant to eat. These foods are sensible and help you to reduce your body to the level you want it to be and maintain it.

Now that you have finished your shopping, imagine yourself in your daily routine, in the morning, waking up having whatever you will have at breakfast time. Remember to eat slowly, taking small bites. Enjoy the color, the taste and the texture of your food.

Remember it takes 20 minutes before that satisfied feeling registers.

Good. You are now having a mid-morning snack. You are concentrating only on eating when you eat. You enjoy eating as a single-focused activity and you now notice the flavor of your food, which helps you to become satisfied with a small portion.

It's now lunchtime and you are enjoying a meal again. Notice how you enjoy getting to eat this often and only a small portion. This way of eating is helping you to increase your metabolism.

It's now time for your mid-afternoon snack. Remembering to eat a small amount of these healthy foods, getting in the habit of eating 5 times a day, these positive power foods.

Moving on to dinner time. You notice you are able to eat calmly. Good. Notice how wonderful it feels to spend the day eating only quality foods that are for your quality body. Feeling a sense of peace and pride and confidence in your ability to maintain proper eating habits.

You take control of your healthy eating behavior right now. Each day becomes easy to naturally eat this way. You feel a sense of accomplishment and excitement because you know you are doing a good thing for your body. You do realize now more than ever that you enjoy eating healthy each day. You enjoy the health benefits you are receiving from eating healthy. It makes you feel good. It gives you energy. It keeps you looking good, looking younger.

You are seeing the results in your body, becoming leaner all the time. It helps you to create a more positive attitude about yourself and about life in general. You want only these kinds of foods from now on because you know they are doing your body good. Your body is becoming more fit and beautiful and pure and natural every day. You feel good about your commitment to yourself and you do your best every day. You love and respect your body. Good.

CHAPTER 23:

Affirmation

What are affirmations?

Affirmations are positive beliefs. We have expectations—both positive and negative—in all areas of life. Many of them are shaped by childhood and come from the experiences that we have had. Depending on how long you have been struggling with your weight, you have also internalized some beliefs.

Typical beliefs related to food and weight are:

- In our family, everyone is fat; that's in the genes.

- I have to eat my plate empty—that's the way it should be.

- I can't refuse food because that's rude.

- I'm a failure because I can't lose weight.

- I have to eat my plate empty.

- Healthy food doesn't taste good.

- Anything that tastes good is prohibited.

- I've always been fat—that's the way it is.

- I am already gaining weight when I look at the cake.

- Sport is murder.

- Eating healthy is time consuming.

- There's no point anyway; I'm just not disciplined enough.

- My everyday life is so stressful, and my body needs sugar.

With the right affirmations, you can change these negative beliefs into positive ones or learn to accept negative events; this helps you to focus and use your energy on your goal without a constant struggle with your inner convictions. So, an affirmation is an encouraging, empowering sentence that we keep saying to ourselves to reprogram our thoughts. Because our thoughts become action!

- • Look out because your thoughts become words.

- • Mind what you're doing, because they're becoming acts.

- • Look at your actions, because they become customs.

- • Watch your customs, because they will become your character.

- • Watch your character, because it becomes your fate.

How do affirmations work?

Every thought can become a reality. So how many times a day do you think about something positive and how often about something negative? It's your decision! We promote what we want with positive thoughts. We demote what we don't wish for with negative thoughts.

So, affirmations don't automatically make you slim, but they do help promote weight loss. They strengthen you on your weight loss path!

The field of brain research is incredibly interesting and complex, and I have already followed some lectures in this area with astonishment. Still, I am absolutely not an expert in this field.

So much has been said: Our brain, like many areas of our body, is incredibly adaptable. You can see from our brain whether the area for negative thoughts is more pronounced (right frontal lobe) or the area for positive thoughts (left frontal lobe). The good thing is that it can also be retrained! Thinking positive can be practiced! So, we should look to the thoughts in which we want to strengthen our brain.

How can you use weight loss affirmations?

Affirmations can be easily integrated into your daily routine. For example, you can speak, think, or write down your affirmations in the morning and evening in bed. The daily repetition is important— the more often, the better!

Put yourself completely in your sentence and in the feeling. How does it feel when the affirmation comes true? Emotions are much, much stronger than mere thoughts. And that is why the formulation of the affirmation is particularly important. Because if this provokes dislike and negative feelings, the whole thing makes no sense.

Think about what negative beliefs you carry around with you in terms of your weight, your body, and your health. Formulate an affirmation that suits you. If this is difficult for you, you can first collect your goals and derive affirmations from them, or you can browse through the pre-prepared affirmations below.

A good affirmation should have the following characteristics:

It must be positive. Cross out negative words like not, never, none, no. "I will never be fat again" is not a good affirmation.

Be short and concise

It should be formulated as a fact. And not as a wish or in the future form. "I will be slim" or "I wish to be slim" is not a good affirmation, since your actions are also waiting for the future.

It has to make you feel good. Like gratitude and joy, if your affirmation doesn't feel good, it may be because you doubt it or it feels like you're lying to yourself. Rephrase your affirmation! The sentence "I am slim" can then become "I can be slim" or "I am learning to be slim."

Change your affirmation. If you start with a weakened affirmation (see point 4) change it as soon as your feeling allows it to a more potent form. And now it takes PATIENCE. Exactly how long is different for everyone. A prerequisite is the repeated repetition of the affirmation and perseverance, at least three weeks, they say!

30 weight loss affirmations you must use from time to time. I deliberately mixed weakened and strong affirmations. The affirmation must suit you, and you can change it for yourself.

1. I am thankful for my body and my mind.

2. I respect my body and its signals of hunger and satiety.

3. I allow myself to eat healthily.

4. I am worth being slim.

5. I only eat what my body needs.

6. I have enough energy and stamina to achieve my goals.

7. I am proud of the person I am.

8. I treat myself to rest and enjoyment.

9. I enjoy moving more and more.

10. I intuitively feel what my body needs.

11. I give my body the necessary nutrients to keep it healthy.

12. I treat my body lovingly.

13. My body is my best friend.

14. I have control over how much I eat.

15. I alone determine what I eat and when I eat.

16. I am willing to learn to eat slowly and carefully.

17. I appreciate healthy eating and its positive effects on my body.

18. I accept my body with everything that goes with it.

19. Step by step, I learn to integrate movement into my everyday life.

20. I am on the best way to Lookout to my needs and to put myself first.

21. I am ready to love my body.

22. I take time for my meals.

23. I believe in reaching and maintaining my well being weight.

24. I know what's good for me.

25. I decide what I want to eat.

26. I like healthy foods and nourish my body.

27. I like to take the time to prepare my food.

28. I am worth cooking healthy and varied meals.

29. I deserve to be loved the way I am.

30. I Lookout to the messages from my body.

Avoid the trip hazard. And now to the most important point: When working with affirmations, there is a big stumbling block—THE stumbling block, so to speak. Many people begin to internalize their affirmations and then stop doing them much too soon. And then they are surprised that they didn't work.

Then you often hear: "Affirmations didn't work for me." Yes, they couldn't either, because they stopped too early.

Depending on the topic and the intensity of your affirmation training, it takes about thirty to ninety days to internalize your affirmations. And in these thirty to ninety days, you have to memorize your affirmations as daily as possible.

Uh, that sounds exhausting? But it is actually not.

Because we can squeeze it in somewhere for ten to twenty minutes every day.

The challenge is rather not to forget it.

It is ultimately a question of how serious you are.

If you are serious, you make sure that you cannot forget it and that you cannot outsmart yourself. So not: "I don't have to remember; I think of it by myself."

Because that is exactly the voice of our inner resistance, who would like to leave everything as it is. And hand on heart: how many times have you simply lost sight of and forgotten something that would have been good for you? How well did your memory work there?

So if you're serious, make sure your affirmation training is foolproof, one hundred percent secure, so you can't forget it.

Imagine that you are very, very forgetful, but you have to take a certain tablet every day; otherwise, you would fall dead as a result. Then how would you make sure that you can't forget your tablet?

How would you remember your tablet in this situation? And then you use exactly the same memory mechanism for your affirmation training. A nice affirmation in this context is also:

"I can afford to think about my affirmation training every day and enjoy it more and more every day."

So now you have everything you need for a successful affirmation training. And now I wish you a lot of fun and many, many positive changes in your life.

CHAPTER 24:

Daily Affirmation

This segment will examine the importance of affirmations. An affirmation is something that you assert. It's a phrase stated factually, making sure that the information is understood. We frequently say affirmations to ourselves without thinking about it. You may consistently say to yourself, "I hate my activity." You may thoroughly consider it repeatedly, and before you know it, you're miserable and hating your activity because the thought affirmed that in your head daily. We have to flip affirmations around and use them to our advantage. Instead of consistently repeating negative things in your mind, aim to repeat positive phrases. We will talk about ways to remember affirmations for your daily lives. It takes minimal exertion to say these sentences, so actualize these strategies into your life ASAP.

The more you think these things, the more genuine they will feel, and the easier it will be to finish your weight loss goals. Saying these things will come naturally to you. We consider imagery a lot regarding our pattern of thought. If you're eager, you think, "I am starving," "I am wiped out," "I am not myself." These are dramatic statements, but they are topics that fly into our heads because that's how our brains are wired. We consistently connect thoughts to make sense of things. We also make absolute statements. You may fail once in a diet and think, "I can't do this." We create these assumptions because that's how our brains come up with an answer.

We must turn that intuition around and, instead, wire our brains to think entirely differently. To create your affirmations, speak in "I can," "I am," "I will," or "I have." statements. Use "I" in each affirmation you do, because this is all about increasing your positivity and creative reasoning, not for another person after you use the "I" phrases. Next, move onto making a positive statement. Never depict what you lack, and attempt to avoid calling attention to your flaws, regardless of whether you are doing it decidedly. Speak in strong absolutes. The following four areas are examples of ones that you can use daily. Whichever area you battle with the most, is the one you ought to incorporate the most affirmations from.

You know your own habits, you can choose any or all of the affirmations to help you with your weight loss

Take 10-15mins undisturbed in a quiet place. Concentrate on relaxing each part of your body in turn, from the toes up to your head

Repeat affirmations slowly and clearly (in your head or speaking our loud) for 10mins.

MOTIVATIONAL AFFIRMATIONS

- I am a champ

- I am the most capable of completing the activity that I have to do

- I am not scared of failing

- Nothing that awaits me causes me to fear

- I have everything expected to take care of business

- I am more impressive than my greatest fear

- Each time I attempt I just get stronger

- I was made for something like this

- Giving up isn't in my nature

- My motivation is moving

- I have more motivation

- I am loaded up with motivation and the longing to continue onward

- The one in particular that is preventing me from the beginning, is myself

- As soon as I start, I will already feel good

- I am ground-breaking

- I can complete whatever task

- I have done great previously, so I can improve going forward

- Finishing something always feels better than not doing it at all

- I am doing this because I can do it.

- I have no choices other than to start

- Getting started will be the greatest challenge

- There is nothing to fear other than not completing this task

- My knowledge is moving

- Making mistakes is natural, and I realize how to learn from them

- I take action when I realize I have to most

Weight Loss Affirmations

- My body is vigorous

- I love my body at any shape

- I feel the best when my body is healthy

- Taking care of my body feels better

- My body has gotten me through so much already

- My body is capable of anything

- I make healthy choices for my body

- I don't rebuff myself and just fill my mind with affection

- My mind feels clearer when I am concentrating on weight loss

- I do not care about the numbers; I care about how I feel

- All that matters is that I'm taking care of my body

- Losing some weight, regardless of how small, is better than losing none

- My life is better when I'm concentrating on my health and weight loss

- Losing weight will help me greatly in the long run

- I am taking care of myself now and later on

- Life is easier when I'm healthy

- I am getting the outcomes I've dreamt about

- Working hard to get thinner feels such better than fantasizing about it

- I love shedding pounds

- Every part of my body is healthy

- People appreciate how happy I am

- I love others more when I adore myself

- I am happy to be alive and healthy

- My body is marvelous

- I love the person I've become throughout my weight loss venture

Healthy Eating Affirmations

- Eating healthy feels better

- Eating healthy tastes great

- It is always better to fill myself with something healthy

- The lousy nourishment I like isn't beneficial for me

- I allow myself to eat unhealthy once in a while, but realize that eating healthy takes priority

- Anything green hydrates me and keeps me full

- I am eating healthy for my entire body

- My heart feels full when I eat healthy foods

- Eating healthy reminds me I love myself

- Exercising is simple when I am eating healthy

- I am fortunate to have so much healthy food around

- I love trying various things with healthy food

- I am a superior cook when I make my healthy meals

- I always feel better after I have eaten healthily

- I don't realize all the advantages of eating healthy has on my body, until later on in the week

- My skin is shining because of the healthy foods I put in my body

- I don't have to eat unhealthy foods, because I realize that I feel good with healthy food in my body

- I don't have to fill my emotions with food

- Food makes me feel good, but healthy food encourages me to feel the best

- I need to eat to endure, so eating healthy is the way to satisfy this need, while also making me feel better

- I allow myself to enjoy now and again, because I realize that garbage food can be useful for my mind sometimes

- I will always return to healthy food and make this my major core interest when cooking and preparing meals

- I am saving cash when I eat healthily

- I monitor my food when I eat unhealthily

- I drink water frequently

Self-Control Affirmations

- I am strong enough to realize how to say no

- I make sure that I say "yes" to doing the things that need to be completed

- I take care of my needs

- I strive to break terrible habits

- I am the one that chooses what I do

- Food doesn't have control over me

- Skipping my activities is just harming me in the long haul

- I am strong enough to know when I have to walk away from something

- I am sufficiently trained to begin

- I recognize what it takes to discover success.

- I am in control of the things that come to me

- I am not afraid of a challenge

- I'm mentally ready to complete what I've started

- I am sufficiently strong enough to say no

- I am brave enough to begin all alone

- I buckle down because I merit the enormous payoff

- My self-control is motivating.

- I am adept at completing things

- It feels so great to accomplish what I set out to do

- I am amazing

- I am strong-willed

- I am obstinate against myself.

- I am my greatest inspiration

- I have been strong in the past and will continue to be into the future

- I am in control

You know your own habits, you can choose any or all of the affirmations to help you with your weight loss

Take 10-15mins undisturbed in a quiet place. Concentrate on relaxing each part of your body in turn, from your toes up to your head

Repeat affirmations slowly and clearly (in your head or speaking our loud) for 10mins.

CHAPTER 25:

Bad Habits and Affirmation

Mindless eating

I have self-control.

My willpower is my superpower.

Nighttime eating

I will make the best choice for me.

I succeed because I have self-control.

Endless snacking

I should have strength and self-control.

I keep my relationships with myself true to religion.

Emotional eating

I do maintain absolute influence over my emotions and feelings.

I now have the complete power of my feelings.

Eating quickly

•I love and care for my body.

•I have the right to have a thin, sound, appealing body.

•I am growing progressively good dieting propensities constantly.

•I am getting slimmer consistently.

• I look and feel incredible.

Eating junk food

• I take the necessary steps to be sound.

•I am joyfully re-imagining achievement.

•I decide to work out.

•I need to eat nourishments that cause me to look and to feel great.

•I am answerable for my wellbeing.

Eating sweets

•I feel incredible since I have lost more than 10 pounds in about a month and can hardly wait to meet my woman companion.

•I have a level stomach.

•I praise my power to settle on decisions around food.

Eating giant portions

•I am cheerfully gauging 20 pounds less.

•I am adoring strolling 3 to 4 times weekly and do conditioning practices, in any event, three times each week

•I drink eight glasses of water a day.

Underestimate food calories

•I am learning and utilizing the psychological, emotional, and otherworldly abilities for progress. I will change it!

•I will make new considerations about myself and my body.

•I cherish and value my body.

Eating while stressed

•I decide to grasp musings of trust in my capacity to roll out positive improvements throughout my life.

•It feels great to move my body. Exercise is enjoyable!

•I utilize deep breathing to assist me with unwinding and handling pressure.

•I am a delightful individual.

Drinking sugary drinks

•I am at ease at my lower weight.

•I discharge the need to reprimand my body.

•I acknowledge and make the most of my sexuality. It's OK to feel arousing.

•My digestion is impressive.

•I keep up my body with ideal wellbeing.

Not doing exercise

Any extra fat dissipates from the body.

All my workouts are hard and focused.

As my body has become thinner, I feel a strong deal of liberty and liveliness.

One of my top goals in my lifetime is to remain healthy and strong.

Exercising every day leaves me feeling awesome!

My body has become thinner and stiffer every single day.

My body is ever tougher and slimmer every day.

My body is getting pretty young and bigger and stronger each day.

My muscles are gaining strength and are much more recognized each day.

My muscles get better and harder every single day.

I become fuller and healthier and happier every single second of the day.

Each exercise in which I engage helps me achieve my ideal body weight.

I develop more muscle each time I work out and lose more fat.

Exercising does as much for my body as it does for my state of mind.

Exercising enhances my positive self-image.

Exercising is the greatest relief pitcher of stress ever thought up.

Exercising helps make my body feel strong and vital.

Not getting enough sleep

I'm physically, mentally, and emotionally stable, and I'm appreciative.

My lifelong priority is to be productive and healthy.

My lifestyle change is to be healthy.

Not listening to your body when you are full

I eat a healthy diet and enjoy being energy-filled.

By healthy eating, going to sleep enough, and exercising, I end up taking care of my body.

My healthful food choices enable me to relax and enjoy deep sleep.

Overeating on weekends

•I acknowledge my body shape and recognize the excellence it holds.

•I am the maker of my future and the driver of my mind.

•I let go of unhelpful examples of conduct around food.

•I permit myself to settle on decisions and choices for my higher great.

Overeating at social occasions

•I have faith in myself and recognize my enormity.

•I permit myself to feel great being me.

•I acknowledge myself for who I am.

•I bring the characteristics of adoration into my heart.

•I have expectation and conviction about what's to come.

Being distracted while eating (TV or PC)

•I love eating fresh food, and it causes me to arrive at my optimal weight.

•I love practicing every day, and it causes me to arrive at my optimal weight.

•I am a genuinely dynamic individual, and that encourages me to arrive at my optimal weight.

•Every day inside and out, I am getting slimmer and fitter.

Impulsive eating when not hungry

•I appropriately bite all the food that

•I eat with the goal that it gets processed

•Properly, and that encourages me to arrive at my optimal weight.

•I inhale deeply without fail, so my digestion is at its ideal rate.

CHAPTER 26:

Your Meditation for a Mindfulness Diet

One of the best ways to transition into a diet that's centered on weight loss is to do so using mindful eating. All too often, we eat well beyond what is needed, and this may lead to unwanted weight gain down the line.

Mindful eating is important because it will help you appreciate food more. Rather than eating large portions just to feel full, you will work on savoring every bite.

This will be helpful for those people who want to fast but need to do something to increase their willpower when they are elongating the periods in between their mealtimes. It will also be very helpful for individuals who struggle with binge eating.

Portion control alone can be enough for some people to see the physical results of their weight-loss plan. Do your best to incorporate mindful eating practices into your daily life so that you can control how much you are eating.

This meditation is going to be specific for eating an apple. You can practice mindful eating without meditation by sharing meals with others or sitting alone with nothing but a nice view out the window. This meditation will still guide you so that you understand the kinds of thoughts that will be helpful while staying mindful during your meals.

Mindful Eating Meditation

You are now sitting down, completely relaxed. Find a comfortable spot where you can keep your feet on the ground and put as little strain throughout your body as possible. You are focused on breathing in as deeply as you can. Close your eyes as we take you through this meditation. If you want to actually eat an apple as we go through this that is great. Alternatively it can simply be an exercise that you can use to envision yourself eating an apple.

Let's start with a breathing exercise. Take your hand and make a fist. Point out your thumb and your pinky. Now, place your right pinky on your left nostril. Breathe in through your right nostril.

Now, take your thumb and place it on your right nostril. Release your pink and breathe out through your nostrils. This is a great breathing exercise that will help to keep you focused.

While you continue to do this, breathe in for one, two, three, four, and five. Breathe out for six, seven, eight, nine, and 10. Breathe in for one, two, three, four, and five. Breathe out for six, seven, eight, nine, and 10.

You can place your hand back down but ensure that you are keeping up with this breathing pattern to regulate the air inside your body. It will allow you to remain focused and centered now.

Close your eyes and let yourself to become more relaxed. Breathe in and then out.

In front of you, there is an apple and a glass of water. The apple has been perfectly sliced already because you want to be able to eat the fruit with ease. You do not need to cut it every time, but it is nice to change up the form and texture of the apple before eating it.

Breathe in for one, two, three, four, and five. Breathe out for six, seven, eight, nine, and 10.

Now, you reach for the water and take a sip. You do not chug the water as it makes it hard for your body to process the liquid easily. You are sipping the water, taking in everything about it. You are made up of water, so you need to replenish yourself with nature's nectar constantly.

You are still focused on breathing and becoming more relaxed. Then, you reach for a slice of apple and slowly place it in your mouth. You let it sit there for a moment and then you take a bite.

It crunches between your teeth, the texture satisfying your craving. It is amazing that this apple came from nature. It always surprises you how delicious and sweet something that comes straight from the earth can be.

You chew the apple slowly, breaking it down as much as you can. You know how important it is for your food to be broken down as much as possible so that you can digest it. This will help your body absorb as many vitamins and minerals as possible.

This bit is making you feel healthy. Each time you take another bite, it fills you more and more with the good things that your body needs. Each time you take a bite, you are making a decision in favor of your health. Each time you swallow a piece of the apple, you are becoming more centered on feeling and looking even better.

You are taking a break from eating now. You do not need to eat this apple fast. You know that it is more important to take your time.

Look down at the apple now. It has an attractive skin on the outside. You wouldn't think by looking at it what this sweet fruit might look like inside. Its skin was built to protect it. Its skin keeps everything good inside.

The inside is white, fresh, and very juicy. Think of all this apple could have been used for. Sauce, juice, and pie. There are so many options when it comes to what this apple may have become. Instead, it is going directly into your body. It is going to provide you with the delicious fruit that can give you nourishment.

You reach for your glass of water and take a long drink. It is still okay to take big drinks. However, you are focused now on going back to small sips. You take a drink and allow the water to move through your mouth. You use this water not just to fill your body but to clean it. Water washes over you, and you can use it in your mouth to wash things out as well.

You swallow your water and feel it as it begins to travel through your body. You place the water down now and reach for another apple slice.

You take a bite, feeling the apple crunch between your teeth once again. You feel this apple slice travel from your mouth throughout the rest of your body. Your body is going to work to break down every part of the apple and use it for nourishment. Your body knows how to take the good things that you are feeding it and use that for something good. Your body is smart. Your body is strong. Your body understands what needs to be done to become as healthy as possible.

You are eating until you are full. You do not need to eat any more than what is necessary to keep your body healthy. You are only eating things that are good for them.

You continue to drink water. You feel how it awakens you. You are like a plant that starts to sag once you don't have enough water. You are energized, hydrated, and filled with everything needed to live a happy and healthy life.

You are still focused on your breathing. We will now end the meditation, and you can move onto either finishing the apple or doing something relaxing.

You are centered on your health. You are keeping track of your breathing. You feel the air come into your body. You also feel it as it leaves. When we reach zero, you will be out of the meditation.

Twenty, 19, 18, 17, 16, 15, 14, 13, 12, 11, 10, nine, eight, seven, six, five, four, three, two, one.

CHAPTER 27:

Work Out Meditation Hypnosis

Sit back comfortably in your chair and take a deep breath in and as you breathe out just close your eyes. Allow your breathing to be normal and natural as you begin to relax right now. Imagine yourself in a moment just feeling completely relaxed. What is it like inside your mind as you go into this relaxing trance?

Just pretend for a moment that you are drifting into a relaxing state of hypnosis and make believe that you are a great subject for hypnosis. What's it like when you are in hypnosis, what is it like when you are relaxing even more deeply now?

Allow that relaxation to spread throughout your body. Allow the muscles around your eyes to relax, allow your jaw to relax. Allow the relaxation to continue to your shoulders, arms, chest and abdomen. Just relax. Allow your spine to relax, your hips, your upper legs, knees, lower legs and feet to just relax completely. Feeling comfortable and relaxed in every way, that's right.

Feel the chair and know that you are completely safe. You may, from time to time, hear noises around you and that's ok, it means that you can just relax. Know that wherever you go, my voice will go with you and the meaning of my words will always be clear to you.

And what would it be like if you allow your mind to relax also. And your body continues to relax comfortably. Notice that it is as if your mind is taking you on a journey inside. And why not just suppose that this session of hypnosis begins to deepen more and more. Notice that you are experiencing your thoughts changing as if you were floating on the breeze. I need to tell you that going into hypnosis is the most resourceful experience. So you must take your time to relax your body and your mind fully straight away or in a moment. You should begin by noticing your breathing, your body can relax too and you really should relax completely.

I know you are wondering why you are so relaxed now and you are wondering why your breathing has changed and perhaps you're even wondering why your trance has deepened as you are breathing naturally, as it takes you deeper still. Allow yourself to do that now, so that your inner mind can take you on a journey inside your inner world so that you find yourself going deeper and deeper into hypnosis.

Realize that your body relaxes automatically in all kinds of fascinating ways and realize that this trance is particularly resourceful for you. You can breathe in and out comfortably and your unconscious mind can absorb all kinds of valuable suggestions and pieces of information. That's right.

As soon as you notice your breathing, you'll realize that you are so completely relaxed that your body has been breathing for you all along; as soon as you make that realization you will begin to go even deeper into a very comfortable trance like state.

And your conscious mind begins to wonder about trance and wonder about this session of hypnosis while your unconscious mind can be constructing patterns and integrating learnings while you consciously feel completely and totally relaxed.

Every time you want to be clear and concise about your fitness objectives, know that you can achieve your goals successfully because you can align your positive thoughts and energy that will support you in what you want to achieve. Because it is part of you and you find it easy to work out consistently. Feeling totally in control of your thoughts and in control of achieving your fitness objectives through consistent, regular exercise because it comes naturally to you and that means that you can be clear about what you want and achieve what you want. This means you are motivated and positive and you can achieve all that you want knowing the positive feelings are yours having now experienced that motivation to work out consistently. That means you can access all of the motivation that is yours by right and every time that you do this you are empowered knowing the control that you have over your life and the motivation to work out regularly and consistently puts you in charge allowing you to create the results that you want and to complete your work out goals easily and effortlessly successfully. Simply by realizing that you can achieve your work out objectives for yourself means that it's an experience that is familiar to you allowing you to know that every time you want to feel motivated to achieve your results, you know that the focus and motivation to work out consistently is there because it is part of you. And feeling positive, it comes naturally to you and that means that you can comfortably do all that you want knowing that you can work out consistently and move towards your exercise goals. Having now experienced that you have successfully achieved your workout objectives that means you can access all of the resources and learnings that are yours by right and every time that you do this you will find it easy to work out consistently and regularly knowing the motivation and positivity is easy to access. Because it's a resource that you can use easily and effortlessly. It's natural for you and your focus gives you confidence in that. Because you are in this session of hypnosis that means that the next time you choose to go into hypnosis you will access deeper levels of trance. You are a wonderful person with such a warm and charismatic personality creating such a positive effect on all those people around you as you realize now the changes that this journey has created for you. I want you to know that you are an incredibly capable and confident individual and that you will achieve all that you want. You have done a good job in making this a valuable and resourceful experience and your unconscious mind has accepted all of the positive suggestions I have given you and you can implement them into your behavior at your own pace.

CHAPTER 28:

How to Meal Plan Your Success

O ne of the biggest challenges with the Binge Code is meal planning. So let's break it down and cover it in detail, so you know exactly how to meal plan for success.

If you are stressed at all about what you are going to eat, I strongly suggest you start meal planning. It can really help alleviate any anxiety that might arise when you need to make food choices right before meal-time when you're feeling hungry.

The key to meal planning is keeping it simple. Especially at the start. Don't worry about gourmet cooking if you're not a great cook. Stick to the basics. If you're not into elaborate sauces or flavors don't worry about them. This is about healing and nourishment. You can worry about being a fancy chef some other time. We're going to start simple and then as we get comfortable with simple, we can work on more elaborate recipes.

Choose a time when you're not hungry and you're not in a triggering environment and create your meal plan.

Decide when you are going to eat.

Include in your meal planning the time of the day when you will eat your meals and snacks (avoiding gaps of longer than 3 hours). Think of this as a general guideline, not a strict rule.

Start with 7 meal recipes

We're going to start by deciding on 7 meal recipes. 2 meal ideas for breakfast, 2 for lunch and 3 for dinner. That's 7 recipes to begin with. If this sounds too restrictive, remember this is just the beginning. Once you're comfortable here you can start to be more adventurous.

Sit down and come up with 2 breakfast meal ideas, 2 for lunch and 3 for dinner. Use a cookbook if you need inspiration but choose simpler, easier to make recipes that you are comfortable with.

You will want to have roughly half of your plate dedicated to carbs, a quarter dedicated to proteins and a quarter dedicated to fats. Aim to include as much real whole foods are possible in the meals.

Brainstorm a few ideas for snack foods that can easily be grabbed and eaten when you're in a rush. Things like protein bars, fruit and nut/seed mixes are great options as they can be stored easily and they cut out on the preparation time too. Try to get into the habit of having some things you can snack on in your bag/car/somewhere that is easily accessible. I would always carry around some emergency snack foods every time I left the house just in case my day didn't go as planned and I found myself stranded without food.

Check your portion sizes

I just used a plate as my guide. One plate was one meal. With snacks, I generally stuck to things that were "snack sized" and portioned already, like a piece of fruit with a portion of cheese, or a graze snack box, or snack-portioned nuts.

Another suggestion might be to use your hands or fists to determine a portion. Your palm determines your protein portion. Your cupped hand determines your carb portion. Your thumb determines your fat portion.

You should settle on the way to measure portions that is general and is reassuring to you.

If you feel that you need to count calories to avoid a binge, you can do that too. As a suggestion, if you're working with 2,200 calories a day, you can break that down to 500 calories per meal, 230 calories per snack.

Another option is to purchase individual portions from the supermarket (be careful they are the correct size; a lot of the serving sizes in these products are much too small).

Ultimately you don't have to measure anything because dieting, strict portion sizes and counting calories never work in the long run. Try counting and measuring only if you need to for now and stop once you have an understanding of what portion sizes are appropriate for you.

Go shopping

Make a list of everything you need to buy for your planned meals and go shopping. Supermarkets can be triggering environments for many, so before shopping for any foods make sure you're not hungry and you're feeling safe. Make it quick - stick to your shopping list and avoid over complicating things for yourself. Avoid going down the candy lane of your supermarket if this is triggering for you. If it's too much for you, perhaps you can order your food online.

Prep your meals in advance

Preparing your meal in advance can be really helpful.

The oven works well for this. For example, you can purchase chicken breasts, some sweet potatoes and extra veg and cook them in the oven. Very simple. Once your food is cooked, portion it out for 5 nights. You may wish to purchase good quality food containers for storing and transporting your food.

Layout the 5 containers for your meals, put some chicken in each one and add in your sweet potatoes and veggies. If you want to add rice or quinoa, then do so. Drizzle with olive oil and serve with avocado for some good fats.

Freeze your prepared food and put only tomorrow's meals in the fridge. Take the following day's meals out of the freezer the night beforehand. This helps to prevent you from bingeing on your prepared food. Do this with a few meals so you're not eating the same thing each night.

If you don't/won't cook, you can consider buying prepared meals from a company that provides this service or ask a family member or a friend to cook for you. Alternatively, you can just cook the meal whenever it's required. Again whatever works best for you.

Think about tomorrow

Life will always find a way to interfere with the best plans. Be prepared for this. Your plan will always need adjustment or modification in the face of change.

The night before (or first thing in the morning), take 5 minutes to think about the next day ahead. Think about appointments and work commitments, anything that can interfere with you eating your planned meals or snacks. Then troubleshoot some solutions.

For example, a lunch meeting at work where they provide a buffet, how are you going to get around that? Think of what you will eat there, or if you can bring your own food, etc. Perhaps you will need to bring a packed lunch?

Leftovers

If you feel that leftover food may be a binge trigger, then I recommend you dispose of your leftover food in the trash as soon as you are finished eating. Some people feel uncomfortable with the idea of throwing food away but it's vital to safeguard your progress in this way. Alternatively, you may want to freeze the food if it is something that you want to keep for another day.

"This sounds too strict!"

This can seem quite regimented. However, it is so important to think of your meal plan as your healing plan. You need to eat regular, balanced, whole foods to heal your body. In time, as you get more comfortable with the program, you can let go of the formality and allow your plan to naturally shape into something that works for you.

CHAPTER 29:

Top Gold Easy and Fast Weight Loss Methods - Without the Crash

Who wouldn't like to shed pounds? Regardless of whether you need to search for an outfit for swimming outfit season or you are stressed over your wellbeing because of your weight, you can get thinner. If you need to get leaner, you need to comprehend that it is something that you will need to focus on and stay with. Some weight reduction plans can say that they will enable you to lose your pounds fast, yet they frequently don't give you the life span that you want, after a brief timeframe those pounds will in general return again.

You will get more fit if the calories you expend are more than the calories you consume. It is that plain and straightforward. Then again, numerous eating regimens with guarantees to fast weight reduction will make you lose your muscles mass just as your fat, basically working in reverse. So, if you are losing anything above two pounds every week, no doubt you are consuming more muscle and water than real fat.

These purported fast weight reduction diets will drag your metabolism down. This makes your body set itself into a starvation mode. This mode comprises of a low metabolism rate to spare; however, much vitality as could reasonably be expected to slow down the fat consuming procedure.

At the point when your body needs calories the main thing it goes to as a reinforcement plan is your muscles, so when your fast weight reduction diet starts to push your body to starvation mode, it will genuinely destroy you. This implies you will lose muscles that you may have picked up from working out and you will turn out to be increasingly drained and tired.

This is an essential reason concerning why many health foods nuts who take an interest in such fast weight reduction and counting calories will put on their weight directly back, in addition to a few. If you need to get in shape securely and reliably, you should do it slowly. You must most likely have the best possible eating regimen, correct exercise program, and will as such.

Eat Right for Easy and Fast Weight Loss

Food has a significant influence on any simple, fast health improvement plan. With the sort of way of life we lead we regularly turn towards fast food joints, burgers, and fries to fulfill our appetite and longings. Eating right won't just guarantee that you get all the imperative supplements, it will likewise guarantee that you lose all the unreasonable weight. Alongside the correct eating regimen, you will also need to exercise regularly to keep up overall fitness and have a healthy body and brain.

Here are a couple of sound tips that will enable you to lose weight rapidly.

•   There are other more beneficial techniques for cooking, similar to pan-searing your food, steaming, flame broiling, and heating. Shallow frying your diet will include additional calories on account of the utilization of overabundance fat and oil. Barbecuing, preparing, and steaming guarantee that the food is keeping its nutrients.

•   Fizzy beverages and colas have a ton of sugar content in them. So ditch shakes, and fake organic product squeezes that can be purchased from a bistro or a fast food joint. Concentrate on water, or even a glass of fresh lime juice and different fluids like herbal teas are great wellsprings of nutrients and liquid.

•   Before you head out shopping, have a rundown of what you require. Arrange them into reliable and undesirable foods. Verify whether you genuinely need the unfortunate stuff, this will enable you to eliminate things that don't furnish you with essential supplements and fiber.

•   To prevent yourself from voraciously consuming food, ensure that you have a specific day where you can enjoy the sorts of food that your body pines for. You could eat a bunch of chips, or you could have a double dollop of your preferred frozen yogurt.

A simple, fast weight reduction is conceivable if you keep a watch over what you eat and exercise regularly.

Fasting and Cleansing

Cleansing is a kind of detoxification strategy that many individuals do - not exclusively to get fit; however, to look healthy and fit. It gives you a solid body, sparkling hair, and clears your appearance. Fasting is the most reliable method for flushing out undesirable substance from the body. Pursue the fasting program each year to make your skin sparkling and shed additional pounds. If you fast on a soup or juice, it is conceivable to lose five 1bs each time. Toward the beginning, fasting on only water can hurt your body since snappy detoxing can cause queasiness and migraines from toxins being flushed out of your body.

Fasting is a method for calorie confinement and cleansing expels squandered material from your body. You should begin your cleaning program through intermittent fasting, which is confined to juice, water, and natural products as it were. Our collection contains various sorts of destructive toxins; fasting is the best way to detoxify them. Today we devour a few kinds of lethal toxin such as the lead in bones; which is multiple times more prevalent than 2000 years prior. Inside cells of the body, you will fine dyes, additives, cushions, concoction flavors, colors, harmful splashes, cancer prevention agents, acidifiers, drying operators, antiperspirants, stabilizers, fungicides, and many different substances. Here, I am imparting the job of fasting alongside detox. How about we begin from the lungs!

Through water, air, and nourishment, there is the retention of a few poisons that are soaking the earth. City lifestyle can fill your lungs with 20 million perilous particles like lead, dioxide, nitrogen, monoxide, PCB, radioactive, x-beams, and many more. Fasting can without much of a stretch clean your lungs from these substances. It is a successful method to scrub your kidneys, liver, colon, and courses, filter blood, free additional weight, flush out destructive poisons, bright tongue, and eyes and new breath. Multi-day fasting can do well to wash down the dominant part of substance from the body. To restart a recuperating procedure, and to remake the immune system, you should keep intermittent fasting five days. Before that, it is smarter to eat health products such as vegetables for three or four days. Along these lines, customary fasting won't demonstrate a shock to your digestion. Have pure juice and some green tea daily. In any case, tomatoes or orange juices are not permitted amid fasting. To make your cleaning procedure quick, you should take fiber supplements with it.

At the point when poisons discharge from your body, you may encounter some side effects like weakness, tension, cerebral pain, discombobulation, a sleeping disorder, body throbs, dull pee, textured skin, putrid sinus and many different issues. Day by day, lemon juice can bring some help from these issues. If regardless you face any inconvenience, you should visit a doctor for a meeting. It is smarter to get the supervision of a specialist amid fasting and cleaning program.

One Trick to Improve the Effectiveness of Any Weight Loss Diet

There are many reasons why you ought to incorporate fasting as a piece of your everyday lifestyle, many of which have nothing to do with eating routine. Fasting as an idea has been around as long as the slopes. However, it has been taken to limits now and made to resemble a solid piece of an ordinary and reasonable wellbeing and weight control plan.

Fasts have been attempted during that time for reasons as assorted as political causes (Bobby Sands rings a bell) and religious fasts. The Bible and many different religions advance fasting as an approach to draw nearer to God and to accomplish enlightenment. There is likewise some physical proof that hardship can prompt an uplifted condition of mindfulness, presumably some of which originates from the absence of extra nourishment the system must process.

Fasts can likewise be utilized as a prelude to therapeutic methods. For example, most specialists suggest a 12-hour quick fast before taking a lipid profile. This is additionally a standard strategy before a medical procedure. Confusions from the mix of nourishment and anesthesia have been known to happen. There is likewise in any event experimental proof that fasting can beneficially affect different parts of your wellbeing. There are the individuals who trust that water fasting cannot just work to detoxify cells and revive organs, yet also can help and potentially help in relieving such maladies and conditions as a cardiovascular ailment, rheumatoid joint pain, asthma, hypertension, type 2 diabetes, lupus and many progressively autoimmune disarrange.

A more up to date pattern as far as utilizing fasting as a guide in a reasonable weight reduction plan is the idea of discontinuous fasts. These are transient fasts enduring 24-36 hours long, which helps add to a total caloric deficit, thus realizing quicker weight reduction. This kind of fasting is easy to execute and can be adjusted to most individual needs.

One problem to know of is the act of extraordinary fasting among youngsters. This can prompt different kinds of nourishment issues, for example, bulimia and anorexia. Hardly any teenagers need to go on outrageous fasts for reasons for weight reduction, and if one does undertake a fast, they ought to be under the supervision of their doctor. When the purposes behind going on a fast have anything to do with strain to be meager or sentiments of low confidence, at that point, it is shrewd to offer insight. Outrageous fasts will, in general, show up when a time of overeating has happened, with the plan being to cleanse the body of all the overabundance nourishment.

Fasting can be a suitable and significant bit of a very much considered weight reduction plan. The utilization of transient fasts utilized alongside a healthy eating regimen can offer extraordinary weight reduction results, just as a portion of the auxiliary advantages of fasting. This joined with all the spiritual and gainful impacts fasting can have on an individual's mind make fasting something you should think about while deciding your course

Conclusion

E very other day, new weight loss techniques are invented. Earlier, it was when workouts were all decorated with leotards and spandex costumes with loud music, then came to the age of yoga, which was quite soon overtaken by power yoga. After this, muscle building was seen as the only way to deal with weight loss. There were countless methods such as these, but the new method of weight reduction by hypnosis is an entirely different experience.

Those who think hypnosis does not require physical labor but loses weight of the mind will be disappointed. Hypnosis helps to lose weight by keeping the mind on bodyweight-loss targets. Nearly all ages and sexes, whether male or female, young or old, have been reported as having trouble controlling weight. There are concerns about increasing obesity problems. The issue is no longer limited to the Hollywood idea of body size or weight loss.

However, the issue is that doctors want their patients to lose weight because heart disease, diabetes, and many other types of problems are rising. But it would appear that these people are not guilty of eating all kinds of fast food and that they are satisfied in their current situation. Doctors don't want their patients to stop eating junk food but want to increase their consumption of food with health benefits. However, most people are not sufficiently motivated to lose weight.

Obesity causes women to become fascinated with yo-yo diets and fading diets. Such diets include the cycle of taking a diet, losing a couple of pounds, but not going on and getting off the diet. As a result, the lost pounds return easier. Again, the dieter starts a new diet, and the cycle goes on and becomes an endless chain. This repeated weight loss and increase will lead to a rough ride in the metabolism of the body. This often profoundly influences the dietitian.

A new approach has been created for this health issue. This involves hypnosis, which motivates the body and mind to concentrate on weight loss. As a result, the body attempts to avoid unhealthy foods and yo-yo diets but continues to focus on losing weight healthily. The psychologist or therapist maintains the patient motivation by the constant hypnosis method towards the health loss program.

The key purpose of hypnosis is to enter the unconscious mind and attempt to control the conscious level of thought. In the meantime, the unconscious handles the automatic items that involve binding the shoes and other associated tasks. The subconscious is the driving power that works on the conscious brain to control our actions and, thus, weight loss without fad diets.

The more you practice the meditations we've given to you, the easier it will be to discover the success you've been waiting for. After a difficult diet, again and again, getting nowhere is an ideal opportunity to accept what isn't right about our mindset. An ideal way to turn your mindset around is to rework it through meditation. Tune in to these at whatever point you're home and find the opportunity. If you're exhausted, why not take a few minutes to relax and pull yourself together? This meditation will be useful when you're feeling anxious. There may be a few evenings you may wake up and have trouble falling back asleep. Any one of these can help you relax while also encouraging you to fall into a weight loss mindset. Make sure you are placing yourself in a place where you can do these meditations safely. Try not to drive with them, and regardless of whether you're taking a plane or other transportation where another person is in control, be cautious. When you do meditation, always do it at home in a safe place. Possibly, you will fall asleep without realizing it. After you've attempted a few different meditations, you can use these methods on planes or anywhere else you may go if you realize that you can stay awake and alert, once you've come out of the meditation or hypnosis. Recall that the meditations won't make you magically get more fit. They will assist you with getting into the correct mindset that will be necessary to finish the diet, or exercise routine you are attempting. They will also assist you with relaxing, and decreasing the pressure that can make this procedure harder. Whatever strategy for eating healthy, you may pick; these meditations and trances will help you stop gorging and think it is easier to eat healthily and practice naturally. You should endeavor to pair this book with others in the same genre, to get the optimal after-effects of meditation. Recollect that it takes more than one attempt and that you should practice it regularly, not once a month. At the point when you can incorporate these snapshots of relaxation into your routine, it will help them work better.

It's time to concentrate on putting your mental health and well-being first, instead of concentrating on how you look outside. It's time to dissect the quick fixes and address the underlying issues and make lasting changes – not because of the time of year, pressure from friends or family, or what the media wants us to think about.

No-one should feel under pressure to adapt to please others. It's time to consider what you really want and whether it's now time to start making adjustments – whatever they may be.

GASTRIC BAND HYPNOSIS

Proven Hypnosis To Lose Weight And Transform Your Body. Control Sugar Cravings And Food Addiction With Guided Meditations For Rapid, Massive And Lasting Weight Loss

CAROLINE LEAN

Table of Contents

Introduction

I f you think you will be happy when you reach your ideal weight but get stuck on a negative view of your body, it will not work.

Have you noticed that when you get up on the wrong foot, you are all day in a bad mood, and you think that the spell is going on because you only get nasty things? On the contrary, with a cheerful mood, people seem more pleasant to you, smiling, you feel light.

You have unknowingly emitted a vibration towards the universe, which sends your thoughts back to you. The positive attracts the positive. The negative brings you a negative result.

This form of energy is transmitted to the universe, and it influences what you will get from your unconscious request.

Above all, do not focus on everything negative about weight, calories, fat, diet, suffering in an intensive sports practice. You just attract them with thought.

On the other hand, if you focus on the result you want to achieve, if you see this evolution step by step, you will modify your lifestyle to make this positive result for you.

How can positive thinking be the most powerful solution for programming our brain and dictating that it make us lose weight easily?

Demons, get out of our heads!

These demons (ideas, beliefs, emotions) build what we are by very powerful influence, the law of coherence. The obsessive desire to be and to appear consistent in our behavior sometimes pushes us to act contrary to our interests.

In other words, unconscious pressures force us to react to agree with what we choose to believe. This self-persuasion applies in all choices, and it is impossible for us that our opinions are different from what we have already decided, even if it means lying to us from time to time.

So choosing to think every day that one is overweight unconsciously leads to doing what it takes to be!

So, high resolution, we are going to start losing weight by diet or any other method!

Yes, but, as soon as we start to feel lighter, the brain panics because it is not consistent with the image of the choice that our mind makes daily (the fact that we think we are overweight).

That is when our demons come to tug us. "I feel better slimmer, but, strangely, I am pushed to crack and eat anything to feel better." Personally, the speech of my mind to allow me to make a gap (a big gap of sugar in general), was "you have made efforts, you can have fun, you will take things back seriously after." It was a big lie to return to an image consistent with my misconceptions about my physique.

Without understanding that the method we are choosing is not the right solution, we blame ourselves for not having succeeded. The snacking trend is reinstalling, and so is the yo-yo.

Making positive affirmations means talking to yourself aloud (preferably when you are alone!). By telling yourself positive words, considering the incredible results, it doesn't cost anything to try!

It is a method of personal development that is used to reprogram your brain to think positively. You can make positive statements for your health, your work or your self-confidence, your relationships, etc.

The goal is to attract happiness by pronouncing it! At first, one does not believe frankly in what one says. The lyrics are even the opposite of what we think, but by dint of saying it, the brain will believe it, and so will we! That is how they will have a real impact on our lives.

CHAPTER 1:

Concepts of Hypnosis

The hypnotic stomach band operates in all the same means as the physical one: your consumption of food is limited by your body to make sure that you feel delighted after minimal dishes. There are simply three vital distinctions between the physical and also the hypnotic band.

1. With a hypnotic band, all modifications are instantly done by proceeding to use the hypnotic trance.

2. With the hypnotic band, there is no physical surgical procedure, and for this reason, no physical threats.

3. The hypnotic band is numerous hundreds of bucks less expensive.

What Happens to Your Body during Hypnosis?

How do you recognize when you have had adequate to consume? Initially, you can feel the weight as well as the area of the food. When your tummy is complete, the food presses versus and also extends the tummy wall surface, as well as the nerve endings in the tummy wall surface, respond. As we saw in Phase 2, when these nerves are promoted, they send out a signal to the mind to obtain the sensation, "I have had sufficient."

Second of all, as the belly fills out and also food gets in the intestinal tract, PYY, as well as GLP-1, is launched and set off a feeling of complete satisfaction in the mind that likewise motivates us to quit consuming.

However, when individuals persistently eat way too much, they end up being desensitized to both the anxious signals and also the same neuropeptide signaling system. Throughout the setup hypnotic trance, we make use of hypnotherapy and even images to resensitize the mind to these signals. Your hypnotic band improves the full effect of these worried as well as neuropeptide messages.

With the benefit of hypnotherapy, we can alter this system and also enhance your level of sensitivity to these signals, to make sure that you feel completely satisfied as quickly as you have consumed sufficient to fill up that tiny bag on top of your tummy.

A hypnotic stomach band makes your body act precisely as though you have gone through the surgery. It restricts your belly as well as modifies the signals from your belly to your mind, so you feel complete swiftly.

The hypnotic band uses several amazing features of hypnotherapy. The hypnotherapy enables us to speak straight to parts of the mind and body that are not under mindful control. Extraordinary as it might appear, in hypnotherapy, we can encourage the body to act in different ways even though our mindful mind has no methods of routing that adjustment.

The Power of Hypnotherapy

There are many more instances of just how the mind can straight and impact the body. We understand that persistent tension can trigger tummy abscess, and also an emotional shock can transform somebody's hair grey overnight. Nonetheless, what I specifically like regarding hypnotherapy treatment is just how the mind impacts the body in a favorable and also restorative mean.

The human being wonders that ideas, as well as hypnotherapy, can trigger extensive physical modifications in your body.

Hypnotic trance, all on its own, has an obvious physical result. One of the most instant results is that topics discover it deeply loosening up. Remarkably, one of the most frequent monitoring that my customers report after I have seen them—despite what we have been working with—is that their family and friends tell them they look more youthful.

Cybernetic Loophole

Your mind, as well as body, remains in regular interaction in a cybernetic loophole: they regularly affect each other as the mind unwinds in hypnotherapy, so as well does the body. When the body unwinds, it really feels far better, and also it sends out that message to the mind, which subsequently really feels far better and unwinds additionally. This procedure minimizes anxiety and also makes much more power readily available to the recovery and even the body's immune systems.

The therapeutic impacts of hypnotherapy do not need hoax or memory loss. The enzymes that generate swelling are not launched. Also, because of this, the melt does not advance to a higher degree of damages, and also there is marginal discomfort throughout recovery.

By utilizing hypnotherapy and also visualization, our bodies make points that are entirely outside their conscious control. Self-control will not make these types of modifications, yet creativity is more powerful than the will. By utilizing hypnotherapy and visualization to chat straight to the subconscious mind, we can make a physical distinction in as low as 20 mins.

With hypnotherapy, we can significantly boost the impact of the mind upon the body. When we fit your hypnotic stomach band, we are using specifically the very same system of hypnotic interaction to the subconscious mind. We connect to the mind with dazzling images. Also, the mind changes your body's responses, improving your physical response to food to make sure that your belly is tightened, and so you feel truly complete after merely a couple of mouthfuls.

What Makes the Hypnotherapy Job So Well?

Some individuals discover it unsubstantiated that hypnotherapy, as well as images, can have such a severe and also effective result.

In some cases, the skeptic and the client, coincide individual. We desire the outcomes, yet we battle to think that it truly will function. At the awareness degree, our minds are aware of the distinction between what we visualize along with physical facts. Nevertheless, one more incredible hypnotic sensation shows that no matter what, our company believes at the mindful degree since hypnotherapy permits our mind to reply to a truth that is entirely independent of what we knowingly assume. This sensation is called "hypnotic trance reasoning."

It is feasible to be hypnotized and also have a hypnotic stomach band fitted and yet to "recognize" with your aware mind that you do not have medical marks as well as you do not have a physical stomach band placed. Hypnotic trance reasoning suggests that part of your mind can think one point, along with one more component, can think the full reverse, and also your body and mind can continue functioning, thinking two various points hold. So you will undoubtedly be able knowingly to understand that you have not paid hundreds of bucks for surgery, and yet at the innermost degree of subconscious command, your body thinks that you have a stomach band as well as will certainly act as necessary. Consequently, your tummy is promoted to indicate "really feeling complete" to your mind after merely a couple of mouthfuls of food. So you feel completely satisfied while you slim down.

How Effective Is Hypnotherapy?

The hypnotherapy we utilize to produce your stomach band utilizes "visualization" and "affect-laden images." Visualization is merely the production of images in your mind. We can all do it. It becomes part of the reasoning. For instance, think about your front door and ask on your own which side the lock gets on. To respond to that concern, you see an image in your mind's eye. It does not matter in any way just how sensible or intense the picture is; it is merely the method your mind functions, and also you view as high as you require to see.

Affect-laden images are the emotional term for psychologically significant photos. In this procedure, we make use of images of psychological's eye that have psychological value. Although hypnotic pointers are useful, they are drastically improved by helpful photos when we are connecting straight to the body. For instance, you might not have the ability to accelerate your heart by merely informing it to defeat quicker. Yet, if you picture basing on a train line as well as seeing a train hurrying in the direction of you, your heart quickens quite swiftly. Your body reacts extremely incredibly to vibrant, purposeful photos.

That is why I will certainly explain your procedure in the hypnotic trance area. It doesn't matter whether you are paying attention purposely; your subconscious mind will undoubtedly listen to all it requires to duplicate the genuine band, in all the same manner in which a dazzling photo of a coming close to train impacts your heart price.

You do not require to hold the images of the functional treatments in your aware mind; as a result of the program throughout a procedure, you are anesthetized and also subconscious. Despite what you knowingly keep in mind, under the hypnotic anesthetic, your subconscious mind utilizes all this info, and even images to mount your stomach band is precisely the appropriate location.

The Power of Context

Contextual signs are one more considerable element of the hypnotic pointer. As an example, when I did my hypnotic performance, the context of the theater, the lights, the stage, and the assumptions of the target market all boosted the hypnotic sensations, despite whether the individuals were knowingly familiar with it.

The same holds with the stomach band. I described in the last phase the prep work that cosmetic surgeons need before the physical stomach band procedure, also, you must adhere to the very same primary treatment too. That will reproduce the physical context for the procedure within your very own body. That makes it easier for hypnotherapy to have an immediate, effective result and also installed the modifications you require to create right into your body.

The doctors ask their people to stroll at the very least 20 mins a day. If you build up all the strolling, you perform in a day, and mostly all people currently do this. Just a few non-active individuals stroll less than this. Nonetheless, if you desire, you can make sure you do it by challenging taking a specific stroll of thirty minutes, as an example by strolling to the following bus quit or to the regional park and also go back. The factor of the strolling is not health and fitness or workout, yet only making sure excellent blood flows in the legs. When you do it, your prep work for your hypnotic stomach band corresponds to the prep work for a medical stomach band.

A silver lining impact, nonetheless, is that it will certainly establish you up for the workout that your body will certainly intend to do when you reduce weight. This might appear strange to you currently, however, as you reach your all-natural healthy and balanced weight, you will undoubtedly turn into one of those individuals that are generally slim, in shape and also really appreciate strolling as well as numerous various other kinds of workout.

CHAPTER 2:

Hypnosis and Weight Loss

E ven if hypnosis has no physical side effects, for it to be effective, it has to be done well and by a certified hypnotist. There are many hypnotists in the market, but getting the right one is a challenge. We shall give you a guide into getting an excellent hypnotist to help in your weight loss journey. We shall also discuss various apps that use hypnosis to aid in weight loss as well as a guide to losing weight through hypnotherapy.

Choosing a Hypnotherapist for Weight Loss

Expanding open, GP, and NHS acknowledgment of necessary treatments, hypnotherapy has explicitly brought about a gigantic increment in the number of individuals offering to prepare. The nature of this preparation fluctuates incredibly, so it is the BSCH's (British Society of Clinical Hypnosis) main goal to give its specialists an abnormal state of preparing and moral practice.

There are various things you are encouraged to search for when searching for a trance inducer to assist you with a specific issue:

- Where was the preparation for them?

- Have they passed an independent audit?

- Do you have academic validity in your preparation?

- Is there a continuous preparing framework or a CPD framework?

- Is there a supervisory framework?

- Do they have protection for expert remuneration?

- Do they pursue a composed morals code?

- Is there a formal grumbling strategy for them?

- Are they individuals from an expert body broadly perceived?

- Can you call an inquiry or grievance to that body?

All BSCH individuals are prepared in high quality. We set particular requirements for experts of hypnotherapy. Inside the online database, you will discover various sorts of participation as laid out underneath all can, in any event, a decent degree of expertise.

- **Associate Member**—qualified trance specialist with a go from a perceived preparing school at the diploma/PG Cert level.

- **Full Member**—qualified trance specialist with a go off in any event diploma/PG Cert level from a perceived school of preparing and extra authorize master preparing (for example, a practitioner or cognitive behavioral level pass).

- **Diplomat**—as a full part, however, on an essential clinical subject with an acknowledged paper.

- **Fellow**—full or diplomatic part moved up to extraordinary administration or accomplishment from inside the general public.

The different accompanying tips will manage you all the while:

Get a referral for yourself. Ask somebody you trust, similar to a companion or relative, if they have been to a trance inducer or on the off chance that they know somebody they has.

1. **Ask for a referral from a qualified organization.** A certified subliminal specialist might be prescribed by your PCP, chiropractor, analyst, dental specialist, or another therapeutic expert. They will likewise work with some information of your medicinal history that can enable them to prescribe a specific trance specialist in your condition.

2. **Search online for a subliminal specialist.** The Register of General Hypnotherapy and the American Clinical Hypnosis Society are phenomenal areas to start an inquiry. Visit roughly about six sites. A private site of trance inducers can offer you a smart thought of what they resemble, regardless of whether they explicitly spend significant time in anything and give some understanding into their systems and foundation. Check to see whether earlier patients have tributes. Ensure the site records the certifications of the trance inducers.

3. **Check the protection with you.** On the off chance that you have psychological well-being protection, you can call them. You can likewise get to this information on the site of your insurance agencies. Call your state mental affiliation or state guiding affiliation and ask for the names of confirmed clinicians or approved master advisors who rundown entrancing as one of their strengths.

4. **If required, think about a long-separation arrangement.** Quality over solace is consistently the best approach with regards to your well-being, on the off chance that in your quick district you experience issues finding a gifted trance inducer, extend your inquiry span to incorporate other neighboring urban communities or neighborhoods.

5. **Ask for accreditation.** No confirmed projects are gaining practical experience in hypnotherapy at noteworthy colleges. Instead, numerous trance specialists have degrees in different regions, for example, drug, dentistry, or advising, and have experienced additional hypnotherapy preparing.

6. Check for training in different fields, for example, medication, brain research, or social work.

7. **Be cautious about the so-called hypnotherapy specialists.** They may have gotten their doctorate from an unaccredited college on the off chance that they don't have a degree in another restorative segment.

8. A believable and proficient trance specialist will have proficient offices, inside and out entrancing information, and evidence of the accomplishment of past clients.

9. Check whether the specialist is part of an association.

10. **Match the specialization of a therapist with your prerequisites.** Hypnotherapy can be a viable pressure and tension treatment. It can likewise profit interminable agony sufferers, hot flashes, and successive migraines. Most advisors will list their strengths on their sites. However, you ought to also inquire as to whether they have any experience managing your particular side effects. On the off chance that you have eternal back agony, for example, endeavor to discover a trance specialist who is likewise a chiropractor or general expert.

11. Ask numerous inquiries. You offer the specialist a chance to find out about you as such. You will likewise have a sentiment of how well the subliminal specialist can tune in to your prerequisites.

    a. How long have they been prepared?

    b. How long have they drilled?

    c. The specialist should have the option to explain the differentiation between things, for example, formal and casual stupor and what awareness levels are.

12. **Say the discoveries you are searching for to the specialist.** A unique treatment plan ought to be imparted to you by the trance specialist dependent on your manifestations. Be apparent about what you plan to achieve. "I need to shed pounds" or "I need to kill ceaseless joint torment." You ought to likewise be posed inquiries about your medicinal history or any past hypnotherapy experience.

    a. Make sure that the trance specialist invites you.

    b. Was the workplace spotless and amicable with the staff?

c. To ensure you locate the correct fit, go on a couple of discussions.

13. **Finding a trance inducer, trust your premonitions.** At that point, feel free to arrange the event that you feel energetic or extraordinary about proceeding. Ensure you know and feel great with their methodology. Get some information about rates or costs and what number of visits your concern typically requires.

14. **Consider pricing around.** Now and then, insurance covers hypnotherapy. However, it contrasts. Check your arrangement to ensure you make an arrangement. If your insurance secures it, copayments can extend from $30 to $50 per visit. A subliminal specialist arrangement could cost $50 to $275 without insurance.

Best Hypnotic Weight Loss Apps

1. **Learning Self Hypnosis by Patrick Browning.** That is a superb application to unwind following a protracted day at employment! I appreciate merely utilizing it for 30 minutes to take a portion of my day by day weight. Of note is that all that you need to do in the application costs additional money.

2. **Digipill.** Digipill enables you to tackle your rest issue and unwind! It is additionally a precise instrument for helping you to get in shape, gain certainty, and significantly more!

3. **Health and Fitness with Hypnosis, Meditation, and Music.** With this basic, however amazing application, you can get fit rapidly and keep sound. It is a helpful device that enables individuals to shed pounds by utilizing trance.

4. **Harmony.** Amicability is a simple method to think and unwind! You can decrease tension with this free instrument, acquire certainty, and significantly more!

5. **Free Hypnosis.** It is a basic, however, fantastic asset for simple unwinding that contains valuable strategies and activities!

6. **Stress Relief Hypnosis: Anxiety, Relax, and Sleep.** For those battling with sleep deprivation and nervousness, this free instrument is flawless.

Step by Step Guide to Hypnotherapy for Weight Loss

1. **Believe.** If you don't figure entrancing will enable you to change your emotions, it's probably going to have little impact.

2. **Become agreeable.** Go to a spot where you may not be stressed. That can resemble your bed, a couch, or an agreeable, comfortable chair anyplace. Ensure you bolster your head and neck. Wear loose garments and ensure the temperature is set at an agreeable level. It might be simpler to unwind if you play some delicate, particularly something instrumental.

3. **Focus on an item.** Discover something to take a gander at and focus on in the room, ideally something somewhat above you. Utilize your concentration for clearing your leader of all contemplations on this item. Make this article the main thing that you know.

4. **Breathing is crucial.** When you close your eyes, inhale profoundly. Reveal to yourself the greatness of your eyelids and let them fall delicately. Inhale profoundly with an ordinary mood as your eyes close. Concentrate on your breathing, enabling it to assume control over your whole personality, much the same as the item you've been taking a gander at previously. Feel progressively loose with each fresh breath. Envision that your muscles disperse all the pressure and stress. Permit this inclination from your face, your chest, your arms, lastly, your legs to descend your body. When you're entirely loose, your psyche ought to be precise.

5. **Display a pendulum.** Customarily, the development of a pendulum moving to and fro has been utilized to energize the center. Picture this pendulum in your psyche, moving to and fro. Concentrate on it as you unwind to help clear your brain.

6. **Start by focusing from 10 to 1 in your mind.** You advise yourself as you check down that you are steadily getting further into

entrancing. State, "10. I'm alleviating. 9. I get increasingly loose. 8. I can feel my body spreading unwinding. 7. Nothing yet unwinding I can feel... 1. I'm resting profoundly."

7. **Waking up from self-hypnosis.** You have accomplished what you need, and you should wake up. From 1 to 10, check back. State in your mind: "1. I wake up. 2. I'll feel like I woke up from a significant rest when I tally down. 3. I feel wakeful more... 10. I'm wakeful, and I'm new."

8. **Develop a plan.** You ought to endeavor in a condition of holding yourself ultimately to go through around twenty minutes per day. While beneath, shift back and forth between portions of the underneath referenced methodologies. Attempt to assault your poor eating rehearses from any edge.

Learn to refrain from emotional overeating. You are not intrigued by the frightful nibble of food you experience.

CHAPTER 3:

Experience of Losing Weight with Hypnosis

Wanted to lose weight and sustain it with hypnosis? You can use the therapist's suggestions long-term. Many patients report that after hypnosis, they were convinced that, for example, fatty foods do not taste good, water tastes better than lemonade, or fruit and vegetables are delicious. The suggestions made in hypnosis make renunciation very easy because it is no longer perceived as negative.

For one to achieve success depends on whether the person concerned is ready for changes, for example, in eating habits. Dieting is also advisable to support hypnosis. However, hypnosis makes it much easier to overcome negative habits and behavior patterns and to establish positive ones, thus, make losing weight a success. Therefore, many more people are successful in losing weight with hypnosis than without this tool.

Step-By-Step Self-Hypnosis for Weight Loss

Hypnosis is an excellent tool that can change your life, just as we have said earlier. I think it's a tool that deserves recognition because most people don't know how to use their brains. That is something that you, unfortunately, do not learn in the school system.

The goal is to act on the automatisms that you do not control by will. If tomorrow I tell you to lose weight all by yourself or to stop having food compulsions, you are going to tell me that you cannot do it because you do not control anything. It is "stronger than you" to power this mechanism without wanting to.

My role is, therefore, to act on your memory, to act on the unconscious automatisms, in other words, program your brain in such a way that it loses weight without you knowing and surprise you to lose weight quickly. That sounds great, right? By doing diets in general, we send the body the message that it is not able to regulate itself by itself and believed for a long time that you had to control with your mind the way you eat, but it doesn't work like that; you did not ask yourself all these questions; it was your body that acted for you. That is also why parents always said: "Finish your plates," "Children don't starve, you must eat," "Eat if you want to grow." However, as a child, you knew your needs perfectly and your limits without anybody having to make you aware of what you needed.

You have to help your body to find its place so that it can regulate itself by itself and make you lose weight easily without thinking about it.

You should also look for the trigger for your weight gain because as long as we have not acted on it, you will continue to loop forever.

Your unconscious is a fabulous reservoir of resources that records all your learning since your birth. When you learned to walk, for example, you fell about two thousand times before you managed to balance. Yet today, you are not aware of walking. It is entirely reasonable—you imprinted this process in your memory without knowing it.

That is the reason why my goal is to accompany your unconscious towards "another thing to do" so that you can slim down easily and sustain success. Take time to know how self-hypnosis works.

Self-hypnosis is getting the brain used to a specific pattern, preparing it in advance because the unconscious will facilitate progress towards something it knows. So, it is better to accustom this part of the brain to something positive—to success—rather than to a disaster. To succeed, you have to do it the right way, and this can be a real boost, especially for weight-related issues.

Addressing Your Unconscious

To start, we will have to define its goal; it is objective. We will, therefore, take the time to list the reasons that push us to make this change by asking the right questions: What do I want? Does it depend only on me? Why is it important to me? What will it bring me? We'll formulate the objective to be achieved by a sentence that we will repeat. Be careful, however, that we do not speak to the unconscious as to anyone. For a good reason, our unconscious remains at seven years of mental age and does not understand specific formulations—for example, negation; when we repeat "I mustn't eat," the only thing the brain hears is "eat."

So, choose your words carefully; you will use a somewhat positive message. We often talk about "losing weight"; as a reflex, we don't like to lose, so we would rather say "gain in lightness." As an example, we could use the following formulations of objectives: "I reach my healthy weight gradually over time" or "I contribute to my well-being by doing exercises daily and by eating healthy."

The idea is to find a sentence that you can understand, remember, and repeat as often as you want.

Visualize to Prepare

Some studies in mental imagery have shown that having a real experience or merely imagining it animates the same areas in the brain. Visualization will, therefore, have a real impact on the pursuit of the objective. Indeed, the unconscious moves more easily towards what it knows. Bringing the brain to life by imagining it will allow it to reproduce it easier.

Each day, you should take time for viewing.

For more efficiency, we will ritualize the process. We will sit quietly without being disturbed, in a comfortable position, and perhaps even with music. The moments before we fall asleep is the ideal time to practice visualization. Since the brain processes information during sleep, exercising the brain during that time will be more effective.

A useful visualization exercise is that of projecting into the future. We can imagine the whole day going from dawn to bedtime once the objective has been reached. How are we going to behave? What will change? Does this new identity look alike? We have to go into detail and imagine what this day would be equivalent.

Another exercise will be that of fetish clothing. When we have a weight goal, we often have a reference garment that we use as a goal. One can thus, imagine oneself with the garment in question. What reaction does our appearance elicit? What are our feelings?

Finally, we identify an exercise that will satisfy those who are keener on weighing. With an ideal figure to reach, we can very well imagine it appearing on the scale and projecting ourselves into the feeling of satisfaction and success that this could provide us.

You will understand if, in weight loss or weight gain, diet and physical activity are essential; the work of the mind through self-hypnosis can be a real ally and make all the difference!

Practical Steps for Self-Hypnosis to Lose Weight

Processing of losing weight through hypnosis is to program our mind in such a way that it can make and accept a suggestion. During hypnosis, our mind is positioned in such a way that it accesses the depths of its subconscious to eradicate beliefs and to think that can interfere with achieving the desired goal. That makes hypnosis to be popular among those who want to lose weight. However, there may be no reason to seek the services of a professional weight-loss hypnosis trainer if this guide is diligently followed. Most of the insurance plans do not shelter the cost of hypnotherapy. Try to follow the guideline of this self-hypnosis to lose weight.

Step 1

Set a perfect weight loss goal for yourself. Aim for an available amount of weight you want to shield and choose a specific time for which you want to achieve weight loss. Always read your goal out loud before you begin.

Step 2

Always try to view yourself in the body size you want to be. Try to imagine yourself in your dream shape and the ideal weight you have been longing for; also, try to view your friends' and family's reaction when they will see you in that body and what they will say. Make sure you make the scene as lively and positive as much as possible to trigger some colors, fragrance, sounds, and feelings.

Step 3

Relax your whole body while closing your eyes as if you are drowning until you feel your whole body immerse and become completely soft. Continue to breathe for three minutes until you can feel a different sensation running through your body, relaxing all parts of it. You will see yourself in a different state of trance.

Step 4

Imagine seeing your ideal body in that trance. Thinking about how you feel in your new body and experience the world around you—how other people will see you and how you will feel good about being healthy and having a physically fit body. Do this for at least two minutes. Then view your body in a new state of balance.

Step 5

Slowly return your body to your current state. Be very intentional to bring back the feelings of positive inner experience with you. If you continue to do this daily, you will be able to train your body and mind to know how good it is to lose weight. The necessary behavioral changes that your body needs to lose weight.

Repeat this process daily for two months and recheck your weight to know the amount of weight you have lost.

How This Works on Your Body

There is a spot—called the door of dreams—between the right and the left part of the brain. This "balance" manner is a tool that you can use to set up motivation, love, self-esteem, indifference, disgust, shrinking stomach... That's the part that helps you to change how you see yourself and transform you to whatever you believe you are; by using it, you become your hypnotist, and session after a session; you will lose weight.

Some hypnotists, but still few, know how to induce a hypnotic trance deep enough to be able to establish motivation, love, self-esteem, indifference, disgust, stomach shrinking in their clients. Also, many other techniques specific to hypnotists allow their clients to lose weight. So, this is why you need to take the self-hypnosis teaching seriously.

You can—and it will undoubtedly happen to you—fall asleep during a session of self-hypnosis; it is either because you are exhausted and your brain does not have the strength to concentrate, or you are motivated. You start dreaming and fall asleep, or the session is too long, and your brain must fall asleep to recharge.

CHAPTER 4:

Mindful Eating Habits

Take Things Slowly

Eating should not be treated as a race. Eat slowly. This just means that you should take your time to relish and enjoy your food—it's a healthy thing! So, how long do you have to grind up the food in your mouth?

Well, there is no specific time food should be chewed, but 18-25 bites are enough to enjoy the food mindfully. This can be hard at first, mainly if you have been used to speed eating for a very long time. Why not try some different techniques like using chopsticks when you are accustomed to spoon and fork? Or use your non-dominant hand when eating. These strategies can slow you down and improve your awareness.

Avoid Distractions

To make things simpler for you, just make it a habit of sitting down and staying away from distractions.

The handful of nuts that you eat as you walk through the kitchen and the bunch of morning snacks you nibbled while standing in front of your fridge can be hard to recall. According to researchers, people tend to eat more when they are doing other things too. You should, therefore, sit down and focus on your food to prevent mindless eating behaviors.

Savor Every Bite

Do not forget that eating is not only about enjoying the food you eat, but your health too, and without feeling guilty and uncomfortable. Relishing the sight, taste, and smell of your diet is indeed worth it.

This can be so easy if you take things gradually and don't rush to perfection. Make small changes towards awareness until you are a fully mindful eater. So, eat slowly and savor the good food you are eating and the proper nutrition you are giving to your body.

Mind the Presentation

Regardless of how busy you are, it is a good idea to set the table—making sure it looks divine. A lovely set of utensils, placement, and napkin made of eco-friendly cloth material is a perfect reminder that you need to sit down and pay attention when you have your meals.

Plate Your Food

Serving yourself and portioning your food before you bring the plate to the table can help you to consume a modest amount, rather than putting a platter on the table from which to replenish continually.

You can do this even with crackers, chips, nuts, and other snack foods. Keep yourself away from the temptation of eating straight from a bag of chips and different types of food. It is also helpful if you resize the bag or place the food in smaller containers so that you can stay conscious of the amount of food you are eating. Having a bright idea of how much you have eaten will make you stop eating when you're full, or even sooner.

Always Choose Quality over Quantity

By trying to select smaller amounts of the most beautiful food within your means, you will end up enjoying and feeling satisfied without the chance of overeating.

With this, it will be helpful if you spend time preparing your meals using quality and fresh ingredients. Cooking can be a relaxing and pleasurable experience if you only let yourself into it. On top of this, you can achieve the peace of mind that comes from knowing what is in the food you are eating.

Don't Invite Your Thoughts and Emotions to Dinner

Just as there are many other factors that affect our sense of mindful eating, as well as the digestive system, it would come as no surprise that our thoughts and emotions play just as much of an important role.

It happens on the odd occasion that one comes home after a long and tiresome day, and you feel somewhat "worked up," irritated, and angry. This is when negative and even destructive thoughts creep in while you are having supper.

The best practice would be to avoid this altogether. Therefore, if you are feeling unhappy or angry in any way, go for a walk before supper, play with your children, or play with your family pet. But, whatever you do, take your mind off your negative emotions before you attempt to have a meal.

Make a Good Meal Plan for Each Week

When you start the diet, it is advised to stick to the meal plan that comes with the diet. There should be a meal plan of 2 weeks or four weeks attached to the diet's guideline. Once you are familiar with the food list, prohibited ingredients, cooking techniques, and how to go grocery shopping for your diet, it will be easier for you to twist and change things in the meal plan. Do not try to change the meal plan for the first two weeks. Stick to the meal plan they give you. If you decide to change it right at the beginning, you may feel lost or feel terrified then. So, it is advised to try and introduce new recipes and ideas after you are two weeks into the diet.

Drink Lots of Water

Staying hydrated is vital to living a healthy life in general. It is not relevant for only diets, but in general, we should always be drinking enough water to keep ourselves hydrated. Dehydration can bring forth many unwanted diseases. When you are dehydrated, you feel very dizzy, lightheaded, nauseous, and lethargic. You cannot focus on anything well. Urinary infection occurs, which triggers other health issues.

The purpose of drinking water is to help you process the different food you are eating and to help digest it well. Water helps in proper digestion; it helps in extracting bad minerals from our body. Water also gives us a glow on the skin.

Never Skip Breakfast

It is essential to eat a full breakfast to keep yourself moving actively throughout the day. It gives you a significant boost, proper metabolism, and your digestion starts appropriately functioning during the day. When you skip breakfast, everything sort of disrupts. Your day starts slow, and soon, you would feel restless. It is essential to have a good meal at the beginning of your day in order to be productive for the rest of the day.

If you are very busy, try to have your breakfast on the go. Grab breakfast in a box or a mason jar and have it in the car or on the bus or transport of any kind you are using to get to your work.

You can also have your breakfast at a healthy restaurant where they serve food that is in sync with your diet.

Eat Protein

Protein is perfect for the body. It helps your brain function better. It can come from both animal and non-animal products. So even if you are a vegetarian or vegan, you can still enjoy your protein from plants. Soy, mushroom, legumes, and nuts are a few examples.

Eating protein keeps you strong and healthy, it increases your brain function.

On the contrary, if you do not eat enough protein for the day, your entire way would be wasted. You will not be able to focus on anything properly.

You would feel dizzy and weak all through the day. If you are a vegetarian or vegan, you can enjoy avocado, coconut, almond, cashew, soy, and mushroom to get protein.

Eat Super Foods

Most people eat foods that do not necessarily affect them in the best way. Where some foods may enhance some people's energy levels, it may impact others more negatively.

The important thing is to know your food. It may be a good idea to keep a food journal, and if you know that certain foods affect you negatively, one should try to avoid those foods and stick to healthier options.

It is a fact that the majority enjoy foods that they should probably not be eating. However, if you wish to eat mindfully and enhance your health and a general sense of well-being, then it would be best to eat foods that will do precisely that.

There are also various foods that are classified as superfoods. These would include your lean and purest sources of protein, such as free-range chicken, as well as a variety of fresh fruits, vegetables, and herbs.

Stop Multitasking While You Eat

Multitasking is defined as the simultaneous execution of more than one activity at one time. Though it is a skill that we should master, it often leads to unproductive business. The development of our economy leads to a more hectic way of living. Most of us develop the habit of doing one thing while doing another. This is true even when it comes to eating.

Smaller Plates, Taller Glasses

This habit changer ties in a little bit with drinking more water; however, it's a bit different. People tend to fill up their plates with food, so the size of the plate matters. If you have a large plate, you're going to put more food on your plate but, if you have a smaller plate, you will have less food on your plate.

Stay Positive

The secret to succeeding in anything is positive. When you start something new, always stay positive regarding it. You need to keep a positive mind, an open mind rather. You cannot be anxious, hasty, and

486 | P a g .

restless in a diet. You need to stay calm and do everything that calms you down. Overthinking can lead to being bored and not interested in the diet very soon. The power of positivity is immense. It cannot be compared with anything else. On the other hand, when you start something with a negative mindset, it eventually does not work out. You end up leaving it behind or failing at it because you had doubts right at the beginning. A doubtful mind cannot focus properly, and the best never comes out from a doubtful mind.

CHAPTER 5:

Stop Emotional Eating

Emotional eating occurs typically when your food becomes a tool that you use in responding to any internal or external emotional cues. It's normal for human beings to tend to react to any stressful situation and the difficult feelings that they have. Whenever you have stressful emotions, you tend to run after a bag of chips or bars of chocolate, a large pizza, or a jar of ice cream to distract yourself from that emotional pain. The foods that you crave at that moment are referred to as comfort food. Those foods contain a high calorie or high carbohydrate with no nutritional value.

Do you know that your appetite increases whenever you are stressed, and whenever you're stressed, you tend to make poor eating habits? Stress is associated with weight gain and weight loss. When you are under intense pressure and intense emotions like boredom or sadness, you tend to cleave unto food. Now that's emotion napping, and it is the way that your body relieves itself of the stress and gets the energy that it needs to overcome its over-dependence on food. Usually get you to the point whereby you don't eat healthy anymore.

Emotional eating is a chronic issue that affects every gender, both male and female, but research has shown that women are more prone to emotional eating than men. Emotional eaters tend to incline towards salty, sweet, fatty, and generally high-calorie foods. Usually, these foods are not healthy for the body, and even if you choose to eat them, you should only consume them with moderation. Emotional eating, especially indulging in unhealthy food, ends up affecting your weight.

Emotional eating was defined as eating in response to intense emotional emotions. Many studies reveal that having a positive mood can reduce your food intake, so you need to start accepting that positive emotions are now part of emotional eating in the same way that negative emotions are part of it too.

Effects of Emotional Eating

So here are some effects of emotional eating:

Intense Nausea

When you are food binging, the food provides a short-term distraction to the emotions that you are facing, and more than often, you will tend to eat very quickly; as a result, you will overeat. That will then result in stomach pains or nausea, which can last for one or two days. So, it is essential to concentrate on the problem that is causing you stress, instead of eating food to solve that problem.

Feeling Guilty

The next one is feeling guilty. Occasionally, you may use food as a reward to celebrate something that is not necessarily bad. It is essential to celebrate the little wings that you have in life, and if food is the way you choose to celebrate it, you should want to eat healthy meals instead of going for unhealthy meals. However, when food becomes your primary mechanism for coping with emotional stress whenever you feel stressed, upset, lonely, angry, or exhausted, then you will open the fridge and find yourself in an unhealthy cycle, without even being able to target to the root cause of the problem that is making you stressed.

Furthermore, you will be filled with guilt. Even after all the emotional damage has passed away, you will still be filled with remorse for what you have done and the unhealthy lifestyle you choose to make at that moment, which will lower your self-esteem. And then, you will go into another emotional eating outburst.

Weight-Related Health Issues

The next one is weight-related health issues. I'm sure that you are aware of how unhealthy eating affects your weight. Many researchers have discovered that emotional eating affects the weight both positively and negatively. Generally, the foods you crave during those emotional moments are high in sugar, high in salt, and saturated fats. And in those emotional moments, you tend to eat anything that you can lay your hands.

Even though some healthy fast foods are available out there, many are still filled with salt, sugar, and trans-fat content. High carbohydrate food increases the demand for insulin in the body, which then promotes hunger more and more, and therefore you tend to eat more calories than you are supposed to consume. Consuming a high level of fat can have an immediate impact on your blood vessels, and it does that in the short-term. If you consume too much fat, your blood pressure will increase, and you will become hospitable to heart attacks, kidney disease, and another cardiovascular disease. Many manufactured fats are created during food processing, and those fats are found in pizza, dough, crackers, fried pies, cookies, and pastries.

Do not be misinformed; no amount of saturated fat is healthy. If you continue to eat this kind of food, you'll be putting yourself in the risks of HDL and LDL, which is the right kind of cholesterol and the wrong kind of cholesterol. And to be frank, both of them will put your heart into the risk of diabetes, high blood pressure, high cholesterol, obesity, and insulin resistance.

How to Stop Emotional Eating Using Meditation

You already know what to eat, and you already know what not to eat. You already know what is right for your body and what is not suitable for your body. If you're not a nutritionist or a health coach or a fitness activist, you already know these things. When you are alone, you tend to engage in emotional eating, and you successfully keep it to yourself and make sure that no one knows about it. It is just like you surrender your control for food to a food demon, and when that demon possesses you, you become angry, sad, and stressed at once, before you know what is happening, you have gone to your fridge, opened it, and begin to consume whatever is there.

As strong as you, once this food demon has possessed you, it will convince you that food is the only way to get out of that emotional turmoil that you are facing. So, before you know what is happening, you are invading your refrigerator and consuming that jar of almond butter that you promised yourself not to consume. And just a few seconds that you open the jar of almond butter, you take the bottle, put it in your mouth, and close the door again. You do it again and again and again, and before you know what is happening, you have leveled the jar up to halfway, and not a dent has been made on the initial in motion that you were eating over.

Now before you know it, if your consciousness catches up with you. You start to feel sad, guilty, and ashamed. The almond butter that you were eating didn't help you that much, not in the way that you wanted it to help you. So, if there is anything you need to realize, you now feel worse than you were one hour ago. And then, you make a promise that you won't repeat this again and that this is the last time that this will happen.

You promised yourself never to share an entrance with that almond butter again, but then you realize that this is what you have been doing to the gluten-free cookies, to that ice cream, and hot chocolate before now. If this is your behavior, then you'll be able to relate to this. Emotional eating is a healthy addition that you must stop. It is more of a habit and one not easy to control. So, there is hope for you if you are engaging in emotional eating today. You have to be able to have control by yourself and over your emotional eating. There are many strategies that you can use to combat that emotional eating, and one is meditation.

Now when it comes to emotional eating and weight management, it is essential to acknowledge the connection between our minds and our bodies. Today we live in a hectic and packed world that is weighing us down. However, mindful meditation can be a powerful tool to help you to be able to create a rational relationship with the food that you eat. One of the essential things about overcoming emotional eating is not to avoid the emotions, but rather to face them head-on, accept them the way they are and agree that they are a crucial part of your life.

Want to stop emotional eating? Then you need to be able to shift your beliefs and worthiness. You need to be able to create a means to cope with unhealthy situations. It is essential to note that meditation will not cure your emotional eating completely. Instead, it will help you to examine and rationalize all the underlining sensations that are leading to emotional eating in your life. For emotional eaters, the feeling of guilt, shame, and low self-esteem are widespread.

Frequently these negatives create judgment in their mind and trigger unhealthy eating patterns, and they end up feeling like an endless self-perpetuating loop. Meditation helps you to be able to develop a non-judgmental mindset about observing your reality. And that mindset will help you and suppress your emotions negative feelings, without even trying to suppress them or comfort them with foods.

Develop the Mind and Body Connection

Meditation will help you to develop the mind and body connection. And once you're able to create that connection, you will be able to distinguish between emotional eating and physical hunger. Once you can differentiate between that, you'll recognize your cues for hunger and safety. You will instantly tell when your desire is not related to physical hunger. Research indicates that medication will help to strengthen your prefrontal cortex, which is the part of the brain that helps you with will power. That part of the brain is the part of the brain that allows us to resist the urge that is within us. Mindfulness will help the urges to eat even when they're not hungry.

By strengthening that prefrontal cortex, you'll be able to get comfortable at observing those impulses without acting on them. Getting rid of an unhealthy habit and start building new ones, you need to be able to work on your prefrontal cortex, and you can only do that with meditation. Once you start meditating, you will begin reaping the benefits. You will learn how to be able to live more in the present. You'll become more aware of your thinking patterns, and in no time, you will be able to become conscious of how you treat food. You'll be able to make the right choice when it comes to food.

CHAPTER 6:

Affirmation for Healthy Diet and Body Image

Affirmation has to be appreciated, and people should believe in them so that they can work well.

However, for this to work well, you must have a strong belief. Your belief will make you comprehend affirmation for a healthy diet.

You can genuinely achieve all affirmations if, at all, you put more effort and faith in managing. Nothing can't be grasped either conceived, and that's why for you to come up with the best affirmation, then a little effort and faith has to be employed. Before you move further with all these, it would be better for you to understand the real functions or rather the real purpose of affirmation. That's what they do in your daily life. It also appears as their primary function and purpose. The statement will highly motivate you and adds you with more power of urge to move ahead. In this, they not only keep you focused on your daily goals but also maintain that positive feeling in you. In that, they can affect your subconscious and conscious mind. Affirmation always has that hidden ability to change your way of thinking and behaving. That's, they can control or have an effect on how you reason, especially about yourself. As a result of this, you are placing in a better position in which you will be able to transform every part of your world, that's both external and inner worlds. In short, affirmation is all about being extremely positive about yourself and having no space of negative thoughts in your life. You can also define it as having positive and straightforward thinking about yourself. You can also talk of it as an essential phrase that helps you in achieving some of your roles.

Affirmations are always honest words and phrases that you take your little time to speak to yourself. These phrases usually capture your physical health level. Everything that you want in life and how you will achieve them revolves around affirmation. Now that you have known this, you should understand all the statements for a healthy diet and body image in detail form. The following declarations have been approved as the most influential and have been grouped into different categories to help you transparently understand them.

Preparing Meals Affirmation

These affirmations are positive phrases you say to yourself while preparing food. They include the following:

Healthy meal planning is a kind of joy. You derive pleasure in making food that has got everything needed in terms of quality. You feel delighted having prepared all these plans, and this will reflect on how you feel about yourself. The right diet that you planned will boost your morale and gives you that anxious feeling about your body. It implies that planning healthy food or somewhat having a healthy diet plan will help you to have the right ingredients for a better meal.

Many studies have found that the proper meal has a positive effect on your body image in that it improves it to a certain level.

"Hi kitchen, forever my center of nourishment." You look at your kitchen as a center of pleasure where you get all forms of nourishment. When you have positive affirmation thoughts like these, you understand that feeling of relaxed. Do this every day by reassuring yourself that, indeed, your kitchen is just a darling to you. That is the only place where you can get that kind of nourishment your body needed. After that, spend as much as possible time in your darling kitchen. And make yourself a healthy diet that will help you improve not only to your inner world but also to the rest of the external world.

Appreciate your healthy diet. Your diet has helped you a lot in making sure that you can prepare those delicious meals. These meals are not only sumptuous but also highly nutritious. Without your healthy diet, then you couldn't have been in a position to prepare food with such qualities. It is better to note that preparing these kinds of food makes you even healthier. Also, this will make you feel even more joyous, relaxed, and at the end of the day, give you that kind of body shape you have always admired. Remember, healthy diet preparation is the cornerstone of your health. Without this, then you are doomed. Appreciate this affirmation and make it your daily phrase.

A healthy diet enables you to have a healthy meal plan. These meal plans have every ingredient required in making healthy food. You will be in an excellent position to choose from the available options. Having decided, you can now prepare that healthy diet. It will be of great help not only to your body but also to the rest of your environs. It will make you feel kind and more so grateful since the vast diet is at your disposal. It's now you to make a choice, and this will give you peace of mind while choosing. All these will get reflected in your body image. Many authors have tried their best to find why people are always grateful here. Many have failed, while others have concluded that there is that kind of pleasure someone derives from having a wide variety of healthy diets to choose on. Remember, these healthy diets that you have eventually chosen will support your healthy life.

Making nutritious and delicious meals are unavoidable. With a healthy diet within your disposal, you can now affirm yourself that you are in a position to make delicious meals. Meals like these are not only delicious but also are critical requirements in building up your body. Prepare them as many times as you can so that you can realize that shape.

You love having more time in your kitchen. Owning a kitchen for yourself is the first step in realizing your body image. Being in a position to have a healthy diet meal plan comes immediately after the latter. In this situation, you are only required to spend some adorable time in your kitchen just preparing that healthy diet. Affirm yourself that you can manage this behavior, putting more effort into it. Time spent on this has not gone to waste as it helps you make healthy meals. The purpose of these meals has many illustrations and explanations in detail. Having that right healthy diet will require lots of your time. This time you will spend it in your kitchen. Make sure that you make this affirmation your day to day routine and practice it correctly.

Feel the worthiness of your time and money spent on your health. Many people invest in their lives. The main objective here is to help improve their health. You are also supposed to do the same. Invest much in your life, and you should feel that worthiness of every input you plant in your life. Look at the money you have been investing in that health sector and make comparisons with the first time you were not affirming yourself. Is there any change? If yes, then you are worth it; that your money hasn't been wasted or gone into waste. Check on time, especially the one you have invested in your life. How does the body react towards that kind of change? If everything has been positive ever since you started investing, then have an assurance that you have clicked on it, and you are worth it. Your spiritual body and external world should reflect the healthy diet that has been for so long. An improvement will add more value and worthiness to everything. Therefore, this affirmation will help you to improve so much that within a short time, your changes will realize. For you to master this, you can take it as a hobby and recite it every time that you are free, then follow your heart.

You are being in a position to have a choice in anything for the family. In all the aspects of life, from west to east, south to north, your family will come first. Having that basketful of a healthy diet, you will be in the right position to choose all kinds of healthy nutrition for your family.

Healthy food should be part of your family. You should be in a clear position to choose healthy food for you and your family. Your family is part and parcel of your life, and providing them with excellent healthy food will be a blessing. Healthy eating leads to a relaxed mind. You should also note that this will always result in improved body image.

Your kids always appreciate new foods. Try having a change in your diet by providing a new diet. Kids still love different diets, and this will help them to improve on their body image. Eating healthy and making sure that everything is well-prepared initiate the morale of eating, a steering wheel towards your achievements of body image. Remember, it is good to note that healthy new meals motivate you and give you the pleasure of preparing.

Learning new things will make you heal your body. You should struggle as hard as possible to learn new kinds of stuff. New ideas might include modern diets, new cooking styles, and so on. Many studies have concluded that new things will always radiate your body. Your body will glow, and at the end of the day, you will be able to realize a good impression and improvement. Your goals will become a lesser issue since achieving them will be much easier. Your body will also feel some sort of relaxation as the process of healing continues. You will be in a position to feel juvenile, and happiness will be part of your day.

You should have the will to nurture yourself. This phrase will help you manage all the processes leading to nurturing yourself. Never lose hope in this process since it might be tedious. Concentrate on every detail that leads to the nurturing of your body image. After realizing this goal, try as hard as possible to get to bigger goals, which include shedding off more pounds of your weight. The will of nurturing will act as a driving force in your process of preparing healthy meals. According to studies carried out some years back, the intention to nurture yourself is more urging to an extent someone would wish to accomplish it first. However, for you to achieve this, then you need to play a little bit with your kitchen. Your kitchen will give you that kind of motivation and maximum pleasure to prepare that meal.

Eating Meals Affirmation

You need to note down that eating meals affirmations are phrases of great motivation that you tell yourself when you have already made the food. You speak these words always while you are just about to eat. The following statements are forming the eating meals affirmation, which you usually use day in day out.

You must appreciate the food. You have already prepared a delicious meal that you are just about to start eating. Before anything, you need to be grateful for having made such a meal. Appreciating your food will increase that urge even to eat more and cook more. It is also resulting in a kind of motivation that will help you in your daily life. Eating healthy food will make you realize some goals.

CHAPTER 7:

Practicing Hypnosis

W e all want time just to relax, dream, and pretend. That refreshes the human body and rejuvenates the soul. It gives us precisely that as we perform our hypnosis: a very intimate moment to enliven and enrich our mind and body. The procedure is over. You need nothing more than a secure and convenient venue.

A Few Simple Rules

There are specific guidelines for hypnosis, and they make sure the method is the most effective and has the most significant advantages. Choose a nice and quiet spot in your home or office when you're about to continue using the recording, where you can relax in a chair, recline or even lay down. Make sure you're comfortable, so you don't have to pay attention to anything else in a spot. Should not listen to your trancework when driving a vehicle or working machinery of some kind, it is essential to agree on a daily period each day or night. Bedtime is a perfect chance to enjoy the trancework, and it can be a fantastic way to get into a restful sleep at this time of the train.

Distractions are possible, and interruptions, instead of making them bother you and pull you off your trancework, using them. To improve the sense of trance, using the sounds of the world around you. E.g., you can hear a noise while doing your hypnosis, and start thinking that this sound distracts you. You then concentrate more on that diversion than on the hypnosis. You may be tempted to combat it—which takes energy off the hypnosis. Instead, when you hear a sound that is disturbing or irritating at first, take control of it by giving it your permission as a background sound to be here. Give it an assignment, such as thinking that "the barking dog's sound helps me go deeper and deeper inside" or "the fan motor sounds like a waterfall that's a soothing background sound." In our private practice in Tucson, there's a day school that inevitably lets the kids play during one of our hypnosis sessions. That is when we say, "Children's music can be a background sound that helps you to go deeper and deeper into yourself now." That is part of our philosophy of "using all."

Distractions also include the sensations you may experience in yourself. You may find yourself feeling, for example, a part of your body that itches. The more you focus on itching or rubbing the itch, the less you concentrate on the trance.

You are merely reminding yourself at those moments that you have permission to move your attention back to your trance or daydream and let the itch dissolve. When working with patients with pain disorders, we show them a similar way of focusing attention away from the "distraction" of pain. We can't control the world around us, after all, or the emotions inside of us; however, we can choose where to focus our attention. If you have trouble letting go of an annoying distraction, you may need to order it to be there as a background sound or vibration, helping you to go inside more easily. Detach yourself from anything your commitment to your hypnosis is interfering with. Let go of some dispute with the world. Only let it be there so you won't see it again sooner or later. When you learn to accept a sensation, noise, or another element that interferes with your hypnosis, you don't let it control you any longer.

Law of Reversed Effect

There is a law of hypnosis, called the Reversed Effect Principle, which states that the more you often attempt to do something, the more it doesn't happen. An example is when you want to tell a name that you think you know—it could be a title of a book, a person, a movie—but at the moment you can't say it, and the harder you set goals, the less it is there.

The name comes as you say, "I will know later" or "It will come to me later," to your subconscious mind. When letting go of the question, "What is the word? What name is it?" You activated your subconscious mind to get the answer right now, and it always does. So, the Reversed Effect Rule is that it only gives you the opposite (the reverse) when you are trying too hard for something.

Simple Techniques

Getting lost in your thoughts and ideas is that a soft trip into the core of yourself is called "going into a trance." Basic self-hypnosis methods involve going into a trance, deepening the trance, using that trance state to give mental-body signals and feedback, and coming out of the trance.

Entering Trance

I will be your mentor when you use the trancework on the audio as you go into a trance. I'll use a form of trance induction that you will find relaxing and concentrating. You undoubtedly saw the spinning watch technique on television, which I have never seen anybody use in thirty-five years of experience. Still, there are many different ways to concentrate your mind on slipping into a trance. You can look at a wall spot, use a breathing technique, or use the gradual relaxation of the body. On the audio trancework, you'll hear a range of induction methods. These are simply the signs or signals you send yourself to say, "I'm going into a trance" or "I'm going to do my hypnosis now." Going into a trance can also be thought of as "making yourself daydream... intentionally." You're letting yourself be immersed in your thoughts and ideas, really distracted, and encouraging yourself to think or visualize what you want to do and what you want to accomplish. There is no "going under." Instead, there is a beautiful experience of going inside.

Deepening the Trance

Deepening your trance lets you digest your thoughts, ideas, and learn more. That is done with progressive relaxation: going "deeper and deeper inside..." with images or scenes, for example, or counting a sequence of numbers.

We want to propose that you create a vertical picture synonymous with moving lower, such as a path leading down a mountain or into a lush green gorge, when you hear the counting from 10 down to 0. You can visualize or envision going further into a scene or location that's much more fun and relaxing for you when you hear me count. We say this with "deepening the trance."

Talking to the Mind of Your Body with Messages and Suggestions

You'll hear my voice speaking two areas of your mind during the trancework. Your conscious thought mind is a part of the soul. That's the part of you that's great at telling time, making change, learning how to read and write; it's the "conscious mind." The thinking mind will continue to do its regular activity of having thoughts throughout the trancework. Right now, you don't have to worry about cleaning your head, or emptying your head, or fully setting your mind in order. Only note that your mind begins to "dream," and your task is only to unplug or disconnect entirely that you don't have to respond to those feelings. You owe them permission to continue streaming. For example, if your "to do" list keeps coming up, just let it float past, instead of focusing on it. The other part of your mind that I'm trying to refer to is what we call your subconscious mind—"sub" as it's below your awareness level of thought. Your subconscious mind can control the trillions of cells in your body, your body chemistry, and all of the body's metabolism, digestion, nervous system, endocrine system, and immune system functions. The mind-body has a tremendous amount of experience, and you gain and acquire additional knowledge in doing the hypnosis so your body's mind can function upon, aligned with your inspiration, beliefs, and expectations, to support you with your weight loss.

You also can adapt and customize the words that are spoken or the pictures that are portrayed to suit you best. The cycle of tailoring is critical. Because it is the self-hypnosis, it must suit you, and all hypnosis is self-hypnosis. Hypnosis, as we have said, is not something that you do. It is something you are being guided to experience, and you are learning it as you experience it. Repetition and training build in your strong ability and knowledge. You can also term it subconscious awareness, as your subconscious mind will do it for you without you having to think about it. So the thoughts and ideas that might have troubled you about your weight, or your weight loss inability, are now being changed into something that supports your perfect body. And the mind-body memorizes, so that rather than the unwelcome effects of the past, it may return to the mind.

For starters, if you believe you're a "yo-yo" dietitian, if you've still recovered the weight you've lost, you can use your trancework to say, "I lose weight every day, and my body knows how to make this a lasting capacity. I'm enjoying my ideal weight." Subconscious awareness, or mind-body experience gained from your trancework, is just like learning to ride a bike or drive a car. As you first heard, there appeared to be a lot of things to pay attention to at the same time, but your mind-body soon focused on this information, and you can drive confidently today, so you don't even have to remind your feet what to do.

CHAPTER 8:

Mind Meditation

The Joyful Mind Meditation

This meditation can be used for a time of stress and anxiety. It will help guide you into a more relaxed state where you can focus on the present and find inner peace. Please use this meditation method when you find your mind racing. That can also be used if you feel like you are about to have an anxiety or panic attack.

"Welcome to the joyful mind guided meditation.

Please find yourself in a quiet area to sit and dim the lighting.

Make sure you are comfortable. Just sit your back straight and relaxed. Loosen any tight clothing that may be restricting you.

Let your hands lie loosely and relaxed into your lap. Close your eyes and take a deep breath. Now, relax.

Now that your eyes are closed, you may begin to connect with your inner self of thoughts and feelings.

Gradually, let the outside world fade from your awareness.

For the next few minutes, allow yourself to enjoy and submerge into this relaxing experience.

You are free from all your responsibilities during this meditation. Any thoughts, tasks, or concerns that you may have do not require your immediate attention. Tuck those thoughts away and focus on your inner thoughts.

You may find that your mind will begin to wander during this meditation. That is okay, and this is normal. Just bring your awareness back to the present and the sound of my voice. These will guide you into a place of inner peace and deep relaxation.

Remember that you are in charge of yourself. If you wish to end this meditation, you can do so by opening your eyes.

Begin to take a slow, long, and deep breath in through your nose. Release that breath through your mouth.

Find your inner self begin to relax.

Begin to take another deep breath in, and exhale.

Notice how calm this type of breathing is. Be aware of the feelings of relaxation starting to spread throughout your body. Starting from your lungs, all the way down to your toes.

Continue to breathe deeply, slowly, and gently. Try not to breathe too quickly.

With each inhale and exhale, your thoughts start to become lighter.

Now, you start to feel a sense of spaciousness inside of you. It will open up slowly.

Keep relaxing.

Let the soft movement of your breath to guide you into an even more relaxed state of being.

Breathe in. Breathe out. Deeper you go into this state of relaxation.

Breathe in. Breathe out. Let your mind gradually slow down. Breathe in. Breathe out. Let it slow down some more.

Breathe in. Breathe out.

You may now begin to enjoy a guided journey into your inner place of joy and serenity.

Allow images and visualizations to form in your mind naturally, as I speak. Do so at your own pace.

Begin to let your expectations drift away from you. Let them go. Allow yourself to experience this meditation journey in whatever form comes naturally to you.

Begin to imagine that you are standing in a green and beautiful grassy field. The field stretches on for miles. You can feel the heat of the sun on your face, slowly warming your body.

You feel the soft and lush green grass, cushioning your bare feet. Right now, you can smell the nature all around you.

You can hear the sounds of nature around you, the rustling of the blowing grass. Birds were singing—the rustling of leaves in the distance.

You feel very much at home in this serene place.

You have the time in the world.

You're safe and happy here.

Take a moment to appreciate your surroundings.

You notice a sizeable luscious tree growing close by.

You begin to walk towards that tree.

Take your time walking. There is no rush whatsoever. Stay in the moment and appreciate the feeling of each step.

As you walk towards the tree, you feel yourself falling more deeply into a state of relaxation.

You are now standing under the tree. It's long branches, and large leaves hang right above your head.

You notice that the tree holds many delicious fruits in all shapes, sizes, and colors.

That is not just an ordinary tree. Its fruits carry special powers.

Reach your arm up and take a piece of fruit from the branches. Watch it for a moment. Notice the color of this fruit, the texture, and the weight. It's quite heavy in your hand.

Take a bite of this fruit.

As you swallow the fruit, it slides down your throat and into your belly. You begin to feel something beautiful happen. A feeling of happiness and peace begins to glow inside of your body.

The sensation starts in your abdomen, and it spreads to your chest and into your heart.

Let go of thinking, and begin to bring all your attention on feeling. Embellish in the sensation of joy, love, and peace. Feel your body gently glowing with these feelings.

Take another bite of the magical fruit, taste it.

This wonderful feeling begins to intensify even more.

Feel yourself begin to radiate this wonderful sensation to love and happiness.

Take another bite of the fruit. Take as many bites as you'd like.

Relax and let yourself drown in this enchanting feeling. Instead of trying, just let it effortlessly take over. Break down any walls that you feel comfortable breaking and let it surround you as much as you like.

Stay with these joyful and peaceful feelings. Enjoy this time of meditation.

You may remain in this relaxed state of meditation for as long as you please. Don't feel rushed to leave."

When you are ready, you may finish this meditation. Simple open your eyes to leave. Take a deep breath and give yourself a few moments to adjust before standing up.

The Spiritual Meditation

This meditation is used for those who want to explore spirituality further. You may not feel any different during this meditation, but you will feel the physical and mental benefits of this practice. During this meditation, you will have to be awake. This technique can lead to sleep. Avoid that to experience spiritual effects.

Before we begin this meditation, think about your spirituality. What gives you meaning in life? You will need to conceptualize a word or a short phrase that gives you meaning. You will repeat those words during the time it takes to exhale a breath. For example, if nature holds deep and strong meaning for you, you may select phrases that relate to it.

"Welcome to spiritual meditation.

Find a comfortable position for you, one that allows you to remain awake.

Let's begin.

Close your eyes. Choose to focus your gaze on a small area. Start by relaxing your muscles and relieving any tension you feel.

When you feel thoughts come to your mind, simply acknowledge them and let it pass. Bring your attention back to your body.

Bring your awareness to your breathing. Notice the way each breath feels; let it be natural. Just observe.

As thoughts arise in your mind, acknowledge them and let it go. Return your attention to breathing.

Breathe slowly, deeply, and naturally.

If you find your thoughts wandering some more, bring your attention to breathing.

Notice how your breath flows gently in and out through your body. It feels effortless.

Interruptions are normal. You may find yourself thinking about other thoughts. Let them go, and focus on breathing.

Now, begin to think about the meaningful words or phrases you've selected. Begin to say this word in your mind as you breathe out.

Each time you exhale, repeat the phrase.

Continue repeating the phrase every time you breathe out.

With each breath, allow distracting thoughts to float by your awareness.

Let any spiritual feeling linger in your body. Don't ignore it, but let it brew deeply inside you. Let is consume your body and let it stay.

Repeat the phrase. Feel the spirituality within you intensify. You may leave this meditation at any moment, simply open your eyes.

Let your body communicate and get comfortable with the feeling of spirituality.

Breathe in. Breathe out. Let your thoughts turn to your body. You were relaxed, peaceful, and calm. Notice how your body feels as it becomes more aware of your surroundings.

Bring your attention back to your thoughts. Bring it back to your regular conscious awareness. You may let the spirituality leave your body.

Stay seated for a few more moments with your eyes open. Enjoy the feeling of reawakening. Savor the relaxation and all the other emotions you've encountered.

Begin to reflect on the experience of spiritual meditation. Be aware of all the feelings during the practice. You should be feeling free from worries.

End this guided meditation by wiggling your toes and then your fingers. Stretch your back and shoulders. When you are ready, you may stand up and continue with your day."

The Gratitude Meditation

The gratitude meditation is used as a conscious effort to appreciate all the things in the world that makes us feel good. It is directly related to opening our hearts and embracing all our blessings. This meditation is very popular amongst Buddhist monks and nuns. It's typically practiced at the beginning and end of their days to pay gratitude to everything that helped them throughout that day, and this also includes their sufferings. Gratitude meditation gives us the power we need to face our problems and weaknesses to acknowledge the darker parts of life. This meditation can be used when you are feeling the burdens of the world. Try this guided meditation when you feel self-pity or hopelessness.

Before you begin this meditation, think about something in your life that you are grateful for; think about where that feeling is held in your body. You can feel thankful for your home, spouse, or even the vacation you just purchased.

"Welcome to the gratitude meditation.

Find a comfortable sitting position and dim the lighting.

I will begin by bringing your awareness to the things you are grateful for in life.

Give the sense of gratitude the chance to come up naturally. When it arises, let yourself sink into that feeling. Surrender yourself to it. Begin to notice how it feels inside your body, how that energy feels. If the feeling of gratitude does not come up immediately, don't try to force yourself, it is okay. Instead, just surrender yourself to your heart and not your head."

CHAPTER 9:

Hypnosis Script

A t this point in the audio, I invite you to make yourself as comfortable as possible in your bed. Please have all the light's turned off and distractions put away. You have already set in a full, hard day of work. Think of sleeping sound and comfortable through the night as a reward for working so hard.

- How was your day today?

- Were you productive?

- How did you feel?

Gently tuck yourself under the cover, and we will begin our journey. Ready?

Inhale deeply. Hold onto that breath for a moment, and then let it go. To begin, I am going to lead you through an induction script for self-hypnosis. By allowing yourself to slip into this state of mind, it will help you just let go of your stress that your holding to, even if it is in your subconscious. I am going to help you tap into these emotions so you can let them go and sleep like you never have before.

All of us are stressed. Honestly, who can sleep when worried? In this state of mind, you probably feel too alert to even think about sleeping. When you are stressed, the adrenal glands in your body release adrenaline and cortisol. Both of these hormones keep you awake and stop you from falling asleep.

In the audio to follow, we will go over letting go of your worries, even if it is just for the night. You are in a safe place right now. Anything you need to get done can wait until tomorrow. You must take this time for yourself. We need a break from reality at some point or another. I invite you now to take another deep breath so we can focus on what is crucial right now; sleep.

To start, I would like you to close your eyes gently, as you do this, wiggle slightly until your body feels comfortable in your bed. When you find your most comfortable position, it is time to begin breathing.

While you're focusing on your breath, remind yourself to breathe slow and deep. Feel as the air fills your lungs and release it comfortably. Feel as your body relaxes further under the sheets. You begin to feel a warm glow, wrapping your whole body in a comfortable blanket.

Before you let go into a deep hypnotic state, listen carefully to the words I am saying at this moment.

Everything is going to happen automatically.

At this moment, there is nothing you need to focus on; you will have no control over what happens next in our session. But you are okay with that. At this moment, you are warm and safe. You are preparing your body for a full night's rest and letting go of any thoughts you may have future or the past. What matters the most is your comfort, your breath, and the incredible sleep you are about to experience.

Now, feel as the muscles around your eyes begin to relax. I invite you to continue breathing deeply and bring your attention to your eyes. They are beginning to feel heavy and relaxed. Your eyes worked hard for you today. They watched as you worked, they kept you safe as you walked around, and they showed other people you were paying attention to them as you spoke. Thank your eyes at this moment and allow them to rest for the night so they will be prepared for tomorrow.

Your breath is coming easy and free now. Soon, you will enter a hypnotic trance with no effort. This trance will be deep, peaceful, and safe. There is nothing for your conscious mind to do at this moment. Allow for your subconscious mind to take over and do the work for you.

This trance will come automatically. Soon, you will feel like you are dreaming. Allow yourself to relax and give in to my voice. All you need to focus on is my voice.

You are doing wonderfully. Without noticing, you have already changed your rate of breath. You are breathing easy and free. There is no thought involved. Your body knows what you need to do, and you can relax further into your subconscious mind.

Now, you are starting to show signs of drifting off into this peaceful hypnotic trance. I invite you to enjoy the sensations as your subconscious mind takes over and listens to the words I am speaking to you. It is slowly becoming less important for you to listen to me. Your subconscious listens, even as I begin to whisper.

You are drifting further and further away. You are becoming more relaxed and more comfortable. At this moment, nothing is bothering you. Your inner mind is listening to me, and you are beginning to realize that you don't care about slipping into a deep trance.

This peaceful state allows you to be comfortable and relaxed. Being hypnotized is pleasant and enjoyable. That is beginning to feel natural for you. Each time I hypnotize you, it becomes more enjoyable than the time before.

You will enjoy these sensations; you are comfortable, peaceful. You are entirely calm.

As we progress through the relaxing exercises, you will learn something new about yourself. You are working gently to develop your sleep techniques without even knowing you are developing them in the first place.

Slip completely into your mental state. When I say number three, your brain is going to take over, and you will find yourself in the forest. This forest is peaceful, calm, and serene. It is safe and comfortable, much like your bed at this moment.

As you inhale, try to bring more oxygen into your body with beautiful, deep breaths. As you exhale, feel as your body relaxes more and more into the bed. Breathing comes easy and free for you. Like you, you are becoming more peaceful and calmer without even realizing it.

As we continue, you do not care how relaxed you are. You are happy in the state of mind. You do not have a care in the world. Your subconscious mind is always aware of the words I am saying to you. As we go along, it is becoming less important for you to listen to my voice.

Your inner mind is receiving everything I tell you. Your conscious mind is relaxed and peaceful. As you find your peace of mind, we will begin to explore this forest you have found yourself in, together.

Imagine lying near a stream in this beautiful and peaceful forest. It is a sunny, warm summer day. As you lay comfortably in the grass beside this stream, you feel a warm breeze gently moving through your hair. Inhale deep and experience how fresh and clean this air is. Inhale again and exhale. Listen carefully as the stream flows beside you. A quiet whoosh noise, filling your ears and relaxing you even further. Listen to me. Your subconscious mind takes hold and listens to everything I am saying. Enjoy the beautiful nature around you. The sunlight shines through the trees and kisses your skin gently. The birds begin to sing a happy tune. You smile, feeling yourself become one with nature.

Each time you exhale, I want to imagine your whole body relaxing more. You are becoming more at ease. As you do this, I want you to begin to use your imagination. You are lying on the grass. It is located in a green meadow with the sun shining down on you. The sun is not hot, but a comfortable warm.

Imagine that beautiful flowers are blooming everywhere around you. Watch as the flowers move gently in the breeze. Their scents waft toward your nose as you inhale deeply and exhale.

Imagine that you begin to stand up. As you do this, you look over your left shoulder gently, and you see a mountain near the edge of the beautiful meadow, a trip up to the top of the mountain to see this beautiful view from a different angle.

As you begin to walk, you follow the stream. Imagine gently bending over and placing your hand, not the cool, rushing water. As you look upon the sea, imagine how clean and cool this water is. The stream flows gently across your fingers, and it relaxes you.

When you are ready, we will head toward the mountain again. As you grow closer to the mountain, the birds begin to chirp. Inhale deep and imagine how the pine trees smell around you. Soon, you begin to climb the mountain at a comfortable pace.

You are enjoying the trip. It is beautiful to be outside with this beautiful nature, taking in all the sights and sounds. The meadow grows smaller as you climb higher, but you are not afraid. The scene is gorgeous from up here, and you are happy at this moment.

As you reach the top, take a deep breath and pat yourself on the back for your accomplishment. Take a look down on the meadow and see how small the trees look.

The breeze is blowing your hair around gently, and the sun continues to shine down on the top of your head. Imagine that you are taking a seat at the very top of the mountain and take a few moments to appreciate this nature. You wish you could always be this relaxed.

When you take your life into your own hands, you will be able to. That is why we are here. Of course, you may be here because you want to sleep, but you can't do that truly unless you learn how to let go of your stress. Through guided meditation and exercises within this audio, you will learn how to become a better version of yourself.

Soon, we will work on deepening your trance. You are beginning to relax further into the meditation and opening your heart and soul to the practice. Remember that you are safe, and you are happy to be here.

CHAPTER 10:

Script 1 – Self-Hypnosis Relaxation Techniques

George taught Bonnie a hundred useful positive affirmations for weight loss and to keep her motivated. She chose the ones that she wanted to build in her program and used them every day. She was losing weight very slowly, which bothered her very much. She thought she was going in the wrong direction and was about to give up, but George told her not to be worried since its completely natural speed. It takes time for the subconscious to collate all the information and start working according to her conscious will. Also, her body remembered the fast weight loss, but her subconscious remembered her emotional damage, and now it is trying to prevent it. In reality, after some months of hard work, she started to see the desired results. She weighed 74 kilos (163 lbs).

According to dietitians, the success of dieting is greatly influenced by how people talk the use of "I should" or "I must" is to be avoided whenever possible. Anyone who says, "I shouldn't eat French fries" or "I have to get a bite of chocolate" will feel that they have no control over the events. Instead, if you say "I prefer" to leave the food, you will feel more power and less guilt. The term "dieting" should be avoided. Proper nutrition should be seen as a permanent lifestyle change. For example, the correct wording is, "I've changed my eating habits" or "I'm eating healthier."

Diets are fattening. Why?

The body needs fat. Our body wants to live, so it stores fat. Removing this amount of fat from the body is not as easy as the body protects against weight loss. During starvation, our bodies switch to a 'saving flame,' burning fewer calories to avoid starving. Those who are starting to lose weight are usually optimistic, as, during the first week, they may experience 1-3 kg (2-7 lbs) of weight loss, which validates their efforts and suffering. However, their body has deceived them very well because it does not want to break down fat. Instead, it begins to break down muscle tissue. At the beginning of dieting, our bodies burn sugar and protein, not fat. Burned sugar removes a lot of water out of the body; that's why we experience amazing results on the scale. It should take about seven days for our body to switch to fat burning. Then our body's alarm bell rings. Most diets have a sad end: reducing your metabolic rate to a lower level. That means that if you only eat a little more afterward, you regain all the weight you have lost previously. After dieting, the body will make special efforts to store fat for the impending famine.

We must understand what our soul needs. Those who desire to have success must first and foremost change their spiritual foundation. It is important to pamper our souls during a period of weight loss. All overweight people tend to rag on themselves for eating forbidden food, "I have overeaten again. My willpower is so weak!"

Imagine a person very close to you who has gone through a difficult time while making mistakes from time to time. Are we going to scold or try to help and motivate them? If we love them, we would instead comfort them and try to convince them to continue. No one tells their best friend that they are weak, ugly, or bad, just because they are struggling with their weight. If you don't say it to someone, don't do so to yourself either! Let us be aware of this: during weight loss, our soul needs peace and support. All bad opinions, even if they are only expressed in thought, are detrimental and divert us from our purpose. You must support yourself with positive reinforcement. There is no place for the all or nothing principle. A single piece of cake will not ruin your entire diet. Realistic thinking is more useful than disaster theory. A cookie is not the end of the world. Eating should not be a reward. Cakes should not make up for a bad day. If you are generally a healthy consumer, eat some goodies sometimes because of its delicious taste and to pamper your soul. I'll give you a hundred positive affirmations you can use to reinforce your weight loss. I'll divide them into main categories based on the most typical situations for which you need confirmation. You can repeat all of them whenever you need to, but you can choose the ones that are more suitable for your circumstances. If you prefer to listen to them during meditation, you can record them with a piece of beautiful, relaxing music.

General Affirmations to Reinforce Your Well-Being

1. Thank you for making me happy today.

2. Today is a perfect day. I meet friendly and helpful people, whom I treat kindly.

3. Every new day is for me. I live to make myself feel good. Today I just pick good thoughts for myself.

4. Something wonderful is happening to me today.

5. I feel good.

6. I am calm, energetic, and cheerful.

7. My organs are healthy.

8. I am satisfied and balanced.

9. Living in peace and understanding with everyone.

10. I listen to others with patience.

11. In every situation, I find the good.

12. I accept and respect myself and my fellow human beings.

13. I trust myself; I trust my inner wisdom.

Do you often scold yourself? Then repeat the following affirmations frequently:

14. I forgive myself.

15. I'm good to myself.

16. I motivate myself over and over again.

17. I'm doing my job well.

18. I care about myself.

19. I am doing my best.

20. Very proud of myself for my achievements.

21. I am aware that sometimes I have to pamper my soul.

22. I remember that I did a great job this week.

23. I deserved this small piece of candy.

24. I have to let go of the feeling of guilt.

25. I release the blame.

26. Everyone is imperfect. I accept that I am too.

If you feel pain when you choose to avoid delicious food, you need to motivate yourself with affirmations:

27. I am motivated and persistent.

28. I control my life and my weight.

29. I'm ready to change my life.

30. Changes make me feel better.

31. I follow my diet with joy and cheerfulness.

32. I am aware of my amazing capacities.

33. I am grateful for my opportunities.

34. Today I'm excited to start a new diet.

35. I always keep in mind my goals.

36. I imagine myself slim and beautiful.

37. Today I am happy to have the opportunity to do what I have long been postponing.

38. I possess the energy and will to go through my diet.

39. I prefer to lose weight instead of wasting time on momentary pleasures.

Here you can find affirmations that help you to change serious convictions and blockages:

40. I see my progress every day.

41. I listen to my body's messages.

42. I'm taking care of my health.

43. I eat healthy food.

44. I love who I am.

45. I love how life supports me.

46. A good parking space, coffee, conversation. It's all for me today.

47. It feels good to be awake because I can live in peace, health, love.

48. I'm grateful that I woke up. I take a deep breath of peace and tranquillity.

49. I love my body. I love being served by me.

50. I eat by tasting every flavor of the food.

51. Being aware of the benefits of healthy food.

52. I enjoy eating healthy food and being fitter every day.

53. I feel energetic because I eat well.

Many people are struggling with being overweight because they don't move enough. The very root of this issue can be a refusal to do exercises due to negative biases in our minds.

We can overcome these beliefs by repeating the following affirmations:

54. I like moving because it helps my body burn fat.

55. Each time I exercise, I am getting closer to having a beautiful, tight shapely body.

56. It's a very uplifting feeling of being able to climb up to 100 steps without stopping.

57. It's easier to have an excellent quality of life if I move.

58. I like the feeling of returning to my home tired but happy after a long winter walk.

59. Physical exercises help me have a longer life.

60. I am proud to have better fitness and agility.

61. I feel happier thanks to the happiness hormone produced by exercise.

62. I feel full thanks to the enzymes that produce a sense of fullness during physical exercises.

63. I am aware even after exercise, my muscles continue to burn fat, and so I lose weight while resting.

64. I feel more energetic after exercise.

65. My goal is to lose weight. Therefore I exercise.

66. I am motivated to exercise every day.

67. I lose weight while I exercise.

List of generic affirmations that you can build in your program:

68. I'm glad I'm who I am.

69. Today, I read articles and watch movies that make me feel positive about my diet progress.

70. I love it when I'm happy.

71. Taking a deep breath to enhance my fears.

72. Today I do not want to prove my truth, but I want to be happy.

73. I am strong and healthy. I'm fine, and I'm getting better.

74. I am happy today because whatever I do, I find joy in it.

75. I pay attention to what I can become.

76. I love myself and I'm helpful to others.

77. I accept what I cannot change.

78. I am contented that I can eat healthy food.

79. I am happy that I have been changing my life with my new healthy lifestyle.

80. Avoid comparing myself to others.

81. I accept and support who I am and turn to me with love.

82. Today I can do anything for my improvement.

83. I'm fine. I'm happy for life. I love who I am. I'm strong and confident.

84. I am calm and satisfied.

85. Today is perfect for me to exercise and to be healthy.

86. I have decided to lose weight, and I am strong enough to follow my will.

87. I love myself, so I want to lose weight.

88. I am proud of myself because I follow my diet program.

89. I see how much stronger I am.

90. I know that I can do it.

CHAPTER 11:

Script 2 – Strengthen the Experience

How Does It Feel Loving Yourself?

Have a look at these characteristics. Are these familiar to you? It is the way it will feel for those who like yourself:

- You genuinely feel happy and accepting your world, even though you might not agree with everything within it.

- You're compassionate with your flaws or less-than-perfect behaviors, understanding that you're capable of improving and changing.

- You mercifully love compliments and feel joyful inside.

- You frankly see your flaws and softly accept them learning to alter them.

- You accept all of the goodness that comes your way.

- You honor the great qualities and the fantastic qualities of everybody around you.

- You look at the mirror while seeing your face smiling (at least all the period).

Many confound self-love with becoming arrogant and greedy. But some individuals are so caught up in themselves they make the tag of being egotistical and thinking just of these. We do not find that as a healthful indulgent, however, as a character that's not well balanced in enjoying love and loving others. It's not selfish to get things your way; however, it's egotistical to insist that everybody else can see them your way too.

The Dalai Lama states, "If you do not enjoy yourself, then you can't love other people. You won't have the capacity to appreciate others. If you don't have any empathy on your own, then you aren't capable of developing empathy for others." Dr. Karl Menninger, a psychologist, states it this way: "Self-love isn't opposed to this love of different men and women. You cannot truly enjoy yourself and get yourself a favor with no people a favor, and vice versa." We're referring to the healthiest type of self-indulgent, that simplifies the solution to accepting your best good.

Have a better look at the way you see your flaws and blame yourself. Self-love and finding an error or depriving yourself aren't in any way compatible. If you suppress or refuse to enjoy yourself, you're in danger of paying too much focus on your flaws, that is a sort of self-loathing. You don't want to place focus on negative aspects of yourself, for holding these ideas in your mind, and you're giving them the psychological energy which brings that result or leaves it actual.

Self-hypnosis can help you use your mind-body to make new and much more loving ideas and beliefs on your own. It helps your mind-body create and take fluctuations in the patterns of feeling and thinking about what has been for you for quite a while, and which aren't helpful for you. The trancework about the sound incorporates many positive suggestions to change your ideas, emotions, and beliefs in alignment with your ideal weight.

An integral goal for all these positive hypnotic suggestions is the innermost feeling of enjoying yourself. In case your self-loving feelings are constant with your ideal weight, then it is going to occur with increased ease. But if you harbor bitterness or remorse, or sense undeserving, these emotions operate contrary to enjoying yourself enough to think and take your ideal weight. Lucille Ball stated it well: "Love yourself first, and everything falls inline."

The hypnotic suggestions about the sound are directions for change that led to the maximum "internal" degree of mind-body or unconscious. However, the "outer" changes in lifestyle activity should also happen. Many weight-loss approaches you have been using might appear to be a lot of work. We suggest that by adopting a mindset that's without the psychological pressure related to "needing to," "bad or good," or even "simple or hard," with no judgment in any way, the fluctuations could be joyous. Yes, joyous.

That produces the whole journey of earning adjustments and shifting easier. The term "a labor of love" implies you enjoy doing this so much, and it isn't labor or responsibility. The "labor" of organizing a family feast in a vacation season, volunteering at a hospital or school, or even buying a present for someone exceptional can appear effortless. Here is the mindset that will assist you in following some weight loss procedures. We want you to just place yourself in the situation of being adored. You're doing so to you. Loving yourself eliminates the job, and that means it is possible to relish your advancement toward a lifestyle that encourages your ideal weight. Think about some action that you like to perform. Imagine yourself performing this action today. Notice that when you're doing something which you like to do, you're feeling energized and enjoyable, and some other attempt is evidenced by enjoyment, "loving what you're doing." Sometimes, we recommend that you also find that as "enjoying yourself doing this." Maybe by directing a more favorable attitude toward enjoying yourself, you'll end up enjoying what you're doing.

Lisa's Brimming Smile

After Lisa and Rick wed, both have been slender and appreciated for their active lifestyles, which included softball and Pilates classes at the local gym. When their very first baby was born, Lisa had obtained an additional fifteen lbs. And now, their second baby came three years after, and she was twenty pounds overweight. Depending on the demands of motherhood depended on fast-frozen foods, canned foods, and table food. Persistent sleep deprivation also let her power level reduced, and she can hardly keep up with the toddlers. Rick, a promising young company executive, took more duties on the job, increasing the"ladder of success," indulging in company lunches, and even working late afternoon. He'd return home late, watched the T.V., and eat leftover pizza.

The youthful couple accepted their old way of life but observed with dismay as their bodies grew tired and old beyond their years. However, they lasted. If their oldest boy entered astronomy, they would become more upset. Small Ricky appeared to be the goal of each germfree, and he started to miss several days of college. If this was not enough, he also attracted the germs to the house to his small brother, mother, and father. It appeared that four of these were with them the whole winter.

The infant was colicky. From the spring, following a household bout with influenza, Lisa's friend supplied the title of a behavioral therapist to whom she explained about the ability to shed some light on the recurrent diseases of Lisa's small boys. In the first consultation, Lisa declared the previous four decades of her household's life, culminating at current influenza where the small boys were recuperating. They were exhausted, tired, not sleeping well, and usually under sunlight. With summer vacation just around the corner, Lisa had been distressed to receive her family back on the right track.

The words of the nutritionist were straightforward: Start feeding yourself along with your household foods, which are fresh and ready in your home. Start buying fruits and veggies, and make some simple recipes using rice and other grains. Learn how to create healthy and wholesome dishes for your loved ones. These phrases triggered Lisa to remember when she had been a kid about the time of her very own small boys. She remembered her mother fixing large fruit salads using lemon. She recalled delicious dishes of homemade soup along with hot fresh bread. Instantly, Lisa knew what she needed to do for her boys. And she'd make it happen. Approximately six months after, we received a telephone call from Lisa. I can hear the grin brimming in her voice. "You cannot think the shift in our loved ones. Ricky has had just one cold in the past six weeks. We are all sleeping much better, and also, the baby is happy and sleeping during the night. Four days per week, we have a family walk after breakfast or after dinner. And guess what? I have lost thirty-five lbs, and I was not dieting! I'm better than I have ever felt."

Giving Forth

Forgiveness is a significant step in enjoying yourself. At any time you forgive, you're "committing forth" or "letting go" of a thing you're holding inside you. Let's be clear about this: bias is simply for you, not anybody else. It's not a kind of accepting, condoning, or justifying somebody else's activities. It's a practice of letting go of an adverse impression that has remained within you too long. It's letting go of any emotion or idea, which can be an obstacle between you and enjoying yourself and getting what you desire.

A lot of us are considerably more crucial and harder on ourselves than we're about others. When you continue with the notions of what you need or shouldn't have completed, you aren't enjoying yourself. Instead, you're putting alert energy to negative beliefs about yourself. Ideas like "I must have taken a stroll" or even "I should not have eaten this second slice of pie" can also be regarded as self-punishing. Sometimes, penalizing yourself, either by lack of overeating or eating, may even lead to a discount for your well-being. By changing your focus to self-appreciation, you go from the negative to the positive, which is quite a bit more conducive to self-loving.

Writing a diary about all choices you make every day may promote self-improvement. By forgiving yourself and forgiving other people, you launch the psychological hold that previous events might have had to you personally, and you also make yourself accessible to appreciate yourself. When you launch the effects of previous encounters by forgiving, then you undergo reassurance and a calm comfort on your body, which helps you take your ideal weight.

Basic Rules of Self – Hypnosis Diet

- No explanations

- No denying

- No criticizing

Negative thoughts, thoughts, and expressions aren't permitted on your understanding (or maybe not for long, anyhow). Remember, there are no mistakes, just lessons. Love yourself, hope on your options, and what's possible.

CHAPTER 12:

Script 3 – How to Use Guided Meditation and Positive Affirmations for Weight Loss

Have you attempted and neglected to get in shape? In this case, you realize how troublesome it very well may be to stay with a weight loss program. What's more, in any event, when you do figure out how to drop those additional pounds, keeping them off is another fight together. In any case, you don't need to spend a mind-blowing remainder doing combating with your willpower with an end goal to get and stay thin.

One of the critical contrasts between those individuals who figure out how to get more fit and keep it off effectively, and the individuals who don't, is that the previous gathering changes their eating and exercises propensities as well as their mindset too. If your mind isn't your ally, getting more fit will be troublesome or inconceivable because you'll be continually undermining your endeavors. How about we investigate required for the sort of mindset that prompts lasting, sound weight loss?

Persistence

Right off the bat, you should show restraint. The individuals who shed pounds gradually and consistently are well on the way to keep it off. So overlook each one of those diet designs that guarantee you can drop 10 pounds or more in seven days—the vast majority of that will be water weight, and will recover right when you begin eating ordinarily. It's just human to need a convenient solution; however, if you need to lose the weight, keep it off and move on without having to battle with your body for an incredible remainder continually, it merits adopting the moderate strategy, since compromising makes weight loss increasingly troublesome and tedious over the long haul.

Adaptability

Adaptability is likewise significant for effective long haul weight loss. If you make amazingly rigid guidelines about what you can and can't eat, you may get more fit, yet risks are that you'll be hopeless. You're probably not going to adhere to those principles for an incredible remainder. What's more, when you have this 'win or bust' sort of mindset, and you disrupt your guidelines even somewhat, it very well may be enticing to go on a hard and fast binge a short time later, because all things considered, you've blitz now! Then again, if you follow reasonable rules while recognizing that there will be times (for example, occasions and unique events) when you'll eat food that isn't a piece of your ordinary diet. At that point, these 'illegal nourishments' will appear to be less appealing because they're not something that you've restricted from your life forever.

Consistency

Consistency is another piece of a fruitful weight loss mindset. That may appear to repudiate the above point. However, it doesn't generally. Interestingly, you eat heartily and follow your activity plan most of the time. Along these lines, you'll stay away from yo-yo and unfortunate practices, for example, the binge/starve cycle. It's the moves you make most of the time that will give you the outcomes you are looking on. When you're focused on building long haul changes in your way of life, instead of searching for a convenient solution, you'll increasingly spur to embrace a moderate and adjusted arrangement that you can try reliably.

Self-Love

It is additionally imperative to have an inspirational mentality towards yourself. Presently in case you're similar to a great many people who need to shed pounds, odds are you don't feel generally excellent about your body and appearance. While you don't need to claim to cherish something that you loathe about yourself, it's likewise significant not to be continually beating yourself up for not being at your actual weight as of now, in general, overheat because of stress, such self-recriminations will most likely cause you to feel even unhappier and significantly increasingly inclined to overeating—thus, the endless loop deteriorates.

So put forth an attempt to concentrate on those things you do like about yourself, and if you have days where you miss exercises or don't eat just as you'd like, be mindful so as not to blame yourself too brutally. Instead, recognize this is something that happens to everyone, and give a valiant effort to put it behind you and start anew merely. Recall that you don't need to eat or practice flawlessly to shed pounds—you need a moderate system that is sufficient.

If you can make these things part of your ordinary mindset, weight loss ought to be more straightforward. It tends to be somewhat testing, particularly in case you're accustomed to having a negative disposition towards yourself and your weight loss endeavors. One thing that can assist you with adopting a progressively empowered mindset all the more effective is to utilize a weight loss meditation recording. If you use a quality chronicle that incorporates brainwave entrainment innovation, you can increase more straightforward access to your subconscious mind and utilize necessary procedures, for example, affirmations and perception, to reconstruct it with new convictions that work for you as opposed to against you.

Such accounts contain dreary hints of specific frequencies, which make it simpler for your brain to enter a profoundly loose and centered state. In such express, the subconscious is increasingly open to the proposal, and any affirmation or perception work that you do will be progressively successful. That is an extraordinary method to assist with changing your mindset from the back to front, regardless of whether you're not knowledgeable about meditation or other mind control procedures. It's justified even despite the little exertion that it takes to do this since rolling out positive improvements throughout your life; for example, getting more fit is such a lot simpler when you have your mind on your side, battle your self-dangerous inclinations—because those desires aren't there anymore.

CHAPTER 13:

Script 4 – How Do I Love My Body If There Is No Reason?

These are all phrases that you should say to yourself as often as possible. As we read them, let them flow through your mind as if they are your own.

Write the words down to remember those further, put notes around your house with the affirmations written on them, or simply find other creative ways to incorporate these affirmations in your life. Let's start reading them now so that you can get these ideas in your head right away.

1. I have a happy and healthy attitude towards life.

2. I love my body; that is why I want the best for it.

3. I love myself; that is why I want to be healthy.

4. My health is my utmost priority.

5. My body is wonderful, and I love myself at the end of the day.

6. I can feel my body getting slimmer every day.

7. I can feel my appetite getting more manageable every day.

8. I believe in my capability to reach my goals of extreme weight loss.

9. Every day I weigh, the scales show significant weight loss.

10. Each day I successfully lose weight without fail.

11. My weight loss program is working like magic.

12. My body is responding immensely to my weight loss efforts.

13. I can feel my body fat melting away.

14. I have developed a high rate of metabolism that helps me reach my ideal weight.

15. I have complete focus on my weight loss journey.

16. Set a goal and achieve it.

17. Every day I wake up challenged and determined to reach my ideal weight goal.

18. Nobody can stop me from getting into the best shape of my life.

19. My determination to lose weight cannot be deterred.

20. My motivation to exercise is exceptional.

21. Every day I am motivated to follow a regular exercise regimen.

22. I am self-motivated and inspired to lose weight and follow a healthy lifestyle.

23. I already have a clear picture in my head of how sexy and beautiful/handsome I look when I finally reach my ideal weight.

24. Being healthy is not only a lifestyle for me but a principle that I am determined to keep.

25. I am choosing to be healthy and fit.

26. I choose to eat healthily and maintain an active lifestyle.

27. I choose to feel fit and sexy.

28. My mind is hard-wired to want only healthy food, and my body automatically feels that need for daily physical activity.

29. My mind only accepts positive thoughts and compliments about my body and resists any negativities that can divert me away from my weight loss goal.

30. I am surrounded by people who help and motivate me during my weight loss journey.

31. I feel grateful for my body and how effectively it responds to my weight loss efforts.

32. I am grateful for my strong will power and ability to manage my weight.

33. I am thankful for the people who are helping me reach my ultimate weight loss goals.

34. I divert myself from restaurants and establishments that can serve as a temptation to practice unhealthy eating habits.

35. I resist processed food, refined sugars, and salty snacks.

36. I have developed healthy eating habits.

37. I keep myself hydrated to aid in my weight loss.

38. I have established a regular exercise regimen that is very easy for me to follow.

39. I have embraced a life of clean and healthy living.

40. I have finally reached my ideal weight.

41. I am successful in my goal of extreme weight loss.

42. I invite all challenges that lead to a greater understanding of myself and my purpose.

43. My essence guides me daily toward better choices for my body.

44. I am blessed by the choices I make.

45. I am blessed by my ability to choose.

46. I have insights bestowed for my greater good.

47. I answer those insights with wisdom and enthusiasm.

48. I have used my intuition to develop sound confidence in my decisions.

49. I am what I have continuously thought and acted too.

50. I am the transformation the world needs right now.

51. I am the living embodiment of belief in action.

52. I use my body for exercise, my mind for belief, and my heart for forgiveness.

53. I have a choice to be who I want to be.

54. With that choice, I choose to let the flow of universal knowledge speak through me as a vessel of assertiveness.

55. I speak back to the universal flow with my actions.

56. I recognize those needs in all their usefulness, and I claim them for the roadmap to my self-appointed weight loss goals.

57. I am what I focus on.

58. I am the truth of my focus.

59. I love myself with a full heart.

60. I love my body with a full heart.

61. I love myself with a full mind.

62. I love exercising with a full spirit.

63. I am the love I need in my life.

64. I am healthy and my ideal weight.

65. I use my skills, knowledge, and resources to make the best food choices for my life.

66. I shine outward from within, and my body is an example of my inner beauty.

67. I welcome the challenge of exercise.

68. I welcome my sense of personal change.

69. I welcome my higher truth to speak through me.

70. I welcome my goals as benchmarks to help me achieve my ultimate level of happiness.

71. I boldly triumph over all obstacles.

72. I am thankful to receive these challenges to use my will to persevere.

73. I am appreciative of the challenges in my life for how they teach me to succeed.

74. I am successful because I have been tested and passed the tests with flying colors.

75. I am surrounded by teachers that offer me a chance to be my greatest self every day.

76. I am continuously thankful for my mentors, who show me how to overcome my doubts.

77. I am grateful for those who know my true worth and challenge me to see it in myself.

78. I move my body to eliminate stress.

79. I gravitate towards healthy decisions.

80. I rest my body after tireless effort.

81. I am the bravery I admire in others.

82. I move into that bravery with a warrior's spirit, ready for the challenges ahead.

83. That truth gives me the power to make wise choices.

84. I am the mountain.

85. I am the climber.

86. I put faith in my tools, for they assist me on my climb.

87. My motivation inspires my climb.

88. My tools assist me in my choice to persevere and succeed on my own.

89. I am the mountain I have conquered.

90. I am a warrior.

CHAPTER 14:

Preparing for Weight Loss

Weight loss affirmations are an extraordinary approach to move your excursion toward your weight loss. You can utilize these positive affirmations for getting more fit to help program your mind with positive propensities.

We all know that weight loss isn't almost that simple. We were utilizing these weight loss affirmations that can even assist the individuals who face obstinate inward obstruction when attempting to thin down.

Weight loss affirmations invite you. Here you will discover day by day affirmations for weight loss, which, whenever utilized regularly, will assist you with getting in shape.

Lasting weight loss or weight control requires an adjustment in the way of life. The affirmations given here will push you to change your way of life gradually.

Make astute and standard utilization of the positive affirmations for weight loss given underneath. As a rule, weight loss or weight control is an immediate capacity of our way of life.

The food we eat, the recurrence of eating, the method of consumption, the physical efforts that we experience, the rest we take, the psychological disposition that we keep up, all over an extensive period—in truth, over our total lifetime—decides our weight or potentially our weight issues. Utilize a reasonable weight-loss affirmation offered underneath to help with your concern.

Most diets work just as long as you work the diet! The other dieting stops, all the weight that has been lost gradually begins returning. This lone implies that except if you change your way of life, you will again have weight issues. Positive affirmations for weight loss will assist you in improving your way of life.

It has been discovered that our body keeps up the weight that our mind is OK with. If for reasons unknown, the brain thinks that it's vital. At that point, the body will begin collecting weight, and very before long will get itself overweight.

For instance, during youth, if you thought that it was useful to be "enormous bodied" for reasons of security, at that point, your subconscious mind will volunteer to make you huge and afterward to keep up your bigness. Weight picked up along these lines is hard to evacuate if the mind isn't managed first.

In such cases, no type of dieting will ever help. For substantial weight loss, it is essential to change our reasoning. You need to make your mind OK with the new weight you want. At times, heftiness is because of some glandular malfunction. In such cases, affirmations or diets may not work. You need to experience clinical treatment for the equivalent if you are overweight; at that point, counsel your doctor for any glandular issues before beginning a diet or affirmations.

Be cautious about the wording of the affirmation. Never state "I am not fat" because for this situation, you are concentrating on your concern, for example, being fat. Furthermore, whatever you center around, develops. Concentrate on the arrangement. So, the state should be, "I am thin" or "I am shedding pounds day by day and getting slimmer and slimmer."

Suppose you are a decided individual, at that point repeating the accompanying affirmations again and again, in any event, a hundred times day by day, ideally before a mirror, for a time of at any rate a half year. It will gradually assist you with taking a gander at and carrying on with an alternate life that is fitter than fatter. As usual, consolidate at least two of these free affirmations for weight loss, or even compose your sound weight loss affirmations, submitting a general direction to the accompanying.

Weight loss can appear to be difficult; utilizing weight loss affirmations to help you in the process can make it simpler. We should feel free to survey this large round to assist you with your weight loss venture.

1. Losing weight works out smoothly for me.

2. I am cheerfully accomplishing my weight loss objectives.

3. I am getting in shape each day.

4. I love to practice frequently.

5. I am eating nourishments that add to my well-being and prosperity.

6. I eat just when I am ravenous.

7. I now unmistakably observe myself at my optimal weight.

8. I love the flavor of healthy food.

9. I am pushing myself to work out; it causes me to feel great.

10. I am turning out to be fitter and more grounded regularly through exercise.

11. I am effectively reaching and keeping up my optimal weight

12. I love and care for my body.

13. I have the right to have a thin, sound, appealing body.

14. I am growing progressively good dieting propensities constantly.

15. I am getting slimmer consistently.

16. I look and feel incredible.

17. I take the necessary steps to be sound.

18. I am a joyfully re-imagined achievement.

19. I decide to work out.

20. I need to eat nourishments that cause me to look and to feel great.

21. I am answerable for my well-being.

22. I love my body.

23. I understand with creating my better body.

24. I am cheerfully practicing each morning when I wake up with the goal that I can arrive at the weight loss that I have been needing.

25. I am subscribing to my weight loss program by changing my eating propensities from unfortunate to sound.

26. I am content with each part I do in my extraordinary exertion to get in shape.

27. Every day, I am getting slimmer and more beneficial.

28. I am building up an appealing body.

29. I am building up a way of life of dynamic well-being.

30. I am creating a body that I like and appreciate.

Positive Affirmations for Losing Weight

1. My way of life eating changes is changing my body.

2. I feel incredible since I have lost more than 10 pounds in about a month and can hardly wait to meet my woman companion.

3. I have a level stomach.

4. I praise my power to settle on decisions around food.

5. I am cheerfully gauging 20 pounds less.

6. I am adoring strolling 3 to 4 times weekly and do conditioning practices, in any event, three times each week

7. Drinking eight bottles of water in a day.

8. I eat products of the soil everyday and taste, for the most part, chicken and fish.

9. I am learning and utilizing the psychological, emotional, and otherworldly abilities for progress. I will change it!

10. I will make new considerations about myself and my body.

11. I cherish and value my body.

12. It's energizing to find my one of a kind food and exercise framework for weight loss.

13. I am a weight loss example of overcoming adversity.

14. I am enchanted to be the perfect weight for me.

15. It's simple for me to follow a solid food plan.

16. I decide to grasp musings of trust in my capacity to roll out positive improvements throughout my life.

17. It feels great to move my body. Exercise is enjoyable!

18. I utilize deep breathing to assist me with unwinding and handle the pressure.

19. I am a delightful individual.

20. I have the right to be at my optimal weight.

21. I am an adorable individual. I merit love. It is ok for me to get more fit.

22. I am a solid nearness on the planet at my lower weight.

23. I discharge the need to reprimand my body.

24. I acknowledge and make the most of my sexuality. It's OK to feel arousing.

25. My digestion is impressive.

26. I keep up my body with ideal well-being.

27. I have faith in my capacity to adore myself for who I am.

28. I acknowledge my body shape and recognize the excellence it holds.

29. I am in charge of my future and the driver of my mind.

30. I let go of unhelpful examples of conduct around food.

31. I permit myself to settle on decisions and choices for my higher great.

32. I bring the characteristics of satisfaction, joy, and happiness into my life as I am currently.

33. I let go of any blame I hold around food decisions.

34. I acknowledge my body for the shape I have been honored with.

35. I let go of connections that are no longer for my higher great.

36. I have faith in myself and recognize my enormity.

37. I permit myself to feel great being me.

38. I acknowledge myself for who I am.

39. I bring the characteristics of adoration into my heart.

40. I have expectation and conviction about what's to come.

41. I am appreciative of the body I have and everything it accomplishes for me.

42. I weigh _____ pounds/kg.

43. Every day inside and out, I am moving toward my optimal weight.

44. I love being genuinely fit, and I lose enough weight with the goal that I am at my optimal weight.

45. My digestion rate is at its ideal, and it causes me to arrive at my optimal weight.

46. I love eating fresh food, and it causes me to arrive at my optimal weight.

47. I love practicing every day, and it causes me to arrive at my optimal weight.

48. I am a genuinely dynamic individual, and that encourages me to arrive at my optimal weight.

49. Every day inside and out, I am getting slimmer and fitter.

50. I appropriately bite all the food that I eat with the goal that it gets processed properly, and that encourages me to arrive at my optimal weight.

51. I inhale deeply without fail, so my digestion is at its ideal rate.

52. Every physical development that I make consumes the additional fat in my body and encourages me to keep up my optimal body weight.

53. I love myself unequivocally.

54. Life is lovely, and I appreciate life by remaining fit and keeping up my optimal weight.

CHAPTER 15:

Daily Mental Workout

This mental training allows you, every day, even for just a few minutes a day, to train your conscious and subconscious mind in the best way, and the best food intake condition. In other words, with this mental training, you mentally project yourself in the best way of eating: slowly, taking small portions each time, chewing until each bite becomes liquid, remaining concentrated solely on the act of eating, and aware of the taste of food. That is not a real self-hypnosis process, but a mental training performed in the self-hypnotic state, in which you will enter quickly. These allow you, with training, to reach the right state in a few seconds and to proceed with training even for a few minutes, several times a day. What matters in this training, even more than in self-hypnotic sessions, is, in fact, repetition. Repeat, repeat, repeat mental training. And then repeat it, repeat it, repeat it. And then repeat it, repeat it, repeat it until it becomes a habit and becomes an unconscious skill.

The secret is all here.

Use this hypnosis not as a step-by-step guided technique but as a basic recipe to be carried out independently: listen to it one or more times without training, then try to do it yourself, without listening to the audio, bring the skills acquired in any place and at any time, and activate training in any situation, whenever you want.

Sit comfortably.

Find a point of your choice in the room or place where you are to fix your gaze.

Fix that point without interruption.

You don't have to move your gaze even an inch. Just go back to fixing the chosen point immediately.

Look carefully at that point.

Continue to watch it carefully, without ever taking your eyes off it.

Feel how tiring it is for your eyes to keep them focused on that single point.

But keep doing it, without distracting yourself, even if your eyes get heavier.

The eyes can burn a little, blink slightly to let them rest, and just stare at that point.

The eyelids become heavier.

Keep looking at that point.

The eyelids become even heavier.

Keep looking at that point.

The eyes are tired, the eyelids drop.

Keep looking at that point.

The image of that point is blurred.

More and more.

The eyelids become even heavier.

More and more.

They are heavy as lead.

The eyes close with exhaustion.

Stay in this pleasant condition for a few seconds.

Then imagine that you are acting like eating.

Imagine eating when you are really hungry.

Imagine observing and smelling the dish with the meal.

Focus on perfumes.

Let yourself be filled with the scents of the food you are about to eat.

With cutlery, take a small portion of food and bring it to your mouth slowly.

Feel the taste of food.

Chew slowly.

Taste the food.

Continue to chew without haste without anxiety.

Continue to chew without feeling the need to swallow.

Continue to chew until the food in your mouth has become completely liquid.

Only then do you swallow.

Feel the food that gently descends into the body and brings health.

Feel the light digestion.

Between bites, always place the cutlery on the plate.

Keep repeating these actions for each bite and imagine eating until you feel full, put down the cutlery, move the plate away, and get up from the table.

Repeat these actions.

Repeat them, repeat them, repeat them.

That is what mental training consists of.

With training, your taste will become more and more sensitive, and you will always feel better the taste of each bite.

With training, you will learn to eat slower and eat less.

Mentally perform these actions without worrying about anything else: your subconscious will act to achieve it.

You can also use the technique to focus on specific aspects you want to improve and to strengthen self-hypnosis techniques. You can use mental training to continue to perceive the sense of satiety, or to refuse to eat compulsively, to eat calmly and serene, in full control and a state of well-being. And so on.

Use this mental training technique together with self-hypnosis techniques and as additional support for your real action on your food balance. And your real level of improvement will accelerate exponentially.

Important Tips for Performing Mental Training

The secret is to repeat, repeat, repeat by mentally performing the repetition to be already doing your best.

Don't worry if you don't seem to be able to imagine well or to visualize clearly: you don't have to worry. Repeat the sequences with confidence: your subconscious is perfectly processing your mental creation.

This mental repetition technique should be performed consistently every day. You can also perform it in cycles, giving yourself goals and periodically suspending it, and then resume it. Do it for a month, then pause, then resume for another month, and so on. Programming depends on you, but its secret, being progressive and parallel to your improvement, is continuous repetition—more continuity in the exercise, more continuity in success.

A final tip: try to perform mental training before your meals. Even if only for five minutes. In this way, you will undoubtedly remember the best actions throughout the meal to nourish yourself better, consciously, transforming each meal into a real exercise in health and well-being.

CHAPTER 16:

Weight Loss Affirmations

I n this chapter, we will learn about weight loss affirmations. They are a great way to stimulate your journey to weight loss. You can use these positive weight loss affirmations to program your mind with positive habits.

We all know that weight loss is not easy. The use of these weight loss affirmations can help people facing stubborn internal resistance when trying to lose weight.

These are the affirmations that you can suggest yourself while practicing self-hypnosis, cognitive-behavioral theory, or sleep learning system. In the first two methods, these affirmations can directly be suggested, and in the third method, you can record these and listen to them while sleeping.

You must be careful while choosing theses affirmations. You should select affirmations that you believe yourself and do not raise an objection when they are suggested to you. The failure happens because if you do not believe yourself, then it will not work for you. Moreover, it is suggested that you use a few affirmations that you think are effective for you. Do not try to suggest all at once. It may retard the effectiveness of the methods. There are also chances that the brain may become confused in case of any two opposite affirmations. So, better select your affirmations very carefully.

List of Affirmations for Excessive Weight Loss

1. Weight loss makes sense to me.

2. I want to reach the goal of weight loss.

3. I love to exercise regularly.

4. I eat foods that contribute to my health and well-being.

5. I only eat when I am hungry.

6. I can see myself clearly with my ideal weight.

7. I love the taste of healthy food.

8. I can control how much I want to eat.

9. I like training. I feel better.

10. Through exercise, I will be stronger and stronger every day.

11. I can reach the ideal weight and maintain it.

12. I love and care for my body.

13. I deserve a slim, healthy, and attractive body.

14. I always have a healthier eating habit.

15. I lose weight every day.

16. It looks good and feels good.

17. Whatever it takes, I need to be healthy.

18. I am happy to redefine success.

19. I decided to train.

20. I want to eat food that looks and feels good.

21. I am responsible for my health.

22. I love my body.

23. I put up with building a better body for myself.

24. When I wake up, I have a great time doing exercise every morning to achieve my desired weight loss.

25. I am working on a weight loss program by changing my diet from unhealthy to healthy.

26. I am happy with everything I do to lose weight.

27. I get thinner and healthier every day.

28. I am developing an attractive body.

29. I develop a lifestyle with life health.

30. I can create a body that I will like and enjoy.

These were general affirmations that you can use in a normal condition. You can move to more specific affirmations later when you feel that now it is time to modify my practice. Some of these affirmations that are given below will help you cope up with weight gain with a more specific approach.

1. Discovering my unique diet and exercise system for weight loss is exciting.

2. I accept and enjoy my sexuality. You can feel it sensually.

3. I am a beautiful person.

4. I am a weight loss success story.

5. I am happy to lose 20 pounds.

6. I am ready to develop new ideas about myself and my body.

7. I choose to trust the ability to make positive changes in my life.

8. I congratulate myself on choosing the right food.

9. I drink eight glasses of water daily.

10. I eat fruits and vegetables every day, mainly chicken and fish.

11. I enjoy walking 3-4 times a week and have at least three tonings exercised a week.

12. I free the need to criticize my body.

13. I have a strong weight in the world due to my low weight.

14. I learn and use mental, emotional, and spiritual skills for success. Ready to change!

15. I love and appreciate my body.

16. I will take care of my body in optimal health.

17. I'm happy that I have the ideal weight.

18. It feels good to move your body. The practice is fun!

19. It feels great to have lost more than 10 lbs in 4 weeks and can't wait to meet my girlfriend.

20. It's easy to follow a healthy diet plan.

21. My lifestyle changes my body.

22. My metabolism is excellent.

23. My stomach is flat.

24. Take a deep breath to relax and deal with stress.

25. My efforts are worth reaching the ideal weight.

You can make your affirmation to suit your routine and efforts. These affirmations in a normal routine or combined with methods that we discussed in this e-book can help reduce the weight quickly without affecting the emotional health.

CHAPTER 17:

Daily Affirmations

This segment will examine the importance of affirmations. An affirmation is something that you assert. It's a phrase stated factually, making sure that the information is understood. We frequently say affirmations to ourselves without thinking about it. You may consistently say to yourself, "I hate my activity." You may thoroughly consider it repeatedly, and before you know it, you're miserable and hating your activity because the thought affirmed that in your head daily. We have to flip affirmations around and use them to our advantage. Instead of consistently repeating negative things in your mind, aim to repeat positive phrases. We will talk about ways to remember affirmations for your daily lives. It takes minimal exertion to say these sentences, so actualize these strategies into your life ASAP.

The more you think these things, the more genuine they will feel, and the easier it will be to finish your weight loss goals. Saying these things will come naturally to you. We consider imagery a lot regarding our pattern of thought. If you're eager, you think, "I am starving," "I am wiped out," "I am not myself." These are dramatic statements, but they are topics that fly into our heads because that's how our brains are wired. We consistently connect thoughts to make sense of things. We also make absolute statements. You may fail once in a diet and think, "I can't do this." We create these assumptions because that's how our brains come up with an answer.

We must turn that intuition around and, instead, wire our brains to think entirely differently. To create your affirmations, speak in "I can," "I am," "I will," or "I have" statements. Use "I" in each affirmation you do, because this is all about increasing your positivity and creative reasoning, not for another person after you use the "I" phrases, next, move onto making a positive statement. Never depict what you lack, and attempt to avoid calling attention to your flaws, regardless of whether you are doing it decidedly. Speak in strong absolutes. The following four areas are examples of ones that you can use daily. Whichever area you battle with the most is the one you ought to incorporate the most affirmations from.

Motivational Affirmations

- I am a champ

- I am the most capable of completing the activity that I have to do

- I am not scared of failing

- Nothing that awaits me causes me to fear

- I have everything expected to take care of business

- I am more impressive than my greatest fear

- Each time I attempt I just get stronger

- I was made for something like this

- Giving up isn't in my nature

- My motivation is moving

- I have more motivation

- I am loaded up with motivation and the longing to continue onward

- The one in particular that is preventing me from the beginning is myself

- As soon as I start, I will already feel good

- I am ground-breaking

- I can complete whatever task

- I have done great previously so that I can improve going forward

- Finishing something always feels better than not doing it at all

- I am doing this because I can do it.

- I have no choices other than to start

- Getting started will be the greatest challenge

- There is nothing to fear other than not completing this task

- My knowledge is moving

- Making mistakes is natural, and I realize how to learn from them

- I take action when I realize I have to most

Weight Loss Affirmations

- My body is vigorous

- I love my body at any shape

- I feel the best when my body is healthy

- Taking care of my body feels better

- My body has gotten me through so much already

- My body is capable of anything

- I make healthy choices for my body

- I don't rebuff myself and just fill my mind with affection

- My mind feels clearer when I am concentrating on weight loss

- I do not care about the numbers; I care about how I feel

- All that matters is that I'm taking care of my body

- Losing some weight, regardless of how small, is better than losing none

- My life is better when I'm concentrating on my health and weight loss

- Losing weight will help me greatly in the long run

- I am taking care of myself now and later on

- Life is easier when I'm healthy

- I am getting the outcomes I've dreamt about

- Working hard to get thinner feels such better than fantasizing about it

- I love shedding pounds

- Every part of my body is healthy

- People appreciate how happy I am

- I love others more when I adore myself

- Being alive and healthy is something to be thankful for

- My body is marvelous

- I love the person I've become throughout my weight loss venture

Healthy Eating Affirmations

- Eating healthy feels better

- Eating healthy tastes great

- It is always better to fill me with something healthy

- The lousy nourishment I like isn't beneficial for me

- I allow myself to eat unhealthy once in a while, but realize that eating healthy takes priority

- Anything green hydrates me and keeps me full

- I am eating healthy for my entire body

- My heart feels full when I eat healthy foods

- Eating healthy reminds me I love myself

- Exercising is simple when I am eating healthy

- I am fortunate to have so much healthy food around

- I love trying various things with healthy food

- I am a superior cook when I make my healthy meals

- I always feel healthier whenever I eat healthily meals

- I don't realize all the advantages of eating healthy has on my body, until later on in the week

- My skin is shining because of the healthy foods I put in my body

- I don't have to eat unhealthy foods, because I realize that I feel good with healthy food in my body

- I don't have to fill my emotions with food

- Food makes me feel good, but healthy food encourages me to feel the best

- I need to eat to endure, so eating healthy is the way to satisfy this need, while also making me feel better

- I allow myself to enjoy now and again because I realize that garbage food can be useful for my mind sometimes

- I will always return to healthy food and make this my major core interest when cooking and preparing meals

- I am saving cash when I eat healthily

- I monitor my food when I eat unhealthily

- I drink water frequently

Self-Control Affirmations

- I am strong enough to realize how to say no

- I make sure that I say "yes" to doing the things that need to be completed

- I take care of my needs

- I strive to break terrible habits

- I am responsible for what I do

- Food doesn't have control over me

- Skipping my activities is just harming me in the long haul

- I am strong enough to know when I have to walk away from something

- I am sufficiently trained to begin

- I recognize what it takes to discover success

- I am in control of the things that come to me

- I am not afraid of a challenge

- I'm mentally ready to complete what I've started

- I am sufficiently strong enough to say no

- I am brave enough to begin all alone

- I buckle down because I merit the enormous payoff

- My self-control is motivating

- I am adept at completing things

- It feels so great to accomplish what I set out to do

- I am amazing

- I am strong-willed

- I am obstinate against myself

- I am my greatest inspiration

- I have been strong in the past and will continue to be into the future

- I am in control

CHAPTER 18:

Guided Meditation for Weight Loss

Meditation Exercise 1: Release of Bad Habits

Concentrate on your back now and notice how you feel in the bed or chair you are sitting in. Have a deep breath, and let your stress just go with the flow to leave your body. Now focus on your neck. Observe how your neck is joined to your shoulders. Lift your shoulders slowly. Breathe in slowly and release it. Feel how your shoulders loosen. Lift your shoulders again a little bit, then let them relax. Observe how your neck muscles are tensing and how much pressure it has. Breathe in and breathe out slowly. Release the pressure in your neck and notice how the stress is leaving your body. Repeat the whole exercise from the beginning. Observe your back. Notice all the stress and let it go with a deep breath. Focus on your shoulders and neck again. Lift your shoulders and hold it for some moments, then release your shoulders again and let all the stress go away. Sense how the stress is going away. Now, focus your attention on your back. Feel how comfortable it is. Focus on your whole body. While breathing in, let relaxation come, and while you are breathing out, let frustration leave your body. Notice how much you are relaxed.

Concentrate on your inner self. Breathe slowly in and release it. Calm your mind and observe your thoughts. Do not go with them because you aim to observe them and not to be involved. It's time for you to let go of that overweight self that you are not satisfied with. It is like your body is wearing a bigger, heavier top at this point in your life. Imagine stepping out of it and laying it on an imaginary chair facing you. Now tell yourself to let go of these old, established eating and behavioral patterns. Imagine that all your old, fixed patterns and all the obstacles that prevent you from achieving your desired weight are exiting your body, soul, and spirit with each breath. Know that your soul is perfect as it is, and all you want is for everything that pulls away to leave. With every breath, let your old beliefs go, as you are creating more and more space for something new. After spending a few minutes with this, imagine that every time you breathe in, you are inhaling prana, the life energy of the universe, shining in gold. In this life force, you will find everything you need and desire: a healthy, muscular body, a self that loves itself in all circumstances, a hand that puts enough nutritious food on the table, a strong voice to say no to sabotaging your diet, a head that can say no to those who are trying to distract you from your ideas and goals. With each breath, you absorb these positive images and emotions.

See in front of you exactly what your life would be like if you got everything you wanted. Release your old self and start becoming your new self. Feel the solid ground beneath you, open your eyes, and return to your normal state of consciousness.

Meditation Exercise 2: Forgiving Yourself

Sit comfortably. Do not cross your feet because this will lock you away from the desired experience. Hold your hands together to connect your logical brain hemisphere with your instinct. Relax your muscles, close your eyes.

Imagine a staircase in front of you! Descend it, counting down from ten to one.

You reached and found a door at the bottom of the stairs. Open the door. There is a meadow in front of us. Let us see if it has grass; if so, if it has flowers, what color, whether there is a bush or tree, and describe what you see in the distance.

Find the path covered with white stones and start walking on it.

Feel the power of the Earth flowing through your soles, the breeze stroking your skin, the warmth of the sun radiating toward you. Feel the harmony of the elements and your state of well-being.

From the left side, you hear the rattle of the stream. Walk down to the shore. This water of life comes from the throne of God. Take it with your palms and drink three sips and notice how it tastes. If you want, you can wash it. Keep walking. Feel the power of the Earth flowing through your soles, the breeze stroking your skin, the warmth of the sun radiating toward you. Feel the harmony of the elements and your state of well-being. In the distance, you see an ancient tree with many branches. That is the Tree of Life. Take a leaf from it, chew it, and note its taste and continue walking along the white gravel path. Feel the power of the Earth flowing through your soles, the breeze stroking your skin, the warmth of the sun radiating toward you. Feel the harmony of the elements and your state of well-being.

You have arrived at the Lake of Conscience, no one in this lake sinks. Rest on the water and think that all the emotions and thoughts you no longer need (anger, fear, horror, hopelessness, pain, sorrow, anxiety, annoyance, self-blame, superiority, self-pity, and guilt) pass through your skin. You purify them by the magical power of water. And you see that the water around you is full of gray and black globules that are slowly recovering the turquoise-green color of the water. You think once again of all the emotions and thoughts you no longer need, and they pass through your skin. You purify them by the magical power of water. You see that the water around you is full of gray and black globules that are slowly obscuring the turquoise-green color of the water. And once again, think of all the emotions and thoughts you no longer need as they pass through your skin, you purify them by the magical power of water. And you once again see that the water around you is full of gray and black globules that are slowly obscuring the turquoise-green color of the water.

You feel the power of the water, the power of the Earth, the breeze on your skin, the radiance of the sun warming you, the harmony of the elements, the feeling of well-being.

You ask your magical horse to come for you. You love your horse, you pamper it, and let it caress you too. You bounce on its back and head to God's Grad. In the air, you fly together, become one being. You have arrived. Ask your horse to wait.

You grow wings, and you fly toward the Trinity. You bow your head and apologize for all the sins you have committed against your body. You apologize for all the sins you have committed against your soul. You apologize for all the sins you committed against your spirit. You wait for the angels to give you the gifts that help you. If you cannot see yourself receive one, it means you do not need one yet. If you did, open it and look inside. Give thanks that you could be here. Get back on your horse and fly back to the meadow. Find the white gravel path and head back down to the door to your stairs. Look at the grass in the meadow. Notice if there are any flowers. If so, describe the colors, any bush or tree, and whatever you see in the distance. Feel the power of the Earth flowing through your soles, the breeze stroking your skin, the warmth of the sun radiating toward you. Feel the harmony of the elements and your state of well-being. You arrive at the door, open it, and head up the stairs. Count from one to ten. You are back, move your fingers slowly, open your eyes.

Meditation Exercise 3: Weight Loss

Sit comfortably. Relax your muscles, close your eyes, and breathe in and breathe out. Do not cross your feet because this will lock you away from the desired experience. Hold your hands together to connect your logical brain hemisphere with your instinct.

Concentrate on your back now and notice how you feel in the bed or chair you are sitting in. Take a deep breath and let your stress leave your body. Now focus on your neck. Observe how your neck is joined to your shoulders. Lift your shoulders slowly. Breathe in slowly and release it. Feel how your shoulders loosen. Lift your shoulders again a little bit, then let them relax. Observe how your neck muscles are tensing and how much pressure it has. Breathe in and breathe out slowly. Release the pressure in your neck and notice how the stress is leaving your body. Repeat the whole exercise from the beginning. Observe your back. Notice all the stress and let it go with a deep breath. Focus on your shoulders and neck again. Lift your shoulders and hold it for some moments, then release your shoulders again and let all the stress go away. Sense how the stress is going away. Now, place your attention on your back. Feel how comfortable it is. Focus on your whole body. While breathing in, let relaxation come in, and while you are breathing out, let frustration leave your body. Notice how much you are relaxed.

Concentrate on your inner self. Breathe slowly and release it. Calm down your mind. Observe your thoughts. Do not go with them because you aim to observe them and not to be involved. It is time to let go of your overweight self that you are not feeling good about. Imagine yourself as you are now. See yourself in every detail. Describe your hair, the color of your clothes, your eyes. See your face, your nose, your mouth. Set aside this image for a moment. Now imagine yourself as you would like to be in the future. See yourself in every detail. Describe your hair and the color of your clothes, eyes, face, nose, and your mouth and imagine that your new self-approaches your present self and pampers it. See that your new self hugs your present self. Feel the love that is spread in the air. Now see that your present self leaves the scene, and your new self takes its place. See and feel how happy and satisfied you are. You believe that you can become this beautiful new self. You breathe in this image and place it in your soul. This image will always be with you and flow through your whole body, and you want to be this new self. You can be this new self.

After spending a few minutes with this, imagine that every time you breathe in, you are inhaling prana, the life energy of the universe, shining in gold.

CHAPTER 19:

Using Affirmations for Weight Loss

A n affirmation is just anything you state or think. We insist on what we expect in life all the time with our musings and convictions. The Universe, at that point, takes back to our encounters that coordinate the vibration of those considerations.

For instance, on the chance that you think discharging weight is troublesome and tiresome, it will be. If you trust it is trying now and again, however feasible, it will be. Your considerations about discharging weight make the nature of your excursion. They either assist you with succeeding or keep you down.

They are utilizing affirmations, just methods intentionally assuming responsibility for your musings. At the point when used with different methodologies, affirmations assist you with making a positive outlook for progress.

On the off chance that subliminal convictions are hindering your advancement, affirmations help kill them. Claims all by themselves, be that as it may, may not be sufficient to remove profoundly established or injury based convictions. These may best be settled through expert self-development work.

Saying positive affirmations doesn't mean you claim to feel energetic. The word positive likewise implies feeling certain and sure. At the point when you assert joyful musings, you reinforce your certainty to feel sure about accomplishing your weight reduction objectives. Notice what is avowed in these familiar ways of thinking about weight reduction:

"It's incomprehensible for me shed pounds."

"I've attempted previously, and nothing's made a difference. I don't perceive how this will be unique."

"It's difficult to get more fit when you're more established."

Do these words originate from somebody who will succeed or come up short? How about we turn these around:

"I can arrive at my weight reduction objectives."

"It doesn't make a difference what occurred previously; I will accomplish my objectives this time."

"Age has nothing to do with it. I can discharge this weight."

See the distinction? Here are some core values to utilize positive affirmations for discharging weight without hardly lifting a finger:

Discharge your connection to constraining convictions

You may hold convictions concerning why you figure you can't discharge weight. These convictions may originate from excruciating youth messages, for example, "You'll never add up to anything," or visually impaired concurrence with the cultural idea, for example, "Everybody knows it's hard to get in shape." Make space for positive affirmations to grab hold by opening your brain to supplant convictions that restrain you with elevating beliefs that help you. Utilize this fast check framework to decide whether a conviction aide or damages you:

"Does this conviction make dread or uncertainty?"

"Is this conviction despite my objectives?

If a conviction doesn't bolster you, change it.

Make affirmations that vibe regular to you

The intensity of affirmation increments when you put stock in them, and they are essential to you. Regardless of whether something doesn't yet feel valid, be that as it may, you can utilize affirmations to move toward whom you need to turn into delicately. For instance, on the chance that you state, "I discharge weight effectively," however where it counts you don't accept that, make an affirmation that feels genuine, for example, "I am available to discharge weight without any difficulty," or, "Although this feels troublesome on occasion, I am equipped for arriving at my objectives."

Use "I am" proclamations at whatever point conceivable

"I am" proclamations are especially incredible because whatever we connect to the words "I am," we become. There is a profound power within us, and it gives specific consideration to whatever follows our "I am" proclamations. So whether you state, "I am a disappointment" or "I am a triumph," you enact a strong force that delivers that outcome. Use "I am" proclamations to mirror the characteristics you need, regardless of whether they don't yet appear valid. As you interface with the fantastic vitality inside you, in time, your "I am" proclamations will create the outcomes you want.

State affirmations in the current state

The Universe hears your musings and convictions truly and reacts in kind. Make affirmations that serve you right now and not in some future date. For instance, on the chance that you state, "I will get thinner," it keeps your advancement slowed down for some unsure future. However, if you state, "I am discharging weight," you confirm progress today.

Use affirmations when you feel loose and tranquil

Affirmations enter our inner mind all the more effectively when we're in a calm state. While it's essential to rehash claims for the day, make some calm time to extend their belongings.

A Daily Practice

Pick a few affirmations from the accompanying rundown. Change them to best suit you or make your own. Express your affirmations three to multiple times, or more, for the day. You may think that it's supportive of keeping in touch with them on 3×5 cards to convey with you, add them to your PC foundation, or stay in touch with them on post-it notes put in apparent areas, for example, your washroom mirror or vehicle.

Make some calm time during the day where you can sit calmly, rehashing them.

State your affirmations with profound inclination, as though you, as of now, have the characteristics you're asserting.

Positive Affirmation Examples

Because of this definition, here are a few instances of positive affirmations:

- I have faith and belief in myself, and trust my shrewdness;

- I am an effective individual;

- I am sure and skilled at what I do.

Recorded underneath are progressively positive affirmation examples, concentrated on explicit territories.

9 Positive Affirmations for Women

Searching for certain plans to make your affirmations? Here are some pleasant examples:

- I decide to be upbeat;

- My life is occurring directly here, at this moment;

- I'm talented and encircled by astounding loved ones;

- I select to transcend negative emotions and jettison negative musings;

- I am versatile, hardy, and brave, and I can't be devastated;

- No one but me chooses how I feel;

- At the point when I have to rest, everything is as it ought to be, and I rest content;

- I am responsible for my contemplations, and I don't pass judgment on myself;

- I acknowledge and love myself, all together and totally.

9 Positive Affirmations for Men

Here are a few affirmations for men, including declarations of self-acknowledgment and positive self-perception. These affirmations depended on a more considerable rundown of 30 claims and were adjusted utilizing the intellectual, social treatment thought of "negative center convictions."

- I am answerable for taking care of me;

- By acting naturally, I carry bliss to others;

- My objectives and wants are as beneficial as everyone else's;

- Through mental fortitude and dangerous work, I can accomplish whatever I set my focus on;

- I'm fine with who I am, and I love who I am turning out to be;

- Through my commitments, I roll out positive improvements to the world;

- My body is astonishing only how it is, and I acknowledge myself along these lines;

- I pick just to encircle myself with steady and great individuals;

- At whatever point I tumble down, I get back up once more.

15 Positive Affirmations for Teens

Social weights and scholarly anxieties can negatively affect adolescents; however, they can pivot negative self-talk and accomplish something positive about what they think and feel. Here are a few affirmations that are appropriate for young people:

- I am a brisk, fit student;

- I have confidence in myself as an individual, and I put stock in all my abilities;

- I am one of a kind and delightful;

- Others regard me for following my convictions;

- On the off chance that a couple of individuals don't acknowledge me, I'm fine with that;

- I excuse others for now and then doing an inappropriate thing, and I pardon myself when I do likewise;

- I am benevolent and acceptable to the individual I find in the mirror;

- I have the right to consider myself to be stunning;

- Whatever troubles come to my direction, I can defeat them;

- I was brought into the world sound, and I develop more grounded each day;

- Today, I am going to confide in myself and my senses;

- I am adequate, and I am fine with only being me;

- I approach others with deference, and they treat me the equivalent;

- I decide to transcend the frightful things that may come to my direction;

- I am working each day on the best me that I can be.

11 Positive Affirmations for Kids

By figuring out how to rehearse positive affirmations at a young age, children can turn out to be substantially more arranged to utilize them when confronting troubles sometime down the road (Bloch, 2015). These are exceptionally straightforward affirmations because the more ignorant they are for little youngsters to recollect, the more probable kids will have the option to rehearse them without a grown-up's assistance.

- I am cherished;

- I am innovative;

- I am benevolent;

- I am fearless;

- I am a mindful individual;

- I will consistently give a valiant effort;

- I am interesting;

- At the point when I set out to accomplish something, I can do it;

- I'll generally help other people;

- I will adapt parts today since I am able;

- I am a significant and essential individual.

Ordinary Positive Affirmations for Students

Understudies may find that affirmations are useful for adapting to the pressure of scholarly life just as their extracurricular and public activities. Here are the examples from the full rundown that you or an understudy you know can use for inspiration or motivation.

- At the point when I get a terrible evaluation, I am persuaded to improve;

- I am resolved, and I focus on the stars;

- I set only requirements for my scholastic accomplishment. By investing energy and exertion, I can achieve what I set out to accomplish;

- I value my school, educators, and cohorts since they all assume a job in helping me develop as a superior individual;

- Indeed, even on days when I don't gain a lot of ground, I am continually learning. On different days, I get stunning ground toward my objectives.

6 Positive Affirmations to Help Relieve Anxiety

A great many people who have experienced nervousness will probably realize how significant it very well may be to cut off pessimistic idea designs before they start winding. These affirmations can be utilized whenever, and even the individuals who don't commonly feel restless may discover them helpful during upsetting minutes.

During times of uneasiness or desperation, this rundown of positive affirmations can be utilized for consoling yourself. A couple of examples propelled by this asset include:

- I am freeing myself from dread, judgment, and uncertainty;

- I pick just to think great musings;

- My tension doesn't control my life. I do.

Some different affirmations identified with nonjudgment and care for nervousness can be found on this rundown. Here are some that draw motivation from the rundown:

- I inhale, I am gathered, and I am quiet;

- I am protected, and everything is acceptable in my reality;

- Inside me, I feel quiet, and no one can upset this tranquility.

CHAPTER 20:

Meditations for Positive Thinking and Self-Love

Often, we spend a lot of time worrying about loving other people. I want you to pause for a moment and ask yourself; do I love myself? Too often, we put ourselves behind everyone else, whether that be a child, a family member, or a significant other. I want you to realize that it's okay to put yourself first every once in a while. I want you to take a few moments right now to remind yourself how much you love you! Having a positive mindset is one way to love yourself. While it may sound like a simple thing to do, it isn't always. When we have a positive mindset, this can help attract positive events into our life. It's much like the law of attraction like will always attract like. When you add positive thinking into your life, you will be able to attract positive things such as harmonious relationships and good fortune.

When you are ready, I would like to go through a few meditation scripts based around positive thinking and self-love. If you are having a rough day and are a bit down on yourself, I hope one of these scripts can help put a smile back on your face. Remember to live in the moment; you cannot be defined by your future or by your past. There is only now, and you have the power over how you feel about it.

Simple Smile Meditation Script

If you are having a rough day, you may have lost your smile. I want you to first begin by finding someplace that is comfortable for you. If needed, slip into some comfortable clothes or perhaps even wrap yourself up in your favorite comforter.

Once in place, I invite you to close your eyes gently and bring your attention to your breath. We will now go through a simple breathing exercise to help create a sense of serenity back to your mind and your body. Leave all of your issues at the door and focus only on your breath.

As you settle in, begin to breathe for four counts.

Inhale... four... three... two... one. Hold... four... three... two... one, and now exhale long and slow for eight counts... seven... six... five... four... three... two... one, wonderful.

Go ahead and repeat this process for a few more breaths. I want you to focus only on your breath and each number as it passes through your head.

Inhale... four... three... two... one. Hold... four... three... two... one, and now exhale long and slow for eight counts... seven... six... five... four... three... two... one, feel as your body is starting to let go of the tension, your mind becomes calm, your heartbeat becoming steady.

Inhale... four... three... two... one. Hold... four... three... two... one, and now exhale long and slow for eight counts... seven... six... five... four... three... two... one, great job.

When you are prepared to move on, go ahead, and bring attention to your face. Is there any tension that you can sense? Answer yourself kindly and allow for any judgments to pass without a second thought. Perhaps there is tension in your jaw, or your lips, or even behind your eyes. That is all perfectly normal, especially if you're not having the best of days.

While you become aware of these areas of tension, allow them to relax and soften. If you feel like it, allow your lips to form into a smile. As you do this, I want you to think of a family, friend, or a memory that you love dearly. Even if you have a hard day, there is always this person that can make you smile, even when you do not feel like it. I want you to take a few moments now to breathe and focus on this happy memory. Allow happiness to wash over you as you breathe.

As your smile becomes more natural, become mindful of how your heart is feeling when you are thinking of this memory. I want you to visualize what your heart is looking like right now, at this moment. Picture your heart pulsating and opening; it's beginning to spread love and positive energy all through your body. Take a few moments and focus on this love that is filling you up.

When you are ready, I would like you to repeat it after me. We will be going over some positive affirmations that will hopefully place your smile back in place. Take another deep breath, and when you are ready, we can begin.

I can allow happiness to come to me.

(Pause)

I'm the only person in charge of my happiness.

(Pause)

I choose to smile, even in the hard times.

(Pause)

I'm happy and grateful for the life I lead.

(Pause)

When I choose to smile, others will smile with me.

(Pause)

I am truly happy and grateful.

(Pause)

If needed, you can repeat these phrases to yourself whenever you need them most. You truly are in charge of your happiness; no circumstance nor person can change that for you. When you are ready, bring your awareness back to your breath. Notice now how much more relaxed your body feels and how a smile comes naturally back to your face. Gently bring your awareness to your space and gently give your body a little shake as you come back to the present moment. Allow your consciousness to awaken gently, smile, and you are ready to carry on with your day.

Guided Meditation for Self-Esteem Script

There are too many moments in our life when we are our own worst critics. If you are constantly bashing your body, putting yourself down, or feel you generally have low self-esteem, this script is going to be perfect for you! Through meditation, you can boost your confidence and your self-esteem. When you feel good about yourself, your body will be able to relax and just live life the way it's meant to be.

As always, I now invite you to relax. You will want to find your most comfortable position and allow all of the tension to begin melting away from your limbs. As you find your breath, I want to paint a picture for you. Simply do nothing right now but allow for your breath to become natural.

As you breathe, I want you to picture a staircase in your mind. Right now, you are standing at the top of these stairs. As you look down at the bottom, there is a pool of relaxation and peace. When you are looking down, I invite you to take a mental note of how you are feeling right now.

Take a deep breath and picture yourself taking a soft step down. With this step, you are already closer to the relaxation pool you want to be floating in. Each step you take down, feel how much more relaxed your body is becoming. Your arms are relaxing; your legs are relaxing; your jaw is becoming loose as you step closer and closer to the bottom of the stairs.

One step at a time, you are making your way down the stairs. Your arms are feeling heavier, your legs are heavier, the relaxation is pulling you down gently, and it feels comfortable. You are safe at this moment, and slipping into the pool of relaxation will be such a relief. Allow for gravity to pull you down gently.

Feel now as your back and your neck are both relaxing, too. Your shoulders being pulled away from being shrugged up into your shoulders, your eyes becoming heavy with relaxation, and every part of your body is becoming calm and relaxed. Go ahead and allow for your mind to drift away from you. Everything is feeling wonderful as you approach the bottom of the stairs.

Now, you are taking the final steps to the bottom of the stairs. Go ahead and admire the pool of relaxation as you gently step in. Allow for your mind to drift as you settle into the calmness of the pool and rest your eyes. Your whole body is loose and relaxed; you haven't a care in the world.

I would like you to allow your mind to drift now. As it does, I would like to go over some positive affirmations for your self-esteem. You can listen to them and repeat them if you would like to. While some may apply to you, others may not. Listen to your mind and your heart as we go over the affirmations. Once we are done, you can allow your mind to continue drifting. Simply breathe, relax, and we can begin.

You are capable of doing so many amazing things with your life.

You are a loving person, and you deserve to be happy.

You are strong, but you do not need to be strong all of the time.

You are worth it.

You have the power to control your emotions.

It's okay to accept yourself.

You need to be kind to yourself.

You are perfect the way you are at this moment.

It's okay to be happy.

It's okay to be proud of yourself.

Now, repeat after me.

I'm capable of doing so many amazing things with my life.

I'm a loving person, and I deserve to be happy.

I'm strong, but I do not need to be strong all of the time.

I'm worth it.

I have the power to control my emotions.

It's okay to accept myself.

I need to be kind to myself.

I'm perfect the way I am at this moment.

It's okay to be happy.

It's okay to be proud of myself.

Allow for your mind to drift and repeat these affirmations as needed. You can repeat them until you believe them. These are all true for you, and you deserve to build your sense of self-assurance and confidence. You will always have yourself. It's up to you to become your biggest cheerleader!

You can, and you will make positive changes in your life. When you increase your self-esteem and gain a positive mindset, you will begin to attract positive events and positive people into your life.

Now, I want you to bring awareness back to your mind. Feel now how much happier and relaxed you feel. Notice how calm you are and take a moment to enjoy this new sensation. Any time you are feeling down on yourself, I want you to repeat these affirmations to yourself. You deserve to feel good. Be in charge of your happiness.

When you are ready to return to your day, take a few more deep breaths. Gently bring your awareness back to your space and return to your day with positivity and gratitude.

Positive Body Image Script

Let's face it; there is always something that we don't approve of on our bodies. I'm here to tell you that you need to stop being so hard on yourself! Everyone else out there is judging you, stop being mean to yourself. You have a heart in your chest, you have lungs that keep you breathing, and you have a body that allows you to get through life. It's time to appreciate everything that you have instead of fretting over the things you don't.

The body cannot function properly without enough sleep. It will affect other organ systems in your body. Stress and sleeplessness may lead to a more severe problem, and other mental health issues may occur. The solution to this problem may be deep sleep hypnosis.

CHAPTER 21:

Meditation for a Mindfulness Diet

V isualization, suggestion combined with meditation, is an easy way to make positive and powerful personal changes. If you combine meditation with positive affirmation, you will begin to change the way you feel, think, and act. This relaxation exercise will help you change and improve the way you feel. However, time is taken to see the effects that differ from person to person. Let's begin.

Sit or lie down comfortably.

Stretch your back, and then put your shoulders backward to open the rib cage.

Feel your shoulder muscles relax.

Close your eyes.

Relax your body and empty your mind.

Take ten slow but deep breaths.

Concentrate on the breath.

Feel it getting slower and deeper.

Feel relaxed as every tension goes away.

Relax your neck and shoulders again.

(Pause a minute for reflection)

Imagine being happy, being successful, winning, being loved, laughing, feeling good.

Relax your forehead, mouth, and eyes.

Let a soft smile appear on your face as you feel a calm enter your mind.

(Pause a minute for reflection)

(Meditation closing)

Then say the following words:

I'm a good person.

I do what is right.

I have integrity.

Whatever life presents is a useful experience that will only make me wiser, stronger, and more tolerant.

I eat and drink good things.

I am what I eat and drink.

I focus on the joy in my life.

I am what I see, touch, and hear positive things.

I am compassionate, loving, and caring.

I am strong enough to understand that the behavior of others is about them, not me.

I help others when I can.

I exercise because I enjoy it.

I smile and laugh because I am happy.

I help other people. After all, they are all good people, like me.

I'm what I say I am.

I am.

Meditative affirmations are a centuries-old way of gaining control over our feelings and behaviors.

Meditation for Positive Thinking

This hypnotherapy experience will allow you to fall asleep easily. At the same time, your calm and relaxed mind can enjoy listening along to a series of beneficial suggestions, all of which are in the form of positive affirmations to enhance your health, wealth, and happiness.

You will find that there is nothing overly complicated in this session. Allow yourself to drift into hypnosis and then away into your dreams.

During this relaxing time ahead, your conscious mind will inevitably wander, but your subconscious mind will continue to listen to my voice.

As you settle in and lay your head on the pillow, you can be reassured that all of these suggestions will speak powerfully to your subconscious mind. It makes no difference whether you remember or forget the pleasant suggestions in this session. You can trust in my voice to permeate your subconscious being while you fall into the deep state of hypnosis.

As you are preparing to relax, take a moment to reassure yourself that all hypnosis is self-hypnosis, which means that you remain in control throughout the entirety of this session. If something from the outside world requires your presence at any time, you can simply open your eyes, and the hypnosis will be over.

But for now, you can continue to relax and allow the noise and distractions of the outside world to continue to fade away gently into the night.

Because this time is the perfect time to let go and let it all drift away

That is the perfect time to relax

If they aren't already, close your eyes lightly.

Throughout this time, there is no need to do anything. There is no need to worry about things that happened today or things that might happen tomorrow. Right now, all you need to do is to be here, in your body, on your bed, letting your mind do what it needs to do to relax for a good night's sleep.

Thank you for taking this time for self-care. You deserve a night of restful sleep and to wake up feeling refreshed and ready for the day. That is one thing that you can do that is just for yourself. No guilt, no worries.

Know that whatever worries you and stops you from sleeping won't be fixed by keeping you awake.

Know that no matter how you slept last night or the night before, you can sleep well tonight. That is the only night that matters.

Just let yourself go.

Lie still as you allow the stress to fade away.

(Pause a minute for reflection)

Each time you find your mind drifting, notice where it's gone and gently tell yourself to come back to being right here, right now. There is no need to judge what your mind is thinking about or that you have become distracted. That is what our brains are designed to do.

Now, take a deep breath.

And exhale.

Take a deep breath.

And exhale.

Take a deep breath and feel the air as it flows through your nostrils, down into your lungs, and fully into your abdomen. Breathe in as deeply as you can.

(Pause a minute for reflection)

As your body relaxes, it may begin to feel heavy. Feel how it rests on the bed. You are supported in this meditation by the things around you. They hold you and allow your mind to do the work needed to unclutter your mind.

Like your breath, your body may hold areas of tension that distract you. When you notice tension, try to relax those muscles. You may find that a small stretch and release of the muscles help reduce the tension. That doesn't have to be a big movement. Just enough to allow your muscles to fall back down into a restful state.

That is something that resets the muscle memory into one of relaxation rather than tension.

Now, take a deep breath.

And exhale.

Deep breath.

And exhale.

(Pause a minute for reflection)

Now, I will count down from 10 to 1.

With each passing number, you will feel yourself falling deeper and deeper into a peaceful state of relaxation.

With each passing number, you will feel your body grow increasingly heavier. Allow this feeling to wash over you, and allow the tension from your muscles to fade away. Allow yourself to relax.

10.

9.

8.

7.

6.

5.

4.

3.

2.

1.

I am learning to relax to the deepest I can go.

I am learning to relax to the deepest I can go.

With each breath, I fall deeper into a state of relaxation.

With each breath, I fall deeper into a state of relaxation.

I slowly release all control.

I slowly release all control.

(Pause a minute for reflection)

(Meditation closing)

I am the architect of my life.

I am unique.

I am happy.

I am successful.

I am positive.

I am special.

I am in full control, relaxed, and comfortable.

I am now in the perfect place, and this is the perfect time to rest and sleep.

I welcome dreams of positivity and abundance.

I welcome relaxation with a heart full of gratitude.

With each breath, I dive deeper into a state of relaxation.

With each breath, I dive deeper into a state of relaxation.

Positive energy comes to me easily and effortlessly.

Positive energy comes to me easily and effortlessly.

The more I let go, the deeper I relax.

The more I let go, the deeper I relax.

Meditation to Cope during Difficult Times

Sit comfortably with your legs crossed and your arms placed on your thigh's palms facing up.

(5 seconds)

Take three deep breaths and exhale completely with each breath.

(30 seconds)

Keeping your breathing deep will allow your body to become relaxed.

(60 seconds)

Now, bring your attention to the challenges you are facing. Without thinking too much about them, just identify them one by one.

(20 seconds)

How are you feeling? Are you mad, sad, stressed, in pain, or sorrowful? Identify the emotions that stand out for you at this moment.

(10 seconds)

Realize that these emotions are a manifestation of the chemical process taking place in your body. Therefore, notice them without judgment or getting involved in them.

(15 seconds)

Do not try to push them away either. Instead, become a curious observer. Notice how intense they are. Are they manifesting on a specific part of the body? For instance, can you feel heaviness at your solar plexus, or do your shoulders feel tight? Is your heart feeling a bit faster? Have you lost your smile and your jaw is tightly clenched and lips tightly closed? Become aware of the parts of the body that these emotions are manifesting.

(30 seconds)

Whatever feelings you are experiencing, you do not need to be ashamed of them just because you perceive them as negative feelings. Be open to them. See them as a way of your body responding to various circumstances and happenings. It is all right, you are human, and you are allowed to feel how you are feeling at this moment.

(60 seconds)

Now, begin to deepen your breaths.

(20 seconds)

Take notice of your hands and tighten them into fists.

(5 seconds)

Make the fists tighter and notice tension build up in your hands.

(5 seconds)

Release the tight grip on your fists and allow your entire hand to become limp.

(5 seconds)

Become aware of your shoulders.

(5 seconds)

Think of how they would feel if they were relaxed. Now, tighten the muscles around the shoulders and then relax them.

(20 seconds)

Take your attention to your face.

(5 seconds)

Narrow your focus to your jaw. Tense your entire jaw. Now allow the jaw to relax and notice as the tension melts away.

(5 seconds)

Now scan your whole body and search for hidden stress in the muscles. Relax every area that you can sense tension.

(120 seconds)

Scan one more time to see if there is any part of the body that is still tensed even if just a little bit. Tighten the body part and allow it to relax.

(60 seconds)

Now scan the whole body from your head to your toes. Take a deep breath in and tightly squeeze all the parts of your body. Hold your breath in and continue to squeeze your muscles some more. Begin to exhale as you relax the entire body.

You are no longer hiding these emotions.

You have taken a step to allow yourself to feel them, but not giving them control over your life.

Remember that allowing yourself to acknowledge these negative feelings is an act of courage.

(10 seconds)

Once again, begin to take deep breaths.

(20 seconds)

With the expansion of every inhale, allow your body to create room in your heart for positive emotions. With the contraction of every exhale, become aware of your ability to cope with difficult times and emotions.

(5 seconds)

Keep breathing in and out as you allow your body to create more space for grace, strength, and courage.

(60 seconds)

Now, allow your breathing to adapt to its normal rhythm and just observe it.

(60 seconds)

Think of a time when you were delighted and at peace. When was it? How was life then? How did you feel? Remember that moment in detail.

(20 seconds)

Allow yourself to relive that moment, and for the emotions, you felt then to fill your body and mind.

(20 seconds)

CHAPTER 22:

Return to Happiness by Loving Your Body and Healing Your Soul

G lad individuals acknowledge and love themselves regardless of what their body resembles, regardless of how they feel. An ideal body isn't preferred or all the more empowering over a body not considered immaculate by the "powers that be." Your magnificence originates from inside.

Consider somebody you know (or knew) who isn't generally all that appealing; however, who appears to adore herself so much that she feels delightful and acts as needs to be. Individuals like that tend to be well known. Curiously, their excellence sparkles so splendidly that they seem, by all accounts, to be alluring to others.

What is your opinion about your body shape? What about your body condition? How is your well-being? Is it true that you are happy with your physical and emotional well-being?

Imagine a scenario in which your body doesn't fit the portrayal of lovely, as indicated by the media. Does that cause you to feel not exactly second rate or ugly? Who sets the incredible gauges for the media?

Individuals in the media don't typically seem as though they seem to look in front of an audience or magazines and films. That is the reason the calling of make-up specialists exists. In my mind, what they do is makeup how this individual will appear to the crowd and fans. When photograph distributing is included, nobody is viewed as they look. All photographs get finished up.

To whose norms do you hold yourself? Consider the possibility that something about you changes. At the point when you discover and characterize your excellence inside, then nothing in your outside world changes how you feel about being you—nothing.

At the point when you love yourself, truly and genuinely love yourself, regardless of how old you develop to be, your sentiments about you won't change. The fascinating piece about adoring yourself is living in a condition of satisfaction. Hardly any individuals get the chance to abide there—the individuals who do remain youthful until the end of time.

Coincidentally, would you like to get familiar with how you can live in bliss now?

Figuring Out How to Love Your Body

Ordinarily, we are assaulted with pictures of models with impeccable bodies. That can be terrible for our self-regard. How might we figure out how to cherish our bodies when we are continually being contrasted with these incredible immaculate bodies? All things considered, or starters, don't stress over what individuals think a solid body is directly for you.

To begin with, you should work out. Research has demonstrated that practicing routinely will help your self-regard. Isn't it so extraordinary? You won't just have a more advantageous trimmer body, yet you will likewise feel incredible about yourself. So, get out and exercise and consume those calories. You don't have to go to the exercise center; you can do it at home, busy working, or outside.

As referenced before, we are encircled by these pictures of models with alleged impeccable bodies. There is nothing of the sort! We, as a whole, ought to have a body that we're agreeable in. Acknowledge your body shape and spotlight on how you can get more advantageous, and that is simply the ideal approach to figure out how to cherish yourself.

The choice is in your grasp. Pardon me for saying this. You can say that you're content with being fat and can acknowledge yourself as a husky individual. However, can you truly? Genuinely? Would you truly like to be unfit, unfortunate, and drowsy constantly? So, take a gander at the advantages and disadvantages, and you'll see that getting fit and sound is consistently the better choice.

Once more, and I feel compelled to pressure this as much as possible, be consistent with yourself. You shouldn't resemble the supermodels to be exceptional. You are an interesting individual with great qualities. So, center around that, and you will before long observe that the more benefits you have, the more joyful you will be.

When you figure out how to adore your body, you will see that you are more joyful with yourself, and you presently carry on with your existence with an increasingly uplifting disposition. Figure out how to acknowledge your body type, get ordinary exercise, and eat a sound diet, and you will see an extraordinary improvement satisfaction.

Five Ways to Love Your Body and Get Fit as a Fiddle

The strain to get fit and sound is in high rigging. Individuals are anxious to locate the ideal approaches to put themselves on the road to success to well-being and bliss.

One misstep that numerous individuals are making anyway is ignoring their body's fundamental needs as they proceed with their journey for that ideal physical make-up. You need to address your physical, emotional, and profound necessities during your excursion to better wellness and the reason you need to figure out how to cherish your body and praise the experience of being **you!**

Adoring your body implies that you can grasp the magnificence existing apart from everything else and acknowledge who and where at present. At the point when you can do this, it will empower you to discover fulfillment and joy at each phase of your workout schedule.

Here are five different ways to adore your body now and begin headed straight toward better well-being:

Lower the Boom on Stress

Stress is probably the greatest foe of your mind and body. Regardless of how seriously you are working out, if you are keeping up elevated levels of pressure, your activity and wellness routine will be disrupted. Lessening pressure is a key component that will show your body you truly care. Yoga and meditation are two strategies that numerous individuals have discovered successful in countering pressure. It may not have a difference as regards what you pick as a way to dispose of the stressors throughout your life as long as it is an action that makes you glad and truly facilitates the distressing requests on your mind and body.

Better Nutrition

You have heard these multiple occasions previously, however, even though everything bears repeating. Your food decisions have a ton to do with how your body looks, feels, and reacts to insightful choices about the nourishments that you will eat. Fuel your body with the freshest veggies and organic products. Hurl out those over handled low-quality nourishments and arranged meal bundles, find the delight of good dieting, and show your body that you truly care.

Work Out with Weights

Exercise is terrifically significant with regards to cherishing your body. The total workout program ought to include oxygen-consuming and anaerobic exercises. You should likewise join weights into your ordinary exercise schedule. Not exclusively will working out with weights consume fat and assist you with getting more grounded; it assembles bone quality, which is an extraordinary reward for your body.

Set Aside Effort for You

Somewhat self-spoiling is a need, not an extravagance. At any rate, once per week, you have to put aside an hour or two just to entertain yourself. An invigorating back rub with hot stones is an ideal method to loosen up. Those tight muscles and hurting joints will be restored, and you will find that you unexpectedly have a "renewed purpose for carrying on with life." A loosening up spa day at a neighborhood salon is, in every case, great, yet you can simply absorb a tub of warm water at your home. Set the state of mind with candles, blossoms, and fragrant oils, and you will rapidly observe the constructive outcome this loosening up time has on your mind and body.

Accept Circumstances for What They Are

Maybe the ideal way you can show your body the amount you love is by turning out to be sensitive to the signs that it gives. You have to tune in to these signs when you are starting any exercise or exercise schedule. Try not to request beyond what your body can give. Find a steady speed as you manufacture your quality and endurance. Try not to contrast yourself as well as other people because your body is novel. Recollect that getting fit as a fiddle is a long-distance race work in progress, and it's anything but a 24-hour run. Take things at a sensible pace and permit yourself to accept the way things are. You will arrive at the end goal in top structure if you work with your body rather than against it, and isn't this a genuine demonstration of affection?

For what reason do you love your body? Do you love your body since, as Beth expressed above, it houses your radiant soul? Do you love your body since it empowers you to encounter the wealth of existence with the entirety of your faculties? Do you love your body since it permits you to make things, embrace others, and appreciate the joy of development? We need to begin the discussion about cherishing your body with the why not the if—to get you to move your speculation toward that path right away. Individuals, ladies specifically, maybe you, the peruse—have spent fearfully numerous valuable snapshots of life condemning and attempting to change your body instead of genuinely adoring and tolerating the endowment of your body!

The test that most ladies face around adoring their bodies is the social molding around the perfect body for ladies. There was a famous advertisement for "The Body Shop," the skin and hair care items organization, which expressed, "There are 3 billion ladies who don't seem as though supermodels and just eight who do." This promotion featured that what is advanced as the perfect, typical body for ladies is the ordinary body for just an extremely little level of ladies. However, this picture is constantly depicted in publicizing, on magazine covers and, in the entertainers, we find in films and on TV.

It is a twisting of reality that winds up creating a circumstance where ladies feel lacking and that there is some kind of problem with their body for not resembling this. It makes ladies judge and attempt to change their bodies by dieting, plastic surgery, and numerous different methods of attempting to get their bodies to resemble the perfect. This social molding is frightful and harms ladies and young ladies. It is poisonous because rather celebrating and adoring their special shape, and they are making a decision about it against the advanced perfect. As per the Social Issues Research Center, "Over 80% of fourth-graders have been on a prevailing fashion diet." It is miserable to see the weight that little youngsters feel to begin to form their bodies into the perfect, as opposed to utilizing this vitality to learn, investigate and simply be cheerful and content acting naturally.

CHAPTER 23:

Self-Image – Weight Loss

By self-esteem, we talk of body image in particular. When people have a bad picture of themselves, it feeds back into the emotional part. The bad the body image of someone, the less likely they are to adopt a healthy lifestyle. Why? Why?

There are a few explanations for this. One is embedded in the feeling: "Why bother? My body is ugly, it's awful, it's still my enemy, why should I bother trying to take care of it?"

And then in this kind of thinking, there is ignorance:

"Oh, even I don't know what is happening. I'm so scared of my body, I don't like how it looks, and I don't know, so right now I will go for good and not just good, but in half an hour."

Most positive emotions add up to a very unhealthy lifestyle right now. When someone's view of the body is out of control and seeks to dissociate them from their bodies, the food aspect is less important. Interestingly, they're not hunting for healthier products, so it just doesn't matter. It's a shame they're struggling to feel better right now.

Let's now look at someone who has a healthy body and a healthy self-image, spiritual or not.

When they are spiritual, a very simple reframe can be used along the lines:

- "You gave this body some stronger or more strength from above. It's your ride. You may want to know how to care for it."

One sort of reframing is the whole concept that your body is your temple. The notion that the body is the main interface with the world can also act as a legitimate reframe for people who have not been similarly inclined. It's like a connection to the internet. Similar to high-speed broadband, if you have a sluggish dial-up modem, it is easy to say the difference. The same is true for the life experience of your subject.

The more you are in touch with your food and physical needs, the more your brain and mind function, and the greater your life experience. You do not have to deal with it. In other words, don't repair it if it's not broken.

One way of finding out whether there is the problem is to ask a set of near-magical questions:

- What do you feel when you look into the mirror?

- Have you ever seen yourself in the mirror of the shower in the nude? Why do you see what you're seeing?

- What do you see at the moment? Describe yourself.

These questions are almost magical because they evoke an answer. Listen in their descriptions to words and especially adjectives. They are likely to have an issue with their self-image if they use derogatory words such as "horrible, gross, bad, unsafe, nasty." You probably have a good self-image if you use overall compassionate words.

You must always pay attention to your emotional tone and features. The vocabulary may be inherently sympathetic, but if the emotional tone is repulsive, for instance, then a secret decision is probably made. You may be socially friendly by saying what you think you want to hear; however, your feelings will betray you.

How to Help People Improve Their Self-Image

There are two main self-image components. The first is sympathy for oneself, and the second is the prejudice of affirmation. Let's deal with these individuals.

Self-compassion is about being good to you. Knowing you're good enough, you're all right. Self-compassion starts where you are from. And if you make poor decisions, you don't want to punish yourself. When you do, cognitive dissonance is formed. Those times you're not going to want to think about because they feel bad. It means you're not going to benefit from them, and the chances are high to repeat them. If it gets very bad, you will manifest a part of yourself that binge eats to punish you.

The bad behavior comes out, and you don't control it. That is more like having an alter ego that eats the binge. That is avoided by self-compassion. It helps it to go. You know you made a bad choice of food and binged, but it's all right. Forgive yourself. You're going to do great tomorrow. And that's the next day.

Feeling caring for yourself doesn't mean you let go. That just means you can make mistakes from time to time. The opposite side is a validation distortion. Whenever you feel bad about your body, you can believe that it is worse than it is. A behavior is: what is the point? You let yourself go, and you become that very thing.

You can hear them say, for example, "Look, I eat well. I am still obese. I'm still overweight. I'm still unattractive."

You want to prove yourself correctly. That is the prejudice of belief and one of the psychological effects most difficult to resolve.

Naturally, methods like the classical double-blind language and another mind-altering language can be used.

When a person has an awful self-image, you might ask them:

- "Which body part do you want? Pick just the part of your body that you like even a little."

- "What part of your body would you say is maybe the nicest?"

- "How much do people compliment you; on what part(s) of your body?"

What are they going to say? Who knows? Yet something they're going to have to claim. You will pick one part of your body. You'll assign them

608 | P a g .

a mission then. Suppose your favorite physical feature is your smile. Tell them to note their smile in the following week and then tell you how much they smile.

What you do is continue to use a confirmatory bias to guide you towards the quantities of stuff you like about your body.

It is the old classic Ericksonian double-blind: which one of your hands now feels lighter?

Which one of your hands now feels most unusual?

The fact that they respond means that they are looking for some kind of information. You search for proof.

You may even ask them to remember which part of their body shocked them, so they like it more than they know.

It is the language of mind-bending at work. You're going to get curious about your body in a way that your connection to your body image searches for things that work.

Let's assume, for starters, that they're overweight. You have other medical conditions as it affects your breathing, your pulse, and your cholesterol levels. No, they haven't got diabetes. It is really important for the reframe below.

You tell me that you are putting all this thing in your body and that, as a result, your body has reached that condition, but you have no diabetes. What did your body manage on earth to keep diabetes away while most people have it? That is a good job. How is your body doing such a good job on earth? It is the secret to self-image to find what they do correctly.

If they're still alive, something's right. If they didn't do anything wrong, then they would have another question. They will be dead, and for that, there's no cure. When you have learned to despise your body early in life, you might continue to relapse and repress.

You may have to make a series of regressions to retrain them to learn how they respond to their bodies. When you like the sound of your voice, you have to know that your body produces the sound.

You can, therefore, thank them. You may revive your singing and your speech and wonder how your body creates it. And what a wonder your body is. That is a powerful Ericksonian trick that tells them that their bodies are unique. It's an amazing creature. When someone starts appreciating his body as an amazing tool, they'd like to take better care of it—a guy who loves his car.

They keep it tidy, tidy, and suspicious, particularly with food or drink, when someone comes too close to it. You appreciate that. And what if everyone decided to care about their body in the same way?

People who love their car do not put in cheap fuel or gasoline. It's their kid. I love it. We love it. And they carefully surround it with the finest materials to hold it in top condition. If someone were to relate to their body with the same sensation of wonder as a car enthusiast, they would like to take extra care of it.

It is the core of the process' self-image, to make them enjoy their bodies again, to see the magic of it.

You can do this with basic facts about your body, which contribute to a confirmatory distortion.

You teach a mentality that eventually leads them to believe their body is a wonderful thing worth taking care of.

CHAPTER 24:

The New Behavior Generator

H ave you ever start doing something that would be valuable or resourceful to you? Is it changing your eating patterns? Is it doing your yard work?

I am notorious for having the second-worst yard on my block. I never want to be the worst yard in the neighborhood; I have just never been a big fan of doing yard work before. I have no problem being the second-worst yard in the neighborhood: I don't get all the negative attention, and I don't have to expend energy to make my yard look nice.

Last year I bought a new house. When I bought the new house, I decided that I was going to, after 50 some years, finally break the mold of having the second-worst yard in the neighborhood and take care of my yard. I bought a hedge trimmer. I bought a weed eater. I bought some buckets to pick up debris. I bought a blower. I bought a big broom. I bought all the accouterments that I would need to be able to take care of my yard and perhaps be able to bump myself up to the owner of the best yard in the neighborhood.

Even though that was my intention when I moved in, I noticed after a few months of living there that I had, once again, returned to my old title of the owner of the second-worst yard in the neighborhood.

So, what I did was the self-hypnosis technique called a New Behavior Generator. It is amazing! Whatever new behavior you would like to generate, you can use this strategy to do so. It will program you to not only act on the behavior but to make it a habit. Park with the kids and our golden doodle, I pulled into my driveway, and I looked at my yard. I was proud of my yard, realizing that my yard was way better than most of my neighbors' yards. It looked so good. And that was because I have been going out there regularly and taking care of my yard.

How does this new behavior generator work? How does one break an old pattern, such as neglecting one's yard work and establish a new pattern? It is easy. Simply close your eyes and access your resourceful state of self-hypnosis. And in that resource state of self-hypnosis, focus on what you truly want to do, the yard looks as good as I possibly could, to make it stand out, to make it something I could be proud of. I envisioned in my mind the result of my efforts.

In my self-hypnosis, after creating a mental 8 x 10 glossy image of my yard being beautiful, I decided to expand that imagery into the scene of a movie. The kind of place where a Hollywood film scout might come and say, "We need a front yard of an average American neighborhood, and we'd love it if we could use your front yard." And so, I imagined my front yard is in a movie, and I imagined myself making a movie, a documentary of me taking care of my yard to make it good enough for a Hollywood movie. And thus, I created a movie in my mind of me trimming the hedges; I created a movie of me sweeping the walkways; I created a movie of me using the blower to remove debris from underneath the bushes in my yard.

I played these movie clips over and over, and gradually amplified the details of each—imagining the sound of the blower, the green of the well-watered leaves, the sound of me using the trimmers to trim the tree. All of these things were elements of my movie. I enjoyed playing that movie, and I amplified, and I paid attention to each of the attributes of me doing the work: I paid attention to the feeling of exercise—it's a good feeling; I paid attention to the feeling of sweat; I paid attention to the feeling of the sun and the vitamin D that was helping my body and my immune system become even stronger. I focused on all of the elements of putting together a complete cinematic compilation of the new behavior that I wanted to engage in.

What I did then is I put myself in three scenarios where I saw myself in that movie doing my yard work before a holiday weekend. I always appreciated in the past when my neighbors before the holiday weekend, Memorial Day, Labor Day, 4th of July, and Thanksgiving would make an effort to make their home look nice. So I pictured myself noticing an impending holiday on the calendar and getting ready to make my yard look nice. I then viewed myself in another scenario where yard work needed to be done after having rain during the rainy season when the yard can become dirty and muddy, and outside debris could be blown onto it. I saw myself cleaning up the mess that needed to be cleaned up following a storm, putting myself in that mental movie.

The third time, of course, is when the Hollywood producers came and said, "We'd like to feature your yard in a movie, make it look nice so that we can use it for a Hollywood movie shoot?" So, I pictured myself in that third scenario, getting ready to have my yard star in a Hollywood movie. And in self-hypnosis, I spent a day or two mentally rehearsing these scenes, these new behaviors in my mind. And guess what? The result has been that over the last several months, I've consistently had what I think is probably one of the best yards in the neighborhood. It was interesting. I was just out talking to my neighbor the other day, and he said, "Your yard always looks so nice." And I thought to myself, thank goodness I know the new behavior generator because I've set aside my old pattern of having the second-worst yard in the neighborhood and now I have the best in the neighborhood.

You can use this new behavior generator yourself. What behavior would you like to generate? Would you like to see yourself setting aside a portion of your paycheck each week and saving a hundred dollars in a savings account? Would you like to see yourself manicuring your nails rather than biting them? Would you like to see yourself responding with empathy and kindness rather than anger? This new behavior generator can be utilized literally with any behavior that you would like to create, but more importantly, that you would like to create an ongoing response.

The process is pretty simple: Close your eyes and create a mental picture, an 8 x 10 glossy photo, of the outcome that's important for you. See yourself in that image with the success that is important to you. Amplify that picture into a movie; it might only be a two or three-minute movie, perhaps a movie of you going through the drive-through window and depositing that paycheck but putting one hundred dollars into your savings account, and then coming home to log onto your online bank account and seeing your balance increase every week.

Next, create that mental movie, whatever it is, and amplify the aspects of the movie that make it real for you. Turn up the volume, make the color brighter, sharper, crisper, clearer. Pay attention to the aspects of it. Is the image far, or is the image near? Allow yourself to associate fully into this image and see yourself doing the tasks in this movie that are important to you. And then see yourself in three different scenarios, generating and using this new behavior. Taking a breath, allow yourself to feel awesome, knowing that what the mind can conceive, the body can achieve. Take in another breath. If your eyes aren't open, open them with a smile on your face, feeling fantastic, knowing that the new behavior generator is a powerful way for you to embrace success and to live your best life. In the sample of saving money, see yourself saving money before purchasing something important. You have saved money over a long enough time, and the result is you can now create a better life for yourself doing the things that you want to do. In your movie, create a scenario where you are doing the task of saving money, and the result is something important or meaningful for you.

It's pretty cool to be able to create that new behavior and to see it in your mind. Perhaps the issue was getting a manicure and maintaining beautiful fingernails rather than biting them off. See yourself out for dinner, passing a plate, and somebody else noticing your beautiful nails. See yourself typing on your keyboard with your nails manicured and clean. See yourself in the third scenario, a third situation, where your nails are the way you would finally like them to be. Generate the new behavior of manicuring your nails and taking care of them regularly, rather than sporadically.

You can create an example, any scenario, any new behavior that would be useful to you. See yourself in three different scenarios or three different situations, manifesting that which you have created. And because we can use the creative mind to put ourselves into scenarios that we create, we can experience this in reality. Anything that exists in our physical world had to be a thought first.

You have generated this new behavior here in self-hypnosis. You have applied it in three different ways to three different scenarios. I do not doubt that by spending some time between now and next week, practicing the new behavior generator as an aspect of your self-hypnosis practice, you will discover that it is easy for you to manifest this, not only in the creative mind but in your real world as well.

CHAPTER 25:

Positive Thinking Meditation

B egin in a place you feel the most comfortable and relaxed. This area should be full of positivity.

Don't use a space where you will be distracted, stressed, or bombarded with negative thoughts. For example, avoid work or common areas where you feel tension or conflict with others. It should be a personal space that means something to you and where you won't feel fear or negativity creeping in.

You were keeping your legs straight out in front of you and arms hanging loosely by your side. If you are feeling stiff or too folded up, you won't be able to explore the positive energy coming into you.

Essential to have the right mindset in a mood where you are overcome or stuck on negative thinking from these thoughts and go into a place where you can healthily and happily start feeling more positive.

Notice your breath. Don't try to transform it in any way; simply feel as the air is coming into your body and as it leaves.

Start by breathing gently, and feel as your body fills with air. Allow this air to come out soft and delicately.

Don't breathe in any pattern yet. Just pay attention to how it naturally flows through you. Feel the fresh air come in, and the stale, warm air come out. You are breathing in good vibes.

You are breathing in happiness, positivity, and pure energy. You are breathing out evil thoughts and feelings that are weighing you down, keeping you stuck in the same toxic mindset.

Allow yourself to heal. Allow yourself to feel positive. It is okay to feel this way. Often, we don't like to stay positive because we might feel guilty. We might tell ourselves that it is not reasonable to remain positive when so many people in the world are angry, sad, and generally pessimistic.

That is not the way it has to be and perfectly acceptable for you to want to be happy. Just because other people might be living or thinking does not mean that you have to allow yourself to feel this same way.

Start to count your breath now. Focus your energy and make it easier to think positively. It's an exercise that you can apply whenever you need to change your pattern of thinking.

Breathe in. Count to five as you feel your lungs fill with air inside your body. As you breathe out, count down from five. Let this air come out slowly. Breathe in now for one, two, three, four, and five.

Breathe out now for five, four, three, two, and one. One more time, we are going to count down from ten. Breathe in for the first five and out for the last five. Continue this pattern as we finish throughout the meditation.

Changing how you think and noticing the one you have now. Let thoughts naturally pass through your mind now. Notice any that might be attached to negativity.

These thoughts are natural. Let them flow in and out as easily as you would any other part of your day. Except for this time, don't let the evil thoughts thrive, or even linger. Simply let it come into your mind and push it out with intention.

Pretend as though you are wading in a body of water, and the negative thoughts are like leaves or debris floating towards you. Each time a blade gets close, push it away gently with your hand. No need to pick it up or throw it. No need to push it away forcefully. Guide this thought away lightly with your fingers.

Each time you notice one of these negative thoughts, stop yourself, and turn it around. These thoughts are fears of what might happen tomorrow. Maybe you are afraid of going into work. Perhaps you are fearful of what somebody might think or do. Perhaps you are scared of a judgment call and making the wrong decision. Maybe it is a freak accident from the past that keeps you up at night. Each time you think of something like this, gently push it away.

Negative thoughts are also regretting that linger from the past. Maybe you are always thinking about what you should or could have done differently. Perhaps you are fearful of all the things that you missed, or you can't stop thinking about one decision you made a long time ago.

Each time one of these thoughts comes into your mind, push it out with tenderness. These thoughts aren't helping you. They aren't going to make you a more productive person. They're just going to keep holding you back. It is time to move forward.

We have to focus on the 'now.' The decisions that you've made cannot be changed. Everything that has already happened did so for a reason.

Notice your mindset and how you might be focusing only on the negative things. A dark and a light side to everything in our life. If you continuously stand in the dark, you will never be able to see all that is in the light.

Each time you have thoughts about what you do not have, remind yourself of all of the things that you do. A negative mindset is one that ignores all the chances for goodness. It is one that chooses not to see these aspects of life.

It is time to use gratitude. Gratitude is the appreciation of the things that you have in life. Both good and evil, you can find underlying recognition. It is not about being thankful for every single thing you have. You are merely noticing how these things have a positive impact on you.

Think of something terrible that has happened to you. What did you learn from this experience? What knowledge did you gain for the future? How were you able to go through this experience and still come out stronger because of it? These experiences are things that we can find benefits from, even if it was something horrible, we never wish to go through again.

There is still at least one lesson you can pull from it. Here we are just trying to find the diamond in the rough.

You are picking out that one small little beam of light through all the darkness. That does not make what happened okay, but it can help to change your mindset.

So, what lessons have you learned?

There is always something, albeit small, that is available to change your perspective for the better. It's up to you to find the gratitude in it. Continue to focus on your breathing as you notice these negative thoughts flowing away and creating a more positive mindset. Notice the negative thoughts slowing down. That makes it easier to focus on that positive energy and the bright light that beams down on your life.

Focus all of it on the good that you already have. Be ready to create more. Breathe in appreciation for everything that you have. Breathe out of any hate or anxiety you feel for the things that you don't have.

Breathe in joy and appreciation for all that surrounds us. Breathe out resentment and jealousy over people who seemingly have more than you. Breathe in the realization that you can get whatever you want. Breathe out the idea that you will be happy only when you have certain things.

Remember, we need to be incredibly appreciative of all that we have. Focus on this rather than focusing on all of the things that you still have to gain. One day, if you achieve all of these things, is that the only time that you are allowed to be happy? You should find a way to be positive all of the time. Don't limit the moments in which you show gratitude or appreciation.

You can be a happy individual at all times in life. You do not have to wait for good things to happen to feel or show happiness. You can do this at any moment. Breathe in the idea that it is okay to be happy. Breathe out any guilt you have over had a positive mindset.

There is no endpoint for happiness.

We were taught to keep a negative outlook, believing we are destined for misery, and only show appreciation for material things or monetary gains. We were instilled with thoughts that we are only allowed to be happy at the end of hard work. Struggle, reap the benefits, repeat. There is no time to focus on the past to interrupt this cycle.

You do not have to live like this. You can enjoy that struggle, and you can appreciate your time as you grow in life—no need to wait for the end to exhale and feel whole. You do not have to wait until you have everything that you've ever wanted to be happy. You are allowed to be happy right now. Breathe in the idea that you are going to focus more on being happy now. Breathe out the idea that we have to have things to feel good. Evil doesn't always mean negative. Negative doesn't always mean bad. We can find appreciation from our greatest struggles. We can pull something of value out from all of the dust once it settles.

There will be struggles. Real-life is not one absent from challenge; an authentic experience is filled with gratitude, positivity, and appreciation for the problem—the chance to improve.

You are making a goal with yourself to do your best to power through any issue. Breathe in the idea that you're going to enjoy the journey. Breathe out the idea that you have to wait until the end of the turbulence to be happy.

Breathe in the idea that you are going to have a positive mindset throughout your entire journey. Breathe out the idea that you have to torture yourself and feel anguish over all of the challenges that you might have to endure. Focus on your breath once again. Notice as the air continues to come into your body, and how easily it leaves.

We can be grateful for this. We can have so much appreciation over the way that our bodies continue to breathe. How grateful are we that we can quickly fill our bodies with air and push it out without any effort! So many individuals are not able to breathe or move as we do. That is a small thing that we can start to understand and cherish. Think about this as you breathe in again. We're going to count down from ten. Breathe in for the first five and breathe out for the last five.

CHAPTER 26:

Affirmations for Losing Weight

Affirmations are statements made to amplify a particular idea. Affirmations are certainly going to help take you through your diet. You are going to want to repeat these affirmations when you are feeling both positive and negative. Whenever you feel like giving up or giving in, repeat these affirmations. Write them down, put notes around your home, and do whatever else is needed to keep you dedicated to your weight loss goals.

This first set of affirmations is going to be great if you are interested in working out and dieting to lose weight. These affirmations can be said while you are working out or while you are eating.

When you are working out, affirmations are going to be helpful to get you to a place where you don't want to give up. If you feel like you just want to throw in the towel, try some affirmations to keep you focused on what matters most—not giving up.

Sometimes, we might mindlessly eat as well. That can be dangerous because it means that we are not focused on eating healthy. That could end up leading to overeating or binge eating. If you want to control your portions, then these affirmations are helpful.

- I know that I have control over whether or not I will lose weight.

- I can get the body that I want.

- It is possible to achieve my dreams.

- I do not have to fantasize about my weight anymore. I have everything it takes to go through this process myself.

- I have no guilt over my past choices.

- Every decision I have made about my health has led me to where I am today.

- I am proud of my body that I have endured.

- I am grateful for the struggle that I have had with my body.

- The challenges I've faced with my health have helped me to be more appreciative of what I have.

- I might wish things were different with my body sometimes, but I know that I am grateful that they are the way they are now.

- I can do so much with my body.

- I know how to treat my body healthy so that I lose weight.

- I am losing weight all the time, not just at certain moments.

- As soon as I start to eat healthily, I feel lighter.

- Whenever I work out, I feel lighter.

- I am constantly losing weight, and it is making my body healthier.

- I know how to focus on healthy breathing.

- My breathing helps me to lose weight even more.

- When I am relaxed, I am happy.

- When I am happy, I am losing weight.

- I do not lose weight because I hate my body. I lose weight because I love my body.

- I am exercising to take care of my health.

- I am making healthy choices not just for me now, but for me later as well.

- I am reaching the weight that I want every day.

- I am continuously closer to getting the things that I have always wanted for my life.

- I am healing myself when I lose weight.

- My mind is improving just as much as my body is.

- I am blessed to have the mind and body that I have.

- I have important parts in my body that I need to be grateful for.

- My body could have less than what it has now, so I am grateful for the things that are present.

- I am focused on pushing through my exercises.

- Every time I want to give up exercising, I push forward because I know it will help me feel healthier.

- I make sure to eat something healthy instead.

- I do not torture my body with things that it cannot take.

- I am putting my body through the challenges needed to get the results that I want.

- I am focused on growing my body, not punishing it.

- I want to teach my healthy body habits, and that is what I am doing.

- I am helping my body be the best body possible.

- That is something that I deserve.

- I am working hard, and I deserve rewards.

- I am not hard on myself when I don't meet a goal that I was hoping for.

- I make sure to put myself first and keep moving on because I know that this is the most important thing that I can do.

- Believing in myself is what matters most.

- I know how to get the healthy body that I want, and there is nothing that is going to stop me.

- I am in charge of achieving my goals in life, and I am the one that is in charge.

Affirmations for Feeling Better

When we are feeling gross, ugly, or discouraged, then we are not feeling great. If you want to stick to a workout regime and lose weight, then you must emphasize feeling better. The better you feel, the easier it is going to be for you to have the confidence needed to make it to the gym, go for a walk, or attend the party.

Losing weight and getting healthy is important for you to feel better, not just to look better. These affirmations are going to be useful for you to understand that as well.

Say these affirmations to yourself when you need to feel better, whether you are lazy or self-conscious.

Listen to these frequently, even every day, to help remind you that you deserve to look good but feel even better.

- I feel better and change myself based on the actions I choose to take.

- I have everything that I need to feel good.

- There is nothing that I can let make me feel bad at the moment.

- I have what it takes to feel good all the time.

- I am completely in control of my emotions.

- Others might do things that make me feel bad, but I am in control of how much I let these things affect me.

- I deserve to feel good in life.

- Others know that I deserve to feel good.

- Other people like being around me.

- Other people want me to feel good.

- I want others to feel good. We should all be feeling good.

- The positive attitude that helps me to feel even better.

- I am always excited and ready to start a new day.

- I look forward to what adventures might be waiting for me tomorrow.

- There is nothing in my life that scares me or holds me back from doing what I want.

- I have the confidence needed to accomplish my wildest dreams.

- I believe in myself, and that is what is going to power me through and help me find the things that I have been looking for.

- I have no problem deciding what I should do because I always know what is best.

- I know how to listen to my body, and I can tell whether it is feeling good or bad.

- I have so much joy that it overflows to others.

- I can spread how good I feel because I have so much positive energy.

- Even when I am in pain, it does not affect my mood.

- I appreciate the pain because I know it is presenting me with a healthy struggle.

- Everything that I will ever need is something that I already have.

- I don't have to be worried about anything making me feel bad because I have the power to change my perspective.

- I feel good and, therefore, I look good.

- I look good and, therefore, I feel good.

- There is nothing else I need to move forward to make me happy. Everything that does make me happy is going just to be an added benefit.

- I know what it takes to feel good.

- I make good decisions all the time so that I feel good all the time.

- I only include positive habits in my life that will help me to feel better overall.

- No one feels as good as I do.

- I care about how I feel because that is what matters first.

- I believe in myself, and that helps me to feel better.

- Whenever I am feeling down, I know how to turn my mood around and feel better.

- Everything that has happened bad in my life has taught me how to feel better.

- I am not afraid of what might be out there because I know that no matter how bad it might be, I will still be able to feel good.

- There are things I can't control in my life, but I know how to do what is important so that I am in control.

- I defeat challenges easily because I feel good about myself.

- I make sure to stand on what is right and fight for a good purpose.

- I always feel good because I choose to, even when things are tough.

- I know that feeling bad does me no good, so I will always focus on how I can feel good.

Conclusion

The more that you allow these types of exercises into your life, the more fit and active your mind will be. Having a healthy body is important, but if your mind isn't healthy first, it will be a much greater struggle.

This process requires willpower, strength, and discipline. Ensure that you can incorporate these into your life to see the results you've only been fantasizing about in the past. Pair this with other meditation books as well to get a variety of brain training that will keep you focused on your biggest dreams.

Your attitude can be one of those major things keeping you from reaching your fitness goals. Being on a healthy kick is not necessary for sustainable weight loss.

Losing weight is surely an amazing goal, but it is extremely hard to reach if there is no good motivation to encourage you to keep going.

It takes some time to reach that ideal weight, both time and effort, and to motivate yourself on this journey, and the best idea is to embrace positive self-talk.

You need to remind yourself of all of the amazing health benefits of losing weight, such as feeling more energized, feeling better about yourself, having a night of better sleep, and much more.

In addition to reminding yourself of all of the amazing health benefits of losing weight, another great idea is to keep a success journal where you will write every single step you have taken and succeeded in.

This way, you are more likely to stay committed to your weight loss journey. To boost your commitment, you also need to embrace some positive affirmations and positive self-talk, which will keep you going.

630 | P a g .

Therefore, the next time you look yourself in the mirror, instead of telling yourself I will never be thin and I will just give up, say to yourself this is going to be amazing, losing those five pounds feels great, and I will keep going.

Both of these statements are self-talk, but the first one is extremely negative self-talk, while the second one is positive self-talk.

These are automatic statements or thoughts to make to yourself consciously. Positive self-talk is an extremely important step as it can influence how you act or how you feel.

Instead of saying to yourself negative statements, embrace positive affirmations that come with some constructive ideas.

Once there, your positive self-talk can act as your guardian angel, destroying that annoying, destructive devil that has been sitting on your shoulder, keeping you from reaching your goals.

If you have battled to stay on the right track in the past, this is mostly due to that annoying negative self-talk, which, once there, brings failure, so you are more likely just to give up.

For this reason, say yes to positive self-talk. The most powerful thing about embracing positive self-talk is that those positive affirmations and positive statements you say to yourself tend to stick in your mind, so you are surrounded by positive feelings and thoughts.